The Vegetarian
Kitchen Table Cookbook

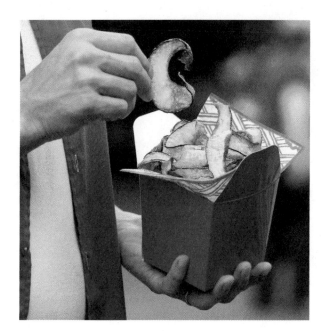

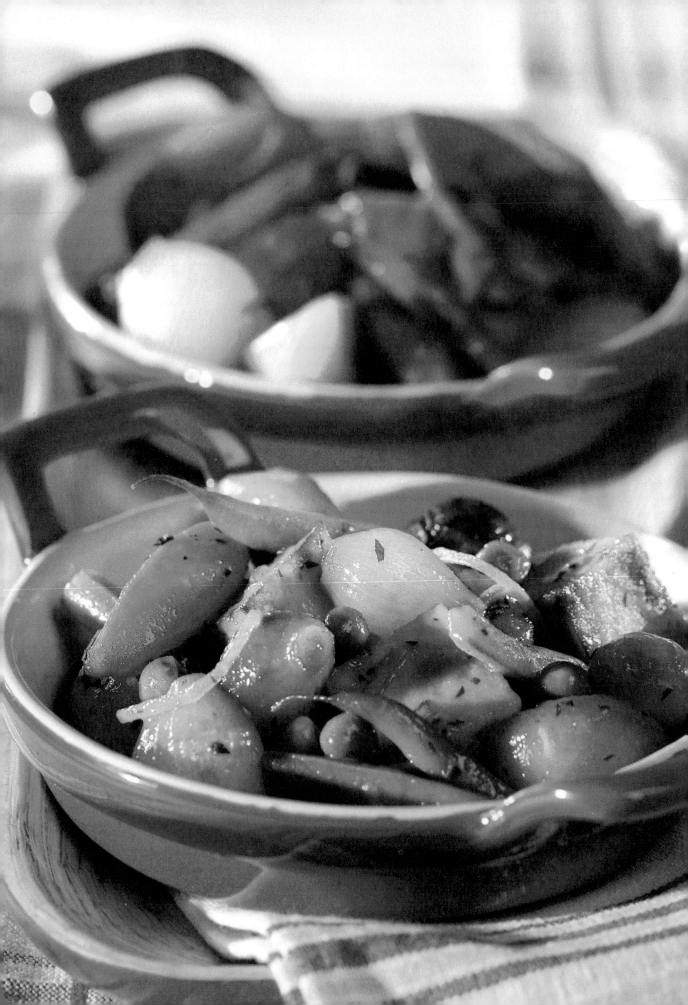

The Vegetarian
Kitchen Table Cookbook

275
Delicious Recipes

Igor Brotto and Olivier Guiriec

Robert
ROSE

The Vegetarian Kitchen Table Cookbook
Text copyright © 2012 Igor Brotto and Olivier Guiriec
Chefs and professors at the Institut de tourisme et d'hôtellerie du Québec
Photographs copyright © 2010 Les Éditions de l'Homme, a division of Groupe Sogides Inc.,
    subsidiary of Groupe Livre Quebecor Media Inc. Montreal (Quebec)
Cover and text design copyright © 2012 Robert Rose Inc.

For complete cataloguing information, see page 320.

Disclaimer

The recipes in this book have been carefully tested by our kitchen and our tasters. To the
best of our knowledge, they are safe and nutritious for ordinary use and users. For those
people with food or other allergies, or who have special food requirements or health issues,
please read the suggested contents of each recipe carefully and determine whether or not
they may create a problem for you. All recipes are used at the risk of the consumer.

We cannot be responsible for any hazards, loss or damage that may occur as a result of
any recipe use.

For those with special needs, allergies, requirements or health problems, in the event of
any doubt, please contact your medical adviser prior to the use of any recipe.

Design and Production: Kevin Cockburn/PageWave Graphics Inc.
Editor: Carol Sherman
Copy Editor: Gillian Watts
Photography: Pierre Beauchemin
Prop and Food Stylist: Luce Meunier
Kitchen and Table Accessories: Linen Chest, La maison d'Émilie (Outremont)
Locations: Jude-Pomme orchard in Oka, the merchants of Jean-Talon Market in Montreal,
    particularly Birri and Chez Michel

Cover image: Mixed Baby Vegetable Fricassee (page 240)
Photo page 1: Squash Chips (page 264)
Photo page 2: Tofu Spring Vegetable Stew (page 165)

We acknowledge the financial support of the Government of Canada through the Book
Publishing Industry Development Program (BPIDP) for our publishing activities.

Published by Robert Rose Inc.
120 Eglinton Avenue East, Suite 800, Toronto, Ontario, Canada M4P 1E2
Tel: (416) 322-6552 Fax: (416) 322-6936
www.robertrose.ca

Printed and bound in Canada

1 2 3 4 5 6 7 8 9 TCP 20 19 18 17 16 15 14 13 12

Contents

Introduction

We don't profess to be strict vegetarians, but we're passionate about food and the art of cooking. The idea of producing a vegetarian cookbook was born of a desire to share classic dishes as well as recipes of our own inspiration, not a wish to impose a particular diet on anyone. On the other hand, we believe that everyone can appreciate a vegetarian dish, no matter what the occasion, in which the best features of the plant kingdom come together in a magnificent variety of forms, colors, aromas and flavors. This is where the word *biodiversity* achieves its fullest sense.

Having both worked in the field of cooking for a long time, we take enormous pleasure in discovering new products and in listening to farmers describe these products to us with passion and pride. They know that we will prepare them with as much love as the farmers put into cultivating them. And at that stage the pleasure of cooking is just beginning. What a joy it is to create happy marriages of high-quality ingredients and products, and what satisfaction there is in preparing a dish that brings out the ingredients' organoleptic qualities without masking their taste or altering their texture! Admittedly, all this requires experience, know-how and a fairly good mastery of culinary techniques, but we have made sure that the recipes in this book are within the capabilities of anyone who enjoys cooking.

People now understand the importance of consuming a variety of foods, reducing portions for better health and seeking out products of superior quality and organic origin. We are sensitive to these considerations, and to the recent evolution we've observed in cooking. Today, for example, dishes are lighter, not as rich as they used to be. Our customers' demands have changed — they now expect to eat healthy and more balanced dishes. More people than ever are turning to vegetarian or vegan cuisine, whether influenced by trends, out of conviction or even to protest the methods of raising livestock, which are often abusive. For all these reasons, the recipes in this book have been created with ingredients that are fresh, impeccable, tasty and absolutely essential to good health.

As much as possible, one should cook with local produce to encourage and raise the status of artisan growers who strive to bring us vegetables and fruits with authentic flavors from one season to the next. Thanks to some adventurous growers, vegetables and fruits that had been long forgotten are appearing in the stalls of public markets and even in large supermarkets. We salute these growers and encourage our readers to buy from them.

In the end, it is our hope that, with this book, we will pass on to you all the passion and excitement that cooking brings out in us.

— *Igor Brotto and Olivier Guiriec*

Photos (clockwise from top left): Cream of Cauliflower Soup with Hazelnut Oil (page 148), Celeriac and Seeds Salad with Maple Foam (page 56), Roman-Style Artichokes (page 96), Fusilli Salad (page 58), Ciabattas with Grilled Vegetables, Goat Cheese and Alfalfa Sprouts (page 175) and Potato and Spinach Roulade (page 112)

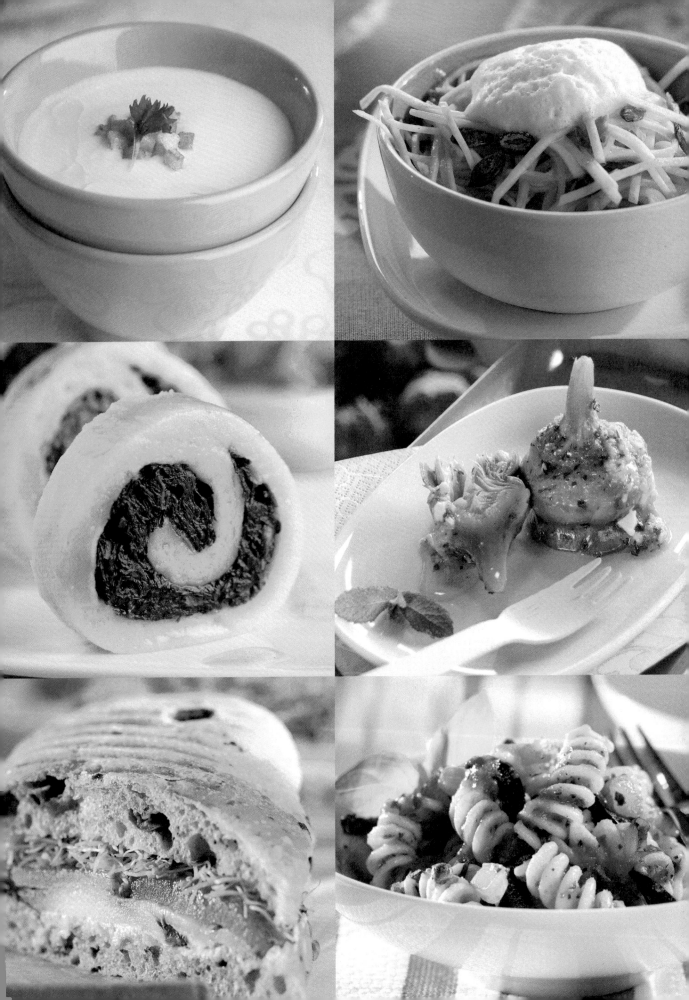

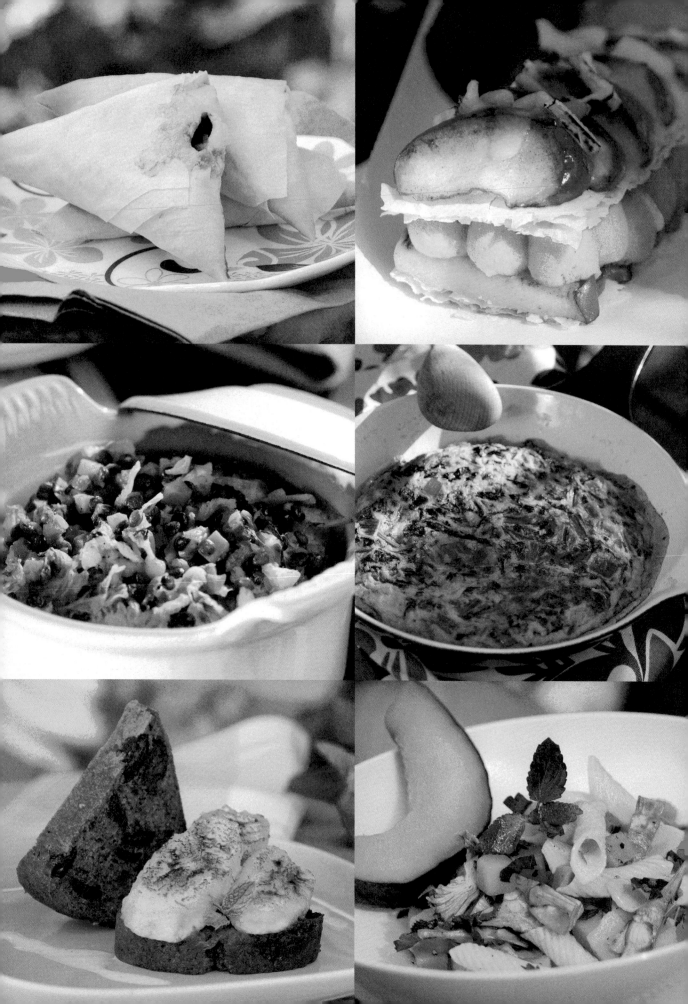

Vegetarianism

The desire to eat healthily, the wish to ward off cardiovascular diseases brought on by a diet high in animal fats, and even respect for the environment are pushing more and more people to turn vegetarian. Vegetarianism comes in a variety of forms that are in some cases associated with religious beliefs or are linked to ecological or ethical convictions. In India, 40 percent of the population is considered to be vegetarian.

Forms of vegetarianism:
- Lacto-vegetarians exclude all meat from their diet but consume milk and dairy products (cheese, yogurt, butter, etc.).
- Ovo-vegetarians avoid all products containing meat, as well as all dairy products. Eggs are permitted.
- Ovo-lacto-vegetarians avoid all meat but consume dairy products and eggs.
- Strict vegetarians exclude all animal products (including cheese, milk, eggs and honey) and eat only plant foods.
- Vegans are individuals who, in addition to being strict vegetarians, try to avoid any products and by-products that come from the exploitation of animals (such as wool, fur, leather, etc.)
- Fruitarians eat only fruits, seeds, nuts and other plant foods, provided that harvesting them does not damage the plants, shrubs or trees.
- Pescetarians are ovo-lacto-vegetarians who also eat products from the sea (fish, crustaceans, shellfish, mollusks).
- Rawtarians or crudivores eat only uncooked foods or those that have been heated to a temperature of no more than 118°F (48°C).

Whatever diet you choose should be adapted to your needs and should not lead to possible nutritional deficiencies. It is also important to respect the products you use. They should be fresh, varied and preferably organic. Of course, cereal grains and legumes are available all the time. Germinating cereal grains and legume seeds is an ancient practice that is still widespread. Sprouted grains and seeds provide a steady supply of varied nutrients that are easily absorbed and essential to the body.

Vegetarianism and the Mediterranean Diet

In the Mediterranean basin, a cuisine based on local products developed over the centuries. While it is not a strictly vegetarian cuisine, many classic recipes from this region emphasize garden produce and highlight traditional fruits such as olives, all thanks to a mild climate, fertile soil and a long summer. The Mediterranean peoples, who lived mainly on what they could grow themselves, developed a daily diet based on products that were readily available, saving meat and fish for important occasions and festivities.

Photos (clockwise from top left): Spanakopita (page 31), Squash and Cortland Apples with Cheese (page 174), Frittata with Rapini and Chard (page 188), Garganelli Salad with Artichokes and Squash (page 57), Banana Chocolate Cake (page 298) and Cabbage Cooked in Butter with Braised Lentils (page 172)

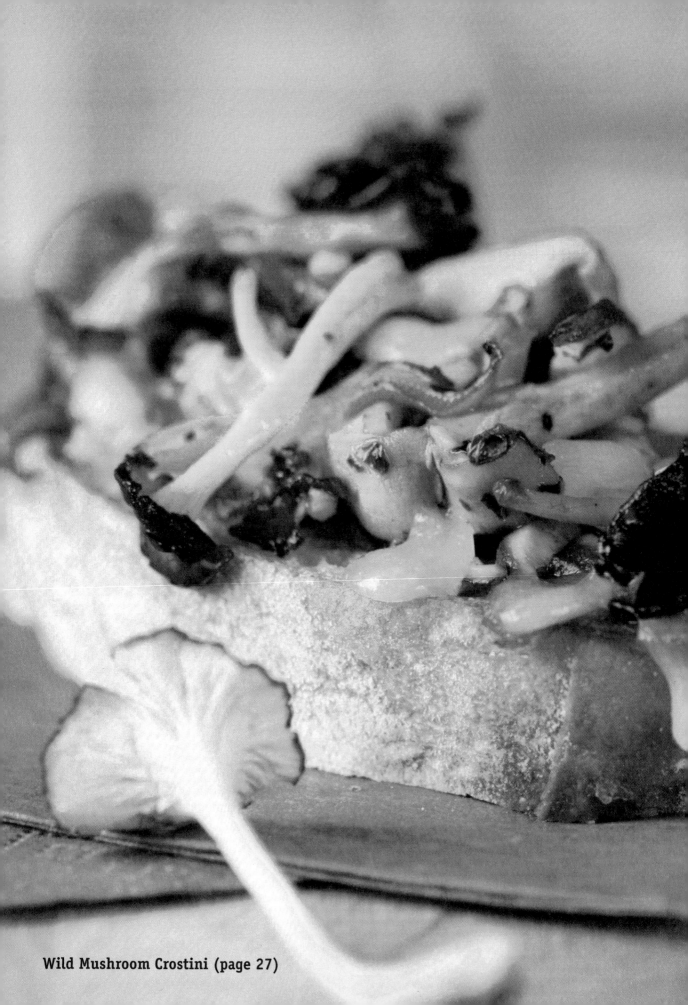

Wild Mushroom Crostini (page 27)

Appetizers

Guacamole

Preparation time
15 minutes

Chilling time
1 hour

4	avocados	4
	Juice of 1 lemon	
1	small tomato, peeled, seeded and diced	1
	Hot pepper sauce	
	Salt	
	Cayenne pepper	
	Tortilla chips	

1. Cut avocado in half lengthwise and remove pit. Using a spoon, scoop out flesh, discarding skins. Place flesh in a bowl and sprinkle lightly with lemon juice, then mash with a fork.

2. Add tomato, hot pepper sauce, and salt and cayenne pepper to taste. Stir to combine. Cover and refrigerate for 1 hour, until chilled, or for up to 4 hours.

3. Serve with tortilla chips.

Avocado Mousse

Serves 4

Preparation time
20 minutes

Cooking time
5 minutes

Chilling time
1 hour

Tip

Agar powder, or agar-agar, is extracted from red algae and used to gel liquids in place of non-vegetarian gelatin. It comes in powder and flake forms and is available at health food and bulk food stores.

Variation

This mousse can be served with crostini or pita bread that has been slightly dried or toasted in the oven.

1	small avocado	1
$\frac{1}{4}$ cup	freshly squeezed lime juice	60 mL
$1\frac{1}{4}$ cups	heavy or whipping (35%) cream	300 mL
$\frac{1}{4}$ cup	granulated sugar	60 mL
1 tsp	agar powder (see Tip, left)	5 mL
$\frac{1}{4}$ cup	water	60 mL
	Tomato Salsa (page 272)	

1. Cut avocado in half lengthwise and remove pit. Using a spoon, scoop out flesh, discarding skin.

2. In a bowl, using an electric mixer, mash together avocado flesh and lime juice until smooth.

3. In a separate chilled bowl, using an electric mixer, whip together cream and sugar until soft peaks form.

4. In a small saucepan, dissolve agar powder in water and bring to a boil over high heat. Boil for 2 minutes. Remove from heat and let cool slightly.

5. Using a whisk, carefully fold whipped cream into avocado purée. Fold in warm agar.

6. Spoon mousse into glasses until three-quarters full. Cover and refrigerate for 1 hour, until chilled, or for up to 4 hours. Spoon a little tomato salsa on top to serve.

Hummus

• **Food processor**

½ cup	drained rinsed canned chickpeas	125 mL
1	clove garlic, chopped	1
2 tsp	freshly squeezed lemon juice	10 mL
	Salt	
1 tsp	toasted sesame oil (see Tips, left)	5 mL
4 tsp	olive oil (see Tips, left)	20 mL
	Chopped fresh parsley	
	Paprika	
	Olive oil	

1. In a food processor, purée chickpeas, garlic, lemon juice, salt to taste, and sesame oil. Add olive oil and process until incorporated. Transfer to a bowl, cover and refrigerate for at least 1 hour before serving or for up to 1 day.

2. Form into a dome on serving dish, then garnish with parsley and paprika to taste. Drizzle with a little olive oil.

Tzatziki

1	cucumber, peeled and cut in half lengthwise	1
	Salt	
1½ tsp	minced garlic	7 mL
1¼ cups	plain yogurt, preferably goat or sheep milk	300 mL
⅔ cup	olive oil	150 mL
2 tsp	vinegar	10 mL
½	bunch fresh dill, chopped	½
	Crudités, pita bread and/or olives	

1. Lightly sprinkle cucumber with salt and let drain. Rinse, then pat dry with paper towels. Shred on the coarse side of a box grater.

2. In a bowl, thoroughly blend garlic, yogurt, olive oil, vinegar and dill. Add grated cucumber and blend thoroughly. Cover and refrigerate for 1 hour, until chilled, or for up to 8 hours.

3. Serve very cold with crudités or pita bread and olives.

Celery with Gorgonzola

Serves 4

Preparation time
15 minutes

4	stalks celery	4
6 oz	Gorgonzola cheese (see Tip, page 20)	175 g
3 oz	mascarpone cheese	90 g
1 tbsp	pink peppercorns	15 mL

1. Peel strings from celery. Cut each stalk into 6 sticks.

2. In a bowl, using a spatula, blend Gorgonzola and mascarpone cheeses into a smooth, creamy mixture.

3. Using a mortar and pestle, crush peppercorns.

4. Spread celery sticks with Gorgonzola mixture and sprinkle with crushed peppercorns.

Buckwheat Blinis

Makes about 54 blinis

Preparation time
1 hour 30 minutes

Cooking time
20 minutes

Tip

Fresh baker's yeast comes in compressed cake form and is available at some health food stores and specialty baking stores. *To use active dry yeast in place of fresh:* In Step 1, heat milk to 105 to 115°F (41 to 46°C) and pour into the bowl. Sprinkle 1⅛ tsp (5.5 mL) or ½ package (¼ oz/8 g) active dry yeast overtop and let stand for 10 minutes or until frothy, then whisk in sugar and flour and let rise as directed.

- Instant-read thermometer

1⅔ cups	milk, divided	400 mL
Pinch	granulated sugar	Pinch
¼ oz	fresh baker's yeast (see Tip, left)	8 g
¾ cup	all-purpose flour, divided	175 mL
2	eggs, separated	2
⅓ cup	buckwheat flour	75 mL
⅛ tsp	salt	0.5 mL
2 tbsp	melted butter, divided	30 mL

1. In a saucepan over medium heat, warm half the milk to 70 to 80°F (21 to 27°C). Pour into a bowl. Add sugar and yeast and stir to dissolve. Whisk in 3 tbsp (45 mL) of the all-purpose flour. Cover bowl with plastic wrap and let rise in a warm, draft-free area for 45 minutes.

2. Add egg yolks, remaining milk, remaining all-purpose flour, buckwheat flour and salt. Gently stir together ingredients just until blended. Cover and let rise for 45 minutes.

3. In a bowl, using a whisk or electric mixer, beat egg whites until soft peaks form. Using a spatula, gently fold whites into batter just until blended, then incorporate 1 tbsp (15 mL) of the melted butter.

4. Preheat a nonstick skillet over medium heat and lightly brush with some of the remaining butter. Drop 1 tbsp (15 mL) batter per blini into skillet. Cook until bubbles form on the top and the underside is golden brown, about 1 minute. Flip and cook until golden, about 30 seconds. Adjust heat as necessary between batches to prevent burning and brush with more melted butter as needed. Serve blinis hot.

Goat Cheese Blinis

Preparation time
2 hours 20 minutes

Cooking time
50 minutes

Tips

Fresh baker's yeast comes in compressed cake form and is available at some health food stores and specialty baking stores. *To use active dry yeast in place of fresh:* In Step 1, heat milk to 105 to 115°F (41 to 46°C) and pour into the bowl. Sprinkle 2¼ tsp (11 mL) or 1 package (¼ oz/8 g) active dry yeast overtop and let stand for 10 minutes or until frothy, then whisk in flour and let rise as directed.

If the blinis are too thick to cook properly in the skillet, you can transfer them to a baking sheet and finish cooking them in a 350°F (180°C) oven.

Sponge

6 tbsp	milk	90 mL
½ oz	brewers' yeast (see Tips, left)	15 g
¾ cup	all-purpose flour	175 mL

Blinis

1⅔ cups	milk	400 mL
2 cups	all-purpose flour	500 mL
½ tsp	salt	2 mL
5	eggs, separated	5
3 tbsp	butter	45 mL
7 oz	firm goat cheese, thinly sliced	210 g
	Hazelnut oil	
	Finely chopped fresh chives	

1. *Sponge:* In a saucepan over medium heat, warm milk to 70 to 80°F (21 to 27°C). Pour into a bowl and stir in yeast to dissolve. Stir in flour until blended. Cover bowl with plastic wrap and let ferment at room temperature for about 1 hour (mixture should be thick and have a yeasty aroma).

2. *Blinis:* In a saucepan over medium heat, warm milk just until lukewarm (70 to 80°F/21 to 27°C).

3. In a deep bowl, combine flour, salt, egg yolks and sponge. Gradually whisk lukewarm milk into batter. Cover and let stand at room temperature for 1 hour.

4. In a bowl, using an electric mixer or whisk, beat egg whites until stiff peaks form. Using a spatula, gently fold whites into batter just until blended.

5. In a large nonstick skillet, melt a small piece of butter over medium heat to thinly coat pan. Pour in 1 tbsp (15 mL) batter per blini and lay a slice of goat cheese on top of each. Cook, without turning, until batter is set, about 3 minutes (see Tips, left). Transfer to a platter and repeat with remaining butter, batter and cheese.

6. Sprinkle with hazelnut oil and chives before serving.

Bruschetta

Tips

Day-old or slightly stale bread makes bruschetta even better. Toast on a grill for the most authentic flavor.

Traditionally the bread slices are rubbed with garlic. But the overpowering taste of raw garlic can ruin the delicate flavor of the tomatoes. It is up to you whether you use it or not.

8	very ripe plum (Roma) tomatoes, finely diced	8
4	large leaves fresh basil, finely chopped	4
¼ cup	extra virgin olive oil	60 mL
1	clove garlic, optional (see Tips, left)	1
4	thick slices country-style bread, toasted (see Tips, left)	4
	Fleur de sel	

1. In a bowl, combine tomatoes, basil and olive oil.

2. If using, cut garlic in half lengthwise and rub cut sides over one side of each toast slice.

3. Place toast slices, garlic side up, if using, on a platter or individual plates. Spoon tomato mixture on top and sprinkle with fleur de sel to taste. Serve immediately.

Bruschetta with Wilted Zucchini and Olives

5 tbsp	extra virgin olive oil, divided	75 mL
1	clove garlic, crushed	1
1½ cups	diced green zucchini	375 mL
1½ cups	diced yellow zucchini	375 mL
	Salt	
¾ cup	pitted kalamata olives	175 mL
8	fresh basil leaves, chopped	8
4	slices country-style bread, toasted	4

1. In a skillet, heat two-thirds of the oil over medium-low heat. Add garlic and cook, stirring, until brown, about 5 minutes. Using a slotted spoon, remove garlic and discard. Increase heat to high and sauté zucchini until starting to brown, about 10 minutes. Transfer to a bowl and lightly season with salt.

2. Crush olives coarsely. Add to zucchini in bowl and stir in basil.

3. Place toast slices on a platter or individual plates. Spoon zucchini mixture on top and drizzle with remaining olive oil. Serve immediately.

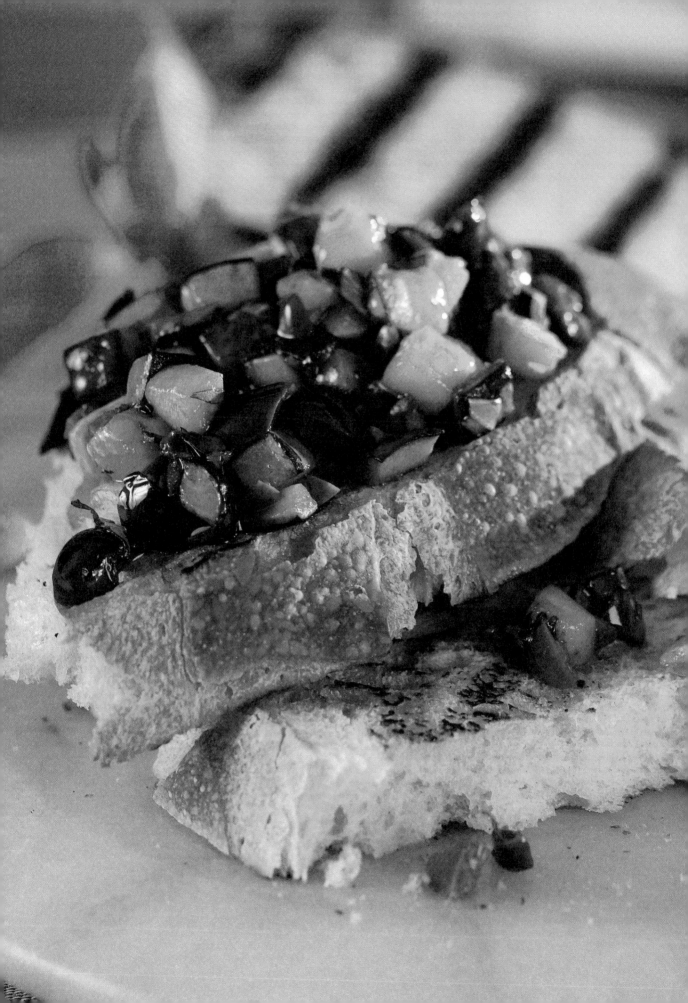

Caponata

Serves 4

Preparation time
1 hour 10 minutes

Cooking time
55 minutes

Variation
The caponata can be served as is, spooned onto crackers or crostini, or with eggs or pasta.

2	eggplants	2
1 tbsp	coarse salt	15 mL
3	stalks celery	3
6 tbsp	olive oil, divided	90 mL
¾ cup	finely chopped onion	175 mL
2 cups	canned tomatoes, drained, juice reserved	500 mL
3 tbsp	red wine vinegar	45 mL
1 tbsp	granulated sugar	15 mL
	Salt and freshly ground black pepper	
1 tbsp	drained capers	15 mL
2 tbsp	coarsely chopped pitted black olives	30 mL
1 tbsp	chopped fresh parsley leaves	15 mL

1. Cut stems from eggplants and dice. Place in a colander and sprinkle with coarse salt. Cover and let drain for 30 to 40 minutes.

2. Peel strings from celery and cut into thin slices. In a pot of boiling salted water, boil celery for 5 minutes, then drain.

3. Rinse eggplant and spread on paper towels to dry.

4. In a skillet, heat 2 tbsp (30 mL) of the olive oil over medium-high heat. Sauté half of the eggplant until light golden, about 10 minutes. Drain on paper towels and set aside. Repeat with 2 tbsp (30 mL) more oil and remaining eggplant.

5. In a large, heavy pot, heat remaining olive oil over medium heat. Fry onion, stirring, until translucent, 5 to 7 minutes. Add tomatoes with about one-third of their juice and bring to a simmer. Simmer for 5 minutes, then stir in vinegar and sugar and add salt and pepper to taste. Reduce heat and simmer gently until thickened, 15 to 20 minutes.

6. Stir in celery, capers and olives. Reduce heat to low, cover and simmer for 30 minutes, stirring occasionally. Make sure there is always a little liquid remaining. If necessary, add a little more tomato juice.

7. Transfer tomato sauce to a bowl and combine with eggplant. Adjust seasoning and add parsley.

Stuffed Grape Leaves

Tips

If fresh grape leaves are not available, you can often find them packed in brine in jars or cans in Mediterranean or Middle Eastern specialty stores or well-stocked supermarkets. If using brined leaves, skip Step 1 and just drain and rinse leaves and pat dry before using in Step 6.

These stuffed leaves can be served as a first course with yogurt or simply sprinkled with lemon juice.

24	fresh grape leaves (see Tips, left)	24
2/3 cup	olive oil, divided	150 mL
2 cups	finely chopped onions	500 mL
1	clove garlic, chopped	1
1/2 cup	long-grain white rice	125 mL
1/4 cup	dried currants	60 mL
	Salt and freshly ground black pepper	
1/4 cup	pine nuts	60 mL
	Juice of 1 lemon, divided	
2 tbsp	finely chopped fresh mint leaves	30 mL
3	bay leaves	3

1. In a large pot of boiling water, in batches as necessary, blanch grape leaves until soft and pliable, 2 to 3 minutes. Rinse in cold water and spread on a plate covered with a clean tea towel.

2. In a saucepan, heat $1/4$ cup (60 mL) of the olive oil over medium heat. Add onions and cook, stirring occasionally, until softened and translucent, about 5 minutes. Add garlic and cook, stirring, for 1 minute. Add rice and cook, stirring, until translucent, about 2 minutes.

3. Stir in currants, $1/2$ cup (125 mL) water and salt and pepper to taste and bring to a boil over high heat. Reduce heat to low, cover and simmer until rice is slightly tender, about 15 minutes (or transfer to a 400°F/200°C oven and bake).

4. Using a fork, gently stir pine nuts, juice of $1/2$ lemon and mint into rice. Let cool.

5. Spread out grape leaves, shiny side down, on work surface, and spoon rice mixture into the center of each leaf, dividing equally. Fold ends of leaves inward before rolling them up to enclose filling. Do not roll too tightly, as rice will expand during cooking.

6. In a large pot, heat remaining olive oil over medium-high heat. Arrange stuffed leaves on the bottom, stacking if necessary. Pour in remaining lemon juice and add water until leaves are covered. Add bay leaves. Place a plate on top of the stuffed leaves to weigh them down and prevent them from opening while cooking. Bring to a simmer. Reduce heat to low, cover and simmer for 1 hour. Let cool in pot, then drain well before serving.

Pumpkin Croquettes with Cheddar Cheese

Makes about 20 croquettes

Preparation time
50 minutes

Cooking time
1 hour

Tip

When buying cheese, read the label carefully and make sure to buy those that are not made from animal rennet.

- Preheat oven to 350°F (180°C)
- Rimmed baking sheet, lined with parchment paper
- Food mill
- Pastry bag with large plain tip
- Candy/deep-fry thermometer

½	large potimarron or sweet pie pumpkin (about 2 lbs/1 kg)	½
5 oz	sharp (aged) Cheddar cheese, shredded (see Tip, left)	150 g
3	egg yolks	3
½ cup	all-purpose flour, divided	125 mL
	Salt and freshly ground black pepper	
2	eggs, well-beaten	2
⅔ cup	bread crumbs	150 mL
6 cups	vegetable oil	1.5 L

1. Remove seeds and strings from pumpkin. Place on prepared baking sheet, cut side down. Bake in preheated oven until tender and easily pierced with a fork, about 45 minutes. While still hot, use a spoon to scoop out the flesh, discarding skin. Immediately pass through food mill into a bowl (you should have about 2¼ cups/550 mL purée). If pumpkin is wet, place in a sieve and gently press to remove excess liquid.

2. Add cheese, egg yolks and 3 tbsp (45 mL) of the flour to pumpkin purée and mash until blended. Add more flour, if necessary, 1 tbsp (15 mL) at a time, to make a dough that just holds its shape when squeezed into a ball. Season with salt and pepper to taste.

3. Spoon into pastry bag and pipe onto a floured surface to form cylinders 1 inch (2.5 cm) in diameter. Slice into rolls about 3 inches (7.5 cm) long.

4. Spread 3 tbsp (45 mL) remaining flour in a thin layer in a shallow dish. Place beaten eggs in another shallow dish. Spread bread crumbs in a third shallow dish.

5. Working with a few rolls at a time, add to flour in dish and shake dish to evenly coat rolls in flour. Gently turn to dip ends, then shake off excess flour. Dip rolls into egg, gently turning and ensuring that egg adheres properly to flour. Add to bread crumbs and turn to evenly coat, then roll them gently on a flat surface to give them a nice shape and to remove excess bread crumbs.

6. In a deep skillet, Dutch oven or deep-fryer, heat oil over medium heat until about 350°F (180°C). Drop rolls, in batches, into hot oil and fry until golden and hot inside, about 2 minutes per batch. Using a slotted spoon, remove from oil and place on a baking sheet lined with paper towels to drain. Adjust heat as necessary between batches. Serve hot.

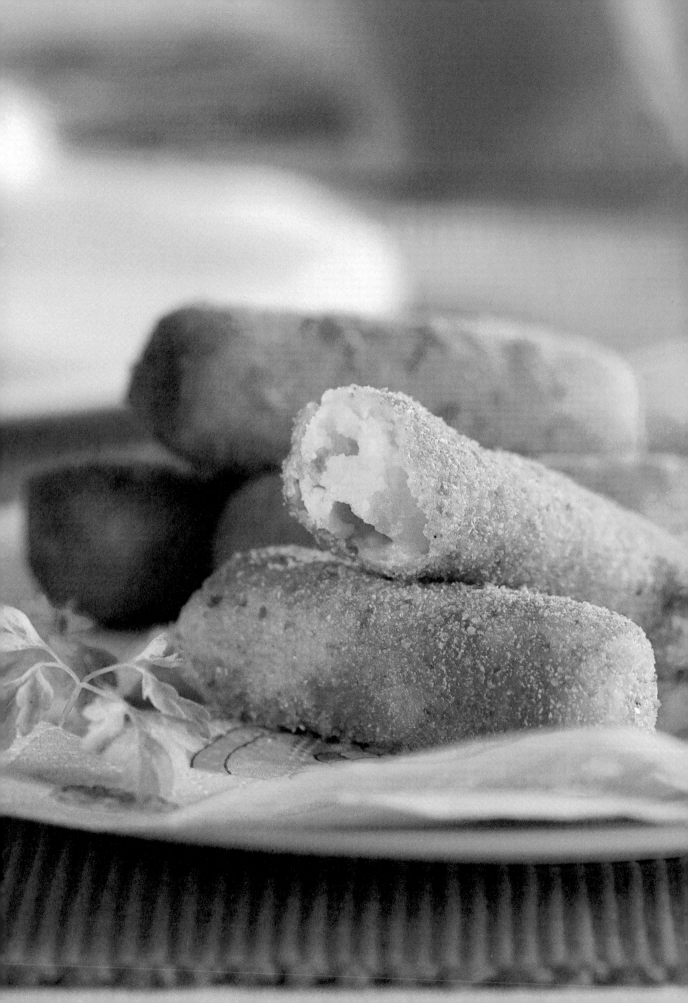

Fingerling Potato Croquettes

Preparation time
30 minutes

Cooking time
35 minutes

Tip

If fingerling potatoes aren't available, you can use small yellow-fleshed potatoes and increase the cooking time in Step 1 as necessary.

Variation

You can add up to 1 cup (250 mL) shredded cheese such as Cheddar to the croquette mixture in Step 2. It should be added before the butter.

- Preheat oven to 350°F (180°C)
- Pastry bag with large plain tip
- Candy/deep-fry thermometer

Croquettes

1 lb	fingerling potatoes, peeled (see Tip, left)	500 g
4 tsp	butter, softened	20 mL
3 or 4	egg yolks	3 or 4
	Salt and freshly ground black pepper	
	Ground nutmeg	

Breading

1¼ cups	all-purpose flour	300 mL
3	eggs, beaten	3
1 cup	bread crumbs	250 mL
6 cups	vegetable oil	1.5 L

1. *Croquettes:* Place potatoes in a large pot and cover with cold salted water. Bring to a boil over high heat. Reduce heat and boil gently for about 15 minutes or until fork-tender. Drain.

2. Place potatoes on a baking sheet and bake in preheated oven for 15 minutes to dry them. Transfer to a large bowl and mash immediately. Add butter, 3 of the egg yolks, and salt, pepper and nutmeg to taste and mash to combine. If mixture seems very stiff, add enough of the remaining egg yolk to make a pliable texture that can be piped.

3. Spoon into pastry bag and pipe onto a floured surface to form cylinders about ½ inch (1 cm) in diameter. Slice into rolls about 2 to 2½ inches (5 to 6 cm) long.

4. *Breading:* Spread flour in a thin layer in a shallow dish. Place beaten eggs in another shallow dish. Spread bread crumbs in a third shallow dish.

5. Working with a few rolls at a time, add to flour in dish and shake dish to evenly coat rolls. Gently turn to dip ends, then shake off excess flour. Dip rolls into egg, gently turning and ensuring that egg adheres properly to flour. Add to bread crumbs and turn to evenly coat, then roll them gently on a flat surface to give them a nice shape and to remove excess bread crumbs.

6. In a deep skillet, Dutch oven or deep-fryer, heat oil over medium heat until about 350°F (180°C). Drop rolls, in batches, into hot oil and fry until golden and hot inside. Using a slotted spoon, remove from oil and place on a baking sheet lined with paper towels to drain. Serve immediately.

Sweet Potato Fritters with Cumin and Sambal

Makes about 20 fritters

Preparation time
15 minutes

Cooking time
110 minutes

- Preheat oven to 350°F (180°C)
- Small food processor or mini chopper
- Food mill, optional
- Candy/deep-fry thermometer

Sambal

2	fresh hot chile peppers (serrano or jalapeño), stems and seeds removed	2
1	clove garlic	1
1 tsp	chopped fresh gingerroot	5 mL
1 tsp	granulated sugar	5 mL
2 tsp	soy sauce	10 mL
	Juice of 1 lime	
2 tbsp	vegetable oil	30 mL

Fritters

1	sweet potato (about 10 oz/300 g)	1
¾ cup	all-purpose flour	175 mL
1 tsp	baking powder	5 mL
1	egg	1
1 tbsp	liquid honey	15 mL
	Salt and freshly ground black pepper	
Pinch	ground cumin	Pinch
4 cups	vegetable oil	1 L

1. *Sambal:* In a food processor, finely chop chile peppers, garlic and ginger. Add sugar, soy sauce, lime juice and vegetable oil and purée until smooth. Set aside.

2. *Fritters:* Bake sweet potato in preheated oven until tender, about 1¹/₂ hours. Peel potato and purée, using a food mill or food processor.

3. In a bowl, combine flour and baking powder. In another bowl, combine sweet potato purée, egg, honey, salt and pepper to taste and cumin. Add flour mixture and stir to combine thoroughly.

4. In a deep skillet, Dutch oven or deep-fryer, heat oil over medium-high heat to about 350°F (180°C). Working in batches to avoid overcrowding, for each fritter carefully drop 1 tbsp (15 mL) batter into hot oil and fry, turning once, until cooked inside and deep golden, about 2 minutes per side. Using a slotted spoon, remove from oil and place on a plate lined with paper towels to drain. Adjust heat as necessary between batches to prevent burning. Serve fritters hot with sambal.

Sweet Mama Squash Hush Puppies

Serves 4

Preparation time
10 minutes

Cooking time
1 hour 15 minutes

See photo, opposite

Tip

We prefer to use Sweet Mama squash for this recipe but you can use another firm orange winter squash such as butternut, acorn, buttercup or sweet potato squash.

• Candy/deep-fry thermometer

1 tbsp	butter	15 mL
1	small onion, finely chopped	1
1 cup	cornmeal	250 mL
1/3 cup	all-purpose flour	75 mL
1 tbsp	baking powder	15 mL
	Salt	
1/2 cup	milk	125 mL
1	egg, beaten	1
3/4 cup	puréed baked Sweet Mama squash or other winter squash (see Tip, left)	175 mL
	Chopped fresh hot chile pepper	
4 cups	vegetable oil	1 L

1. In a skillet, melt butter over medium heat. Add onion and cook, stirring, until softened, about 5 minutes. Let cool.

2. In a bowl, combine cornmeal, flour, baking powder and salt to taste. Form a well in the center and pour in milk, egg and squash purée. Stir until well blended. Stir in onion and add chile pepper to taste.

3. In a deep skillet, Dutch oven or deep-fryer, heat oil over medium heat until about 350°F (180°C). In batches, carefully drop 1 tbsp (15 mL) of batter per hush puppy into hot oil and fry, turning once, until golden brown and hot inside, about 3 minutes. Using a slotted spoon, remove from oil and place on a baking sheet lined with paper towels to drain. Serve hot.

Pissaladière

Serves 4

Preparation time
15 minutes

Cooking time
40 minutes

Tip

The package sizes of frozen puff pastry vary among brands. If your package is larger than 13 oz (400 g), it will still work for this recipe; you'll just get a slightly larger rectangle.

• Preheat oven to 400°F (200°C)

4 tsp	olive oil	20 mL
2 lbs	onions, thinly sliced (about 6)	1 kg
2 tbsp	chopped fresh thyme	30 mL
	Salt and freshly ground black pepper	
13 oz	puff pastry (see Tip, left)	400 g
1/3 cup	quartered kalamata olives	75 mL

1. In a large skillet, heat oil over medium heat. Add onions, thyme, and salt and pepper to taste. Cook, stirring, for 2 minutes. Reduce heat to low and cook, stirring often, ensuring that onions do not brown, until very soft, about 20 minutes. Set aside to let cool.

2. On a baking sheet, roll out puff pastry dough into a rectangle about 1/8 inch (3 mm) thick. Arrange onions in a thin layer on top of dough. Sprinkle olives on top. Bake in preheated oven until pastry is crisp and golden, about 20 minutes. Cut into squares and serve hot.

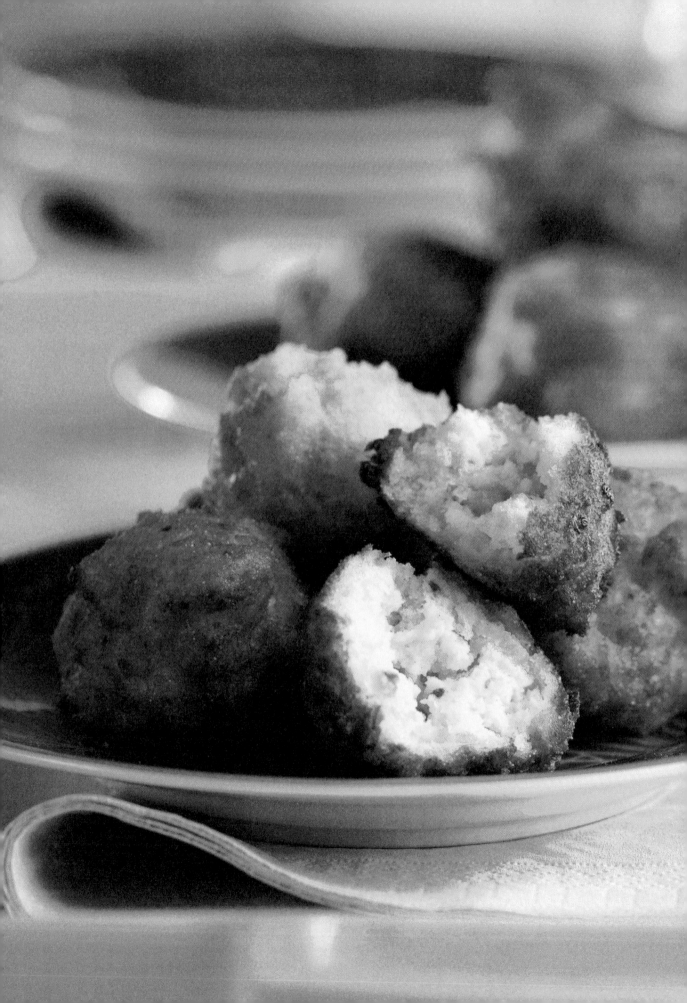

Vegetable Tempura

Serves 4

Preparation time
15 minutes

Cooking time
10 minutes

Variation
You can add a little chopped fresh cilantro to the tempura batter.

- Candy/deep-fry thermometer

1 cup	ice cold water	250 mL
8 oz	tempura flour	250 g
	Salt	
	Hot pepper flakes	
3	stalks celery, peeled and cut into large sticks	3
1 cup	broccoli florets, blanched	250 mL
1	small zucchini, cut into sticks	1
	Vegetable oil	

1. In a bowl, gradually stir cold water into tempura flour to make a thin batter. Season with salt and hot pepper flakes to taste. Let stand for 10 to 15 minutes.

2. In a deep skillet, Dutch oven or deep-fryer, heat 4 inches (10 cm) of oil over medium-high heat until about 350°F (180°C). Working in batches to avoid overcrowding, dip each vegetable individually in tempura batter, then carefully drop into hot oil. Fry, turning once, until batter is golden, about 3 minutes. Using a slotted spoon, remove from oil and place on a baking sheet lined with paper towels to drain. Salt to taste and serve immediately.

Fried Onion Rings

Serves 4

Preparation time
15 minutes

Cooking time
10 minutes

- Candy/deep-fry thermometer

1 lb	onions	500 g
1½ cups	milk	375 mL
	Salt	
1¼ cups	all-purpose flour	300 mL
1 cup	panko bread crumbs	250 mL
	Vegetable oil	
	Mayonnaise	

1. Cut onions into rings about 1/8 inch (3 mm) thick.

2. In a bowl, combine milk and salt. In another bowl, combine flour and bread crumbs.

3. In a large saucepan, Dutch oven or deep-fryer, heat 3 inches (7.5 cm) of oil to 350°F (180°C). Working in small batches, dip onion rings in milk mixture and let excess drain off. Dip into crumb mixture, turning to coat, then shake to remove excess crumbs. Fry, turning once, until crispy, golden brown and onions are tender. Using a slotted spoon, remove from oil and place on a baking sheet lined with paper towels to drain. Serve immediately with mayonnaise for dipping.

Stuffed Jalapeño Peppers

Serves 4

Preparation time
15 minutes

Cooking time
25 minutes

● Preheat oven to 450°F (230°C)
● Large baking dish

2 tbsp	extra virgin olive oil	30 mL
1/2	Spanish onion, finely chopped	1/2
1	zucchini, julienned	1
12	jalapeño peppers	12
	Salt	
4 oz	Cheddar cheese, shredded	125 g

1. In a skillet, heat olive oil over high heat. Add onion and zucchini. Reduce heat to medium and cook, stirring, until soft and golden brown, about 5 minutes. Set aside.

2. Cut peppers in half lengthwise. Cut out seeds and membranes, leaving stems intact.

3. Stuff each pepper half with onion and zucchini mixture and place in baking dish. Top with Cheddar cheese. Bake in preheated oven until peppers are tender and cheese is melted, about 20 minutes.

Wild Mushroom Crostini

Serves 4

Preparation time
15 minutes

Cooking time
25 minutes

Tip
Preferred mushrooms for this recipe are chanterelles, morels, pieds-de-mouton, black trumpets, porcini and other boletes.

● Preheat oven to 350°F (180°C)

8 oz	mixed wild mushrooms (see Tip, left)	250 g
3 tbsp	extra virgin olive oil	45 mL
1	clove garlic, minced	1
	Salt and freshly ground black pepper	
2 tbsp	chopped fresh parsley	30 mL
3 oz	Montasio, friulano or fontina cheese, diced	90 g
4	slices country-style bread, toasted	4

1. Slice or quarter mushrooms depending on their shape and size.

2. In a skillet, heat olive oil over medium-high heat. Sauté garlic until fragrant, about 30 seconds. Add mushrooms and sauté until liquid is released and mushrooms are browned. Season with salt and pepper to taste.

3. In a small bowl, combine mushrooms, parsley and cheese. Place toasts on a baking sheet and spoon mushroom mixture on top, dividing equally.

4. Bake in preheated oven until topping is hot and cheese is melted, about 10 minutes. Serve immediately.

Steamed Dumplings

Makes 30 dumplings		
Preparation time 50 minutes		
Cooking time 20 minutes		

• Steamer basket

¼ cup	extra virgin olive oil	60 mL
1	carrot, diced	1
1	red bell pepper, diced	1
1	yellow bell pepper, diced	1
1	zucchini, diced	1
30	round wonton wrappers, about 3 inches (7.5 cm)	30

Ginger Sauce

2 tbsp	tamari	30 mL
2 tbsp	water	30 mL
2 tbsp	rice vinegar	30 mL
2 tbsp	minced fresh gingerroot	30 mL

Spicy Garlic Sauce

¼ cup	fish sauce	60 mL
6 tbsp	water	90 mL
	Chopped garlic	
	Chopped fresh hot chile pepper	
	Juice of 1 lime	
⅓ cup	packed brown sugar	75 mL

1. In a large skillet, heat olive oil over high heat. Add carrot, red and yellow bell peppers and zucchini and sauté until slightly tender, about 5 minutes. Transfer to a bowl and let cool.

2. Working with one wonton wrapper at a time, place on a work surface and spoon 2 tsp (10 mL) sautéed vegetables in the center. Moisten edges with water and fold into half-moon shape. Pleat edges to make decorative folds. Place on a baking sheet and cover with a damp towel. Repeat with remaining wonton wrappers and filling.

3. *Ginger Sauce:* In a bowl, combine tamari, water, rice vinegar and ginger. Pour into 4 small individual bowls, dividing equally.

4. *Spicy Garlic Sauce:* In a bowl, combine fish sauce, water, chopped garlic and fresh hot chile pepper to taste, lime juice and brown sugar, stirring until sugar is dissolved. Pour into 4 separate small bowls.

5. In a steamer basket set over a pot of boiling water, steam dumplings until wrappers are tender and filling is hot, about 8 minutes. Serve dumplings hot with the two sauces for dipping.

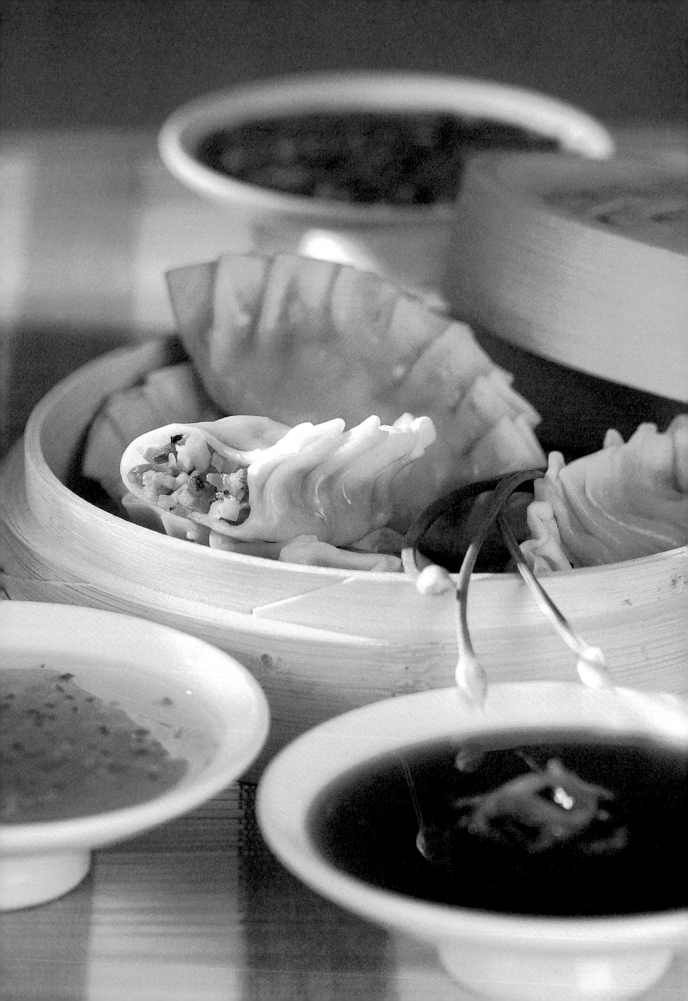

Spicy Lentil Samosas

**Makes
45 samosas**

Preparation time
45 minutes

Cooking time
50 minutes

- Food mill or food processor
- Candy/deep-fry thermometer

2 tbsp	extra virgin olive oil	30 mL
1/4 cup	finely chopped onion	60 mL
1 tbsp	chopped fresh gingerroot	15 mL
1/2 cup	dried brown lentils, rinsed	125 mL
1 1/2 cups	water	375 mL
	Salt	
2 tsp	ground turmeric	10 mL
	Ground cumin	
	Ground cinnamon	
1	bird's-eye chile pepper, minced	1
1/4 cup	chopped fresh cilantro	60 mL
15	large (12 inches/30 cm) square spring roll wrappers	15
1	egg, beaten	1
4 cups	vegetable oil	1 L

1. In a saucepan, heat olive oil over medium heat. Add onion and ginger and cook, stirring, until golden, about 5 minutes. Add lentils and water. Lightly season with salt and bring to a boil. Reduce heat to low, cover and simmer until lentils are tender, about 20 minutes. Pass mixture through food mill or process in a food processor to obtain a fairly thick purée. (Therefore it is important not to add too much water when cooking.)

2. Transfer purée to a bowl, if necessary, and stir in turmeric and a pinch each of cumin and cinnamon, then season with salt to taste. (These spices should enhance the flavor in a very delicate way without dominating.) Stir in chile pepper and cilantro.

3. Separate spring roll wrappers and cut each one into three equal rectangles. Keep wrappers covered with a damp cloth while working.

4. Place 1 tsp (5 mL) of lentil filling about 1/2 inch (1 cm) from edge on one end of a wrapper rectangle. Fold at a 45-degree angle to enclose filling in a small triangle. Continue to fold triangle, following its shape, along the strip. Once opposite end is reached, moisten the last 1/2 inch (1 cm) of wrapper with beaten egg to seal the triangle. Place on a baking sheet and cover with a damp tea towel. Repeat procedure with remaining wrappers and filling.

5. In a deep skillet, Dutch oven or deep fryer, heat oil to 400°F (200°C). In batches to avoid crowding, fry samosas, turning once, until deep golden and hot inside, about 4 minutes. Using a slotted spoon, remove from oil and place on a baking sheet lined with paper towels to drain. Serve hot.

Spanakopita

Preparation time
35 minutes

Cooking time
20 minutes

Tips

Your phyllo sheets should be about 16 by 12 inches (40 by 30 cm), making each strip about 16 by 3 inches (40 by 7.5 cm). If you have different size phyllo sheets, cut them to make approximately the same size strips. If the sheets are too short, double the number of strips and overlap them to make them longer.

Do not prepare spanakopitas too far in advance, especially if you refrigerate them, as the dough will become soggy. They can be frozen and then put directly in the oven before the meal, increasing the baking time to 20 to 25 minutes from frozen.

• **Preheat oven to 350°F (180°C)**

5 tsp	olive oil, divided	25 mL
8 oz	fresh spinach, trimmed	250 g
½ cup	finely chopped onion	125 mL
2	eggs, beaten	2
6 oz	feta cheese, crumbled	175 g
	Salt and freshly ground black pepper	
	Ground nutmeg	
8	sheets thawed phyllo pastry (see Tips, left)	8
¼ cup	butter, melted (approx.)	60 mL

1. In a skillet, heat 2 tsp (10 mL) of the oil over medium-high heat. Add spinach and cook, stirring, just until wilted. Transfer to a cutting board and chop coarsely. Transfer to a bowl.

2. In same skillet, heat remaining oil over medium heat. Add onion and cook, stirring, until softened but not browned, about 3 minutes. Add to spinach and let cool.

3. Stir eggs and feta cheese into spinach mixture and season with salt, pepper and nutmeg to taste.

4. Place one sheet of phyllo pastry on a cutting board and cut it lengthwise into four strips (keep remaining phyllo covered with a slightly damp tea towel to prevent it from drying out). Lightly brush butter on one strip of phyllo, then stack another strip on top. Repeat to make another stack of 2 strips.

5. Place 1 tbsp (15 mL) of spinach mixture on one end of the strips. Fold at a 45-degree angle to make a triangle. Continue to fold along the length of the strip of dough, maintaining its triangular shape. Before the last fold, lightly brush melted butter on the edge of the strip, then seal it. Lightly brush outside of triangle with butter. Place seam side down, at least 1 inch (2.5 cm) apart, on baking sheet. Repeat with remaining filling and phyllo to make 16 triangles total.

6. Bake spanakopitas in preheated oven until golden and crispy, about 15 minutes.

Imperial Rolls

Preparation time
35 minutes

Cooking time
2 to 3 minutes
per batch

Marinating time
4 hours

- Candy/deep-fry thermometer

1 oz	dried shiitake or Chinese black mushrooms	30 g
½ cup	julienned carrot	125 mL
½ cup	julienned celery	125 mL
¼ cup	finely chopped onion	60 mL
2	cloves garlic, chopped	2
½ cup	bean sprouts	125 mL
2 tbsp	soy sauce	30 mL
1 tbsp	rice vinegar	15 mL
	Salt and freshly ground black pepper	
2 oz	rice vermicelli	60 g
30	6-inch (15 cm) square spring roll wrappers	30
	Vegetable oil	
1	head leaf lettuce, separated into leaves	1
1	bunch fresh mint	1

Sauce

½ cup	fish sauce	125 mL
2	cloves garlic	2
	Minced hot chile pepper	
4 tsp	rice vinegar	20 mL
4 tsp	warm water	20 mL
	Granulated sugar	
	Julienned carrot	

1. In a small bowl, cover mushrooms with warm water and let stand until softened. Drain well and trim off stems if necessary, then thinly slice caps.

2. In a bowl, combine carrot, celery, onion, garlic, mushrooms, and bean sprouts. Stir in soy sauce and rice vinegar, then add salt and pepper to taste. Cover and let marinate at room temperature for 4 hours.

3. Meanwhile, in another bowl, soak rice vermicelli in very hot water until tender, for 5 minutes or according to package directions. Drain well and add to marinated vegetables.

4. *Sauce:* In a bowl, combine fish sauce, garlic, chile pepper to taste, vinegar, water and sugar to taste. Add julienned carrot to garnish. Set aside.

5. Working with one spring roll at a time and keeping the others covered with a damp tea towel, place wrapper on work surface with one corner toward you, so it resembles a diamond. Place a heaping tablespoon (15 mL) of the noodle mixture about 2 inches (5 cm) from the bottom point. Fold bottom corner up to cover filling. Brush remaining edges with water. Fold in both edges toward center, then roll up into a cylinder. Place, seam side down, on a baking sheet and cover with a tea towel. Repeat with remaining filling and wrappers.

6. In a deep skillet, Dutch oven or deep fryer, heat 3 inches (7.5 cm) of oil to 375°F (190°C). In batches, fry rolls, turning once, until deep golden and hot inside, 2 to 3 minutes. Using a slotted spoon, remove from oil and place on a baking sheet lined with paper towels to drain.

7. Arrange lettuce leaves on a platter and mint leaves in a bowl. Arrange rolls on another platter. To eat, place a few mint leaves on top of each lettuce leaf, then wrap around roll and dip in the sauce.

Fresh Spring Rolls

Makes 12 rolls

Preparation time
35 minutes

Standing time
2 hours

Tip
Be sure to keep rolls well wrapped and slightly damp to prevent their drying out. Well-wrapped rolls can be refrigerated for up to 4 hours before serving.

6 oz	rice vermicelli	175 g
12	round rice paper wrappers	12
12	lettuce leaves	12
¾ cup	julienned carrot	175 mL
¾ cup	julienned cucumber	175 mL
1	mango, julienned	1
2	packages enoki mushrooms	2
¼	bunch fresh cilantro	¼
1	bunch fresh mint	1
Sauce		
1	clove garlic, chopped	1
5 tsp	granulated sugar	25 mL
½ cup	fish sauce	125 mL
⅓ cup	freshly squeezed lime juice	75 mL
½	carrot, julienned	½
2	hot chile peppers, chopped	2
⅔ cup	boiling water	150 mL

1. In a bowl, soak rice vermicelli in hot water until tender, for at least 2 hours or according to package directions. Rinse with cold water to chill, then drain well.

2. *Sauce:* In a large bowl, combine garlic, sugar, fish sauce, lime juice, carrot and chile peppers. Pour boiling water over top. Cover and set aside.

3. *Prepare rolls:* Dip each rice paper wrapper into a shallow dish of warm water, just until softened and flexible. Gently shake off excess water and place on work surface, making sure wrappers do not touch each other (it's best to work with two or three at a time). Lay a lettuce leaf on top of each. Add a few vermicelli noodles in a line across the bottom third of the circle, leaving a 1-inch (2.5 cm) border at each side, then top with carrot, cucumber, mango and mushrooms. Fold sides of circle toward center over filling, then, starting at the bottom, roll over once to enclose filling, pulling tightly. Add 3 cilantro leaves on top of filling, roll one-half turn and add 2 or 3 mint leaves, then roll up and place seam side down, at least 1 inch (2.5 cm) apart, on a baking sheet lined with a damp tea towel. Cover with a slightly damp tea towel and plastic wrap.

4. When ready to serve, pour sauce into a small bowl and cut rolls in half. Serve in individual dishes or on a tray.

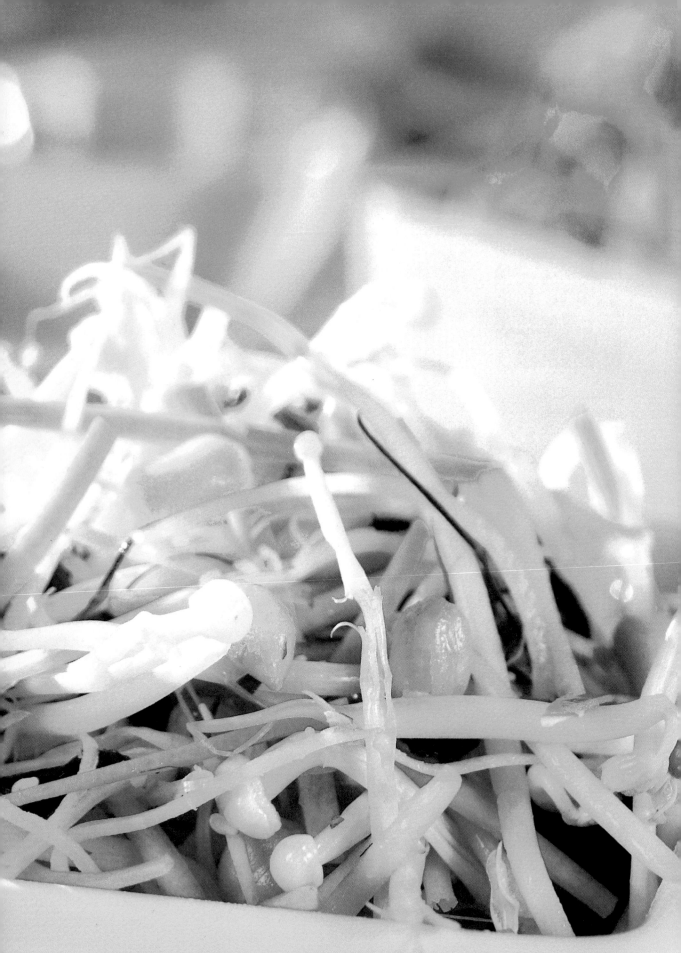

Japanese Salad (page 72)

Salads

Layered Beets, Goat Cheese and Artichokes

Serves 4

Preparation time
2 hours

Cooking time
1 hour 30 minutes

Tips

Do not assemble ahead of time, as the beets will color the cheese.

We love Chèvre des Neiges cheese, a triple-cream goat milk Brie cheese from Quebec, for this recipe. It is very creamy and gets extra flavor from the goat milk. If you can't find it, a regular Brie cheese or another soft goat milk cheese would work as well.

Mizuna lettuce is a tender, peppery-flavored green that is also known as Japanese greens or spider mustard. You can use arugula or other peppery greens if mizuna is not available.

1	large red beet	1
10 oz	triple-cream goat milk Brie cheese, rind removed (see Tips, left)	300 g
2 tsp	heavy or whipping (35%) cream	10 mL
	Salt and freshly ground black pepper	
2 tbsp	olive oil, divided	30 mL
	Juice of 1 lemon, divided	
2	cooked artichoke bottoms or drained canned artichoke hearts, finely diced	2
2 tbsp	chopped skinned toasted hazelnuts	30 mL
	Finely chopped fresh chives to taste	
2 cups	mizuna lettuce (see Tips, left)	500 mL
	Chopped toasted hazelnuts for garnish	

1. Place beet in a large saucepan, add salted water to cover and bring to a boil over high heat. Reduce heat and boil gently until the skin is easy to remove and beet is tender, about 1 hour and 30 minutes. Place in cold water and let cool. Cut crosswise into twelve $1/8$-inch (3 mm) slices. Using a cookie cutter, trim each slice into a perfect circle, discarding scraps or reserving for another use.

2. Using a wooden spoon, mash cheese, cream, and salt and pepper to taste until smooth.

3. In a skillet, heat 1 tbsp (15 mL) each of the oil and lemon juice over medium heat. Add artichokes and cook, stirring, until heated through. Season with salt and pepper to taste.

4. Place the cookie cutter used to cut the beets on an individual serving plate. Place a slice of beet at the bottom.

5. Spoon goat cheese mixture into a pastry bag. Pipe cheese on top of beet, filling cookie cutter halfway. Add another slice of beet. Pipe another layer of cheese, then top with another slice of beet, taking care not to exceed the height of the cookie cutter. Press lightly, then remove the cookie cutter. Assemble three more plates in the same way.

6. In a small bowl, combine remaining oil, lemon juice, artichokes, hazelnuts, chives, and salt and pepper to taste. Toss a little of the dressing with the mizuna lettuce and place some lettuce on top of each stack.

7. Drizzle remaining dressing over assembled stacks. Sprinkle a few chopped toasted hazelnuts on top.

Endive Flowers with Tomatoes and Mangos

Serves 4

Preparation time
15 minutes

Cooking time
5 minutes

See photo, opposite

Tips

Ataulfo mangos are a small variety with golden yellow skin and deep, golden yellow, smooth-textured flesh. They have an intense mango flavor and are worth seeking out for this recipe.

For this recipe you can use inexpensive balsamic vinegar sold in supermarkets.

● Preheat oven to 375°F (190°C)

3 cups	cubed day-old bread	750 mL
	Olive oil	
2	large Belgian endives	2
1	large ripe tomato, cut into ¾-inch (2 cm) cubes	1
2	Ataulfo mangos, cut into ¾-inch (2 cm) cubes (see Tips, left)	2
	Salt and freshly ground black pepper	
¼ cup	extra virgin olive oil	60 mL
1 tbsp	balsamic vinegar (see Tips, left)	15 mL
	Fresh chives, finely chopped	

1. Place bread cubes on a baking sheet and drizzle lightly with olive oil. Toast in preheated oven for about 5 minutes or until golden and crisp. Set aside.

2. Remove outer leaves of endives, using inner portions for another purpose or discarding. Arrange on individual serving plates to resemble a flower.

3. In a bowl, combine tomato and mangos with croutons. Add salt and pepper to taste. Sprinkle with extra virgin olive oil and balsamic vinegar.

4. Spoon mixture equally into endive arrangement. Garnish with chives and serve.

Endive Salad with Pecans

Serves 4

Preparation time
15 minutes

Tip

Endives are grown in the dark to prevent them from turning green. The lack of color keeps the leaves sweet and mild. Be sure to choose endives that are as white as possible for the best flavor for this salad.

½ cup	plain full-fat yogurt	125 mL
	Juice of 2 lemons	
	Salt and freshly ground black pepper	
1 lb	Belgian endives, leaves separated (see Tip, left)	500 g
2 tsp	chopped fresh chervil	10 mL
2 tsp	finely chopped fresh chives	10 mL
1 cup	pecan halves, chopped	250 mL

1. In a large bowl, combine yogurt, lemon juice, and salt and pepper to taste. Add endive leaves, chervil, chives and pecans. Toss gently to coat (being careful not to break the endive leaves). Serve immediately.

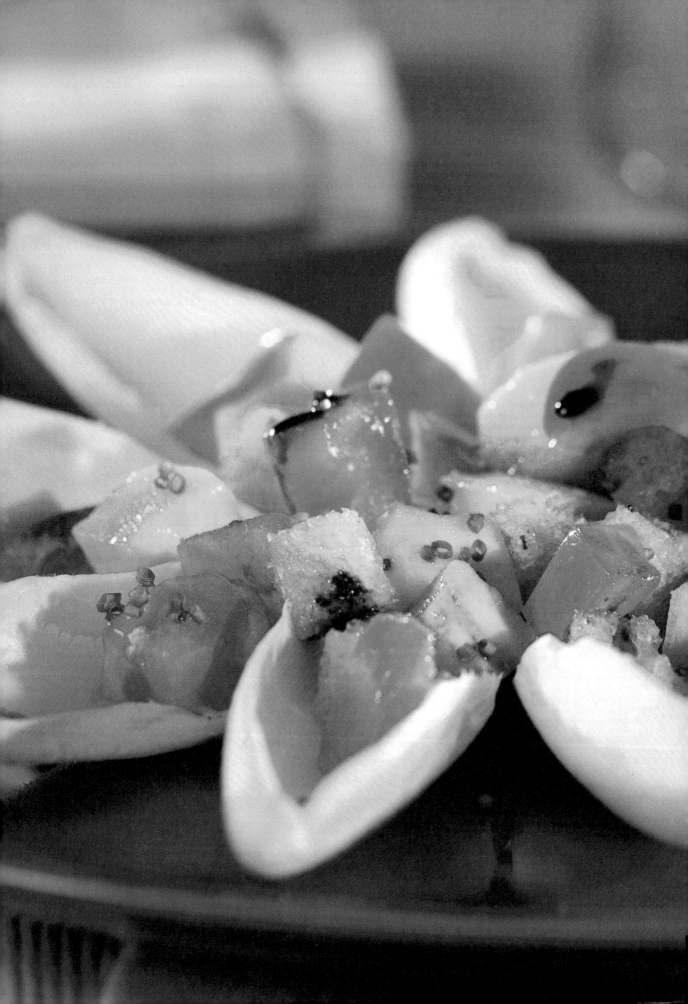

Woodsy Mixed Sprout Salad

See photo, opposite

Tip

You can use your favorite wild or exotic mushrooms in place of the girolles or chanterelles. Trim off any tough stems from mushrooms, and if they're large, cut into thick slices before cooking.

1¼ cups	lentils	300 mL
1¼ cups	pumpkin seeds	300 mL
1¼ cups	adzuki beans	300 mL
1¼ cups	barley	300 mL
⅓ cup	mustard seeds	75 mL
¼ cup	butter	60 mL
1 tbsp	olive oil	15 mL
1 cup	girolle (golden chanterelle) mushrooms	250 mL
1 cup	chanterelle mushrooms (see Tip, left)	250 mL
3 tbsp	finely chopped French shallots	45 mL
1	bunch fresh Italian flat-leaf parsley, chopped	1
1	bunch fresh cilantro, chopped	1
¾ cup	sliced almonds	175 mL
	Salt and freshly ground black pepper	

1. In a large bowl, cover lentils with at least 4 inches (7.5 cm) cold water. Cover and let soak overnight. In separate bowls, repeat with pumpkin seeds, adzuki beans, barley and mustard seeds.

2. Rinse and drain lentils and transfer to a large glass jar. Let jar stand in a cool (59 to 68°F/15 to 20°C) dark place for about 3 days or until sprouts are desired length. Repeat with pumpkin seeds, adzuki beans, barley and mustard seeds, using separate jars for each. Each day, empty lentils, etc. into a sieve and rinse and drain. Rinse jar, then return lentils to jar. Sprouting time will vary for the different beans and seeds. Plan for about 72 hours. (Although it is better to slightly cook the beans and seeds before using them, some can also be eaten raw, except the mustard seeds.)

3. In a large skillet, heat butter and oil over high heat. Sauté mushrooms for about 5 minutes or until liquid is released and mushrooms are brown. Add shallots, parsley and cilantro.

4. Add mushroom mixture while still warm to sprouts. Add almonds. Toss well and season with salt and pepper to taste. Serve slightly warm.

Carrot and Orange Salad

1 lb	carrots, peeled and shredded	500 g
⅔ cup	orange juice	150 mL
3 tbsp	freshly squeezed lemon juice	45 mL
	Salt and freshly ground black pepper	
½ cup	blanched almonds	125 mL
½ cup	raisins	125 mL
1 tbsp	chopped fresh parsley	15 mL

1. In a large bowl, combine carrots, orange juice, lemon juice, and salt and pepper to taste.

2. Add almonds, raisins and parsley. Cover and refrigerate until chilled, for at least 1 hour or for up to 4 hours. Serve chilled.

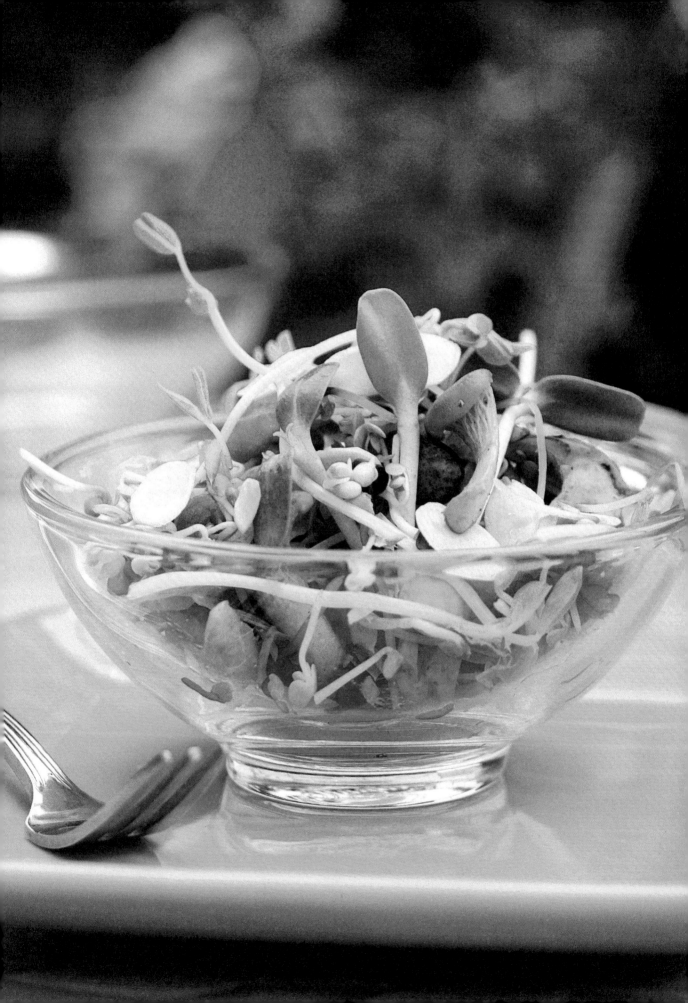

Marinated Beet Salad with Honey Dressing

Serves 4

Preparation time
1 hour 45 minutes

Cooking time
1 hour 30 minutes

Marinating time
2 hours

1	medium red beet, leaves trimmed off	1
1	medium yellow beet, leaves trimmed off	1
2 tsp	white vinegar	10 mL
	Salt	

Honey Dressing

1 tbsp	vegetable oil	15 mL
2 tsp	liquid honey	10 mL
1 tsp	apple cider vinegar	5 mL
	Salt and freshly ground black pepper	
1½ cups	mesclun greens	375 mL
1 tsp	finely chopped fresh chives	5 mL

1. Place red beet and yellow beet in two separate saucepans. Add water to cover. Stir 1 tsp (5 mL) of the vinegar into each and season with salt. Bring to a boil over high heat. Reduce heat and boil gently until the skin is easy to remove and beets are tender, 1 to 1½ hours. (Cooking time will vary according to the size of the beets.) Drain and let cool. Trim off remaining stems and tap roots and peel off skins.

2. *Honey Dressing:* In a small bowl, combine oil, honey, vinegar, and salt and pepper to taste.

3. Cut beets crosswise into thin ⅛-inch (3 mm) slices and place in separate dishes. (You do not want the red beets to color the yellow ones.) Drizzle each with about 1½ tsp (7 mL) of the dressing and marinate for at least 2 hours or for up to 8 hours.

4. In a bowl, combine greens, chives and remaining dressing.

5. *To serve:* Arrange a few slices of red beets on each of four individual serving plates, add some mixed salad greens and then slices of yellow beet. Repeat twice for each ingredient.

Papaya, Tomato and Mango Salad

Serves 4

Preparation time
10 minutes

Tip
For this recipe you can use inexpensive balsamic vinegar sold in supermarkets.

¼	papaya, cut into ¾-inch (2 cm) cubes	¼
1	large tomato, cut into ¾-inch (2 cm) cubes	1
1	mango, cut into ¾-inch (2 cm) cubes	1
1	head Boston lettuce, torn into bite-size pieces	1
	Salt and freshly ground black pepper	
3 tbsp	extra virgin olive oil	45 mL
	Balsamic vinegar (see Tip, left)	

1. In a large bowl, combine papaya, tomato, mango, lettuce, and salt and pepper to taste. Add oil, plus vinegar to taste. Stir well and serve immediately.

Caesar Salad

Serves 4

Preparation time
20 minutes

Cooking time
5 minutes

Tip

This recipe contains raw egg yolks. If you are concerned about the safety of using raw eggs, you may want to avoid this recipe.

Variation

You can replace romaine lettuce with 8 cups (2 L) baby spinach leaves.

● **Preheat oven to 375°F (190°C)**

1 cup	cubed day-old country bread ($\frac{1}{2}$-inch/1 cm cubes)	250 mL

Caesar Dressing

1	egg yolk (see Tip, left)	1
$\frac{1}{2}$ tsp	Dijon mustard	2 mL
	Juice of 1 lemon	
	Hot pepper sauce	
$\frac{1}{4}$ cup	vegetable oil	60 mL
$\frac{1}{4}$ cup	extra virgin olive oil	60 mL
1 tsp	chopped drained capers	5 mL
$\frac{1}{2}$	clove garlic, minced	$\frac{1}{2}$
	A few leaves chopped fresh Italian flat-leaf parsley	
$\frac{1}{2}$	head romaine lettuce, torn into bite-size pieces	$\frac{1}{2}$
3 tbsp	freshly grated vegetarian-friendly Parmesan cheese (see Tips, page 51)	45 mL
	Shaved vegetarian-friendly Parmesan	

1. Spread bread cubes on a baking sheet and toast in preheated oven for about 5 minutes or until golden and crisp. Set aside.

2. *Caesar Dressing:* In a large bowl, whisk together egg yolk, mustard, lemon juice and hot pepper sauce to taste. Gradually drizzle in vegetable oil and olive oil, whisking constantly, to make a mayonnaise. Add capers, garlic and parsley.

3. Add lettuce, croutons and grated Parmesan to dressing and toss to coat. Garnish with shaved Parmesan.

Cucumber Salad

Serves 4

Preparation time
25 minutes

Chilling time
1 hour

Variation

You can also add 8 oz (250 g) cubed cooked potatoes to this salad.

2	English cucumbers	2
$\frac{3}{4}$ cup	sour cream	175 mL
1 tbsp	red wine vinegar	15 mL
1 tbsp	Dijon mustard	15 mL
	Salt and freshly ground black pepper	
1 tsp	chopped chives	5 mL

1. Peel cucumbers, slice in half lengthwise and scoop out seeds. Cut cucumbers crosswise into $\frac{1}{4}$-inch (0.5 cm) slices.

2. In a large bowl, combine sour cream, vinegar, mustard, and salt and pepper to taste.

3. Add cucumbers and toss to combine. Sprinkle with chives. Cover and refrigerate for at least 1 hour, until chilled, or for up to 4 hours. Serve chilled.

Artichoke and King Oyster Mushroom Salad

See photo, opposite

Serves 4

Preparation time
20 minutes

Tip

Chicory is a curly green or greenish yellow bitter salad green. It is also known as niçoise lettuce, curly chicory, chicory endive or frisée. The young, more tender baby chicory is best for this salad.

8	baby artichokes	8
	Juice of 1 lemon, divided	
1	head baby chicory, chopped (see Tip, left)	1
1	king oyster mushroom, thinly sliced	1
3 oz	Grana Padano cheese, thinly shaved	90 g
¼ cup	extra virgin olive oil	60 mL
	Salt and freshly ground black pepper	
	Finely chopped fresh chives	

1. Remove the two outer layers of artichoke leaves. Cut off the upper half of the leaves to remove the indigestible tips and peel the stem. Scoop out the fuzzy purple choke. As you work, place trimmed artichokes in a bowl of water combined with half of the lemon juice to prevent browning.

2. In a large bowl, combine chicory, mushroom and cheese.

3. Just before serving, drain artichokes and slice thinly lengthwise. Add to bowl with chicory mixture along with olive oil. Season with salt and pepper to taste. Arrange salad in individual dishes and garnish with chives.

Fiddlehead Salad

Serves 4

Preparation time
50 minutes

Cooking time
15 minutes

• **Preheat oven to 400°F (200°C)**

1 lb	fiddleheads	500 g
1 cup	hazelnuts	250 mL
¼ cup	olive oil	60 mL
4 tsp	apple cider vinegar	20 mL
1 tsp	chopped fresh tarragon	5 mL
	Salt and freshly ground black pepper	
	Cayenne pepper	
2	tomatoes, seeded and finely diced	2
½ cup	finely chopped French shallots	125 mL

1. Wash fiddleheads thoroughly, changing the water several times. In a large pot of boiling water, boil fiddleheads for about 5 minutes or until tender-crisp. Drain and rinse under cold running water to cool. Drain well.

2. Place hazelnuts on a baking sheet and toast in preheated oven for 8 to 10 minutes or until toasted and fragrant. Rub in a tea towel to remove the skins.

3. In a large bowl, combine oil, vinegar, tarragon, and salt, black pepper and cayenne pepper to taste. Add fiddleheads, hazelnuts, tomatoes and shallots and toss to coat. Adjust seasoning to taste and serve.

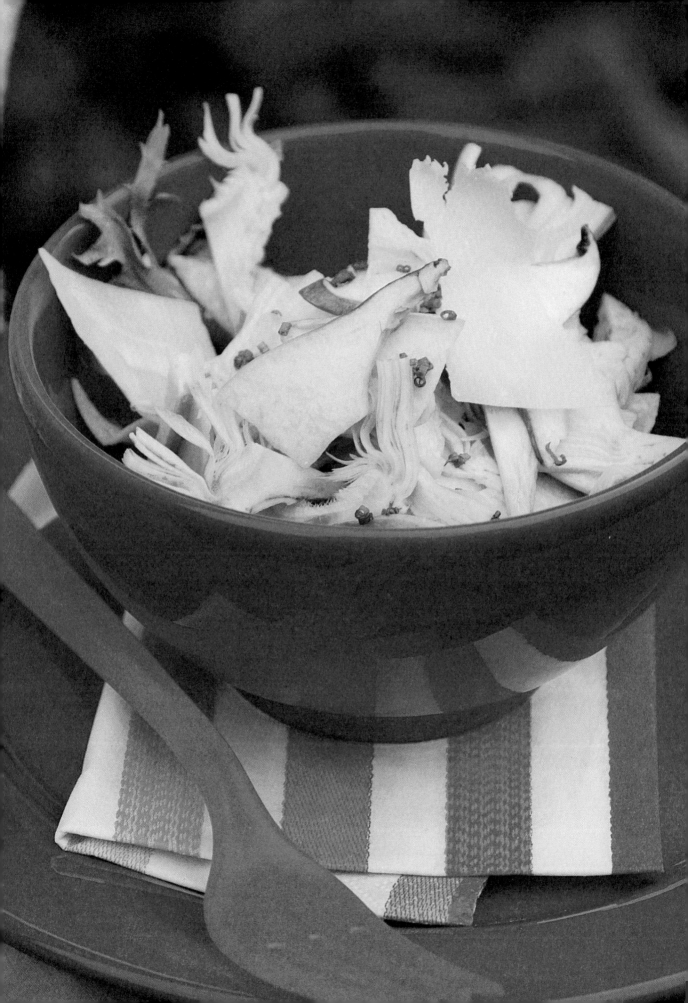

Green Bean and Legume Salad

10 oz	green beans	300 g
¾ cup	diced seeded tomatoes	175 mL
½ cup	canned chickpeas, drained and rinsed	125 mL
½ cup	canned kidney beans, drained and rinsed	125 mL
2	French shallots, finely chopped	2
1	red onion, finely chopped	1
1	clove garlic, chopped	1
⅓ cup	olive oil	75 mL
¼ cup	red wine vinegar	60 mL
1	bird's-eye chile pepper, chopped	1
2 tsp	chopped fresh cilantro	10 mL
2 tsp	chopped fresh parsley	10 mL
	Salt and freshly ground black pepper	

1. In a large saucepan of boiling salted water, boil green beans until tender-crisp, 3 to 4 minutes. Drain and rinse immediately in cold water until chilled. Drain well.

2. In a bowl, gently combine green beans, tomatoes, chickpeas and kidney beans. Add shallots, red onion, garlic, olive oil, vinegar, chile pepper, cilantro, parsley, and salt and pepper to taste.

3. Cover and marinate in the refrigerator for 2 hours before serving.

Green Bean Salad with Balsamic Vinaigrette

1 lb 5 oz	green beans, trimmed	650 g
4 tsp	balsamic vinegar (see Tip, left)	20 mL
	Salt	
¼ cup	olive oil	60 mL
	Freshly cracked peppercorns	
¼ cup	diced Vidalia onion	60 mL
¼ cup	julienned red bell pepper	60 mL
¼ cup	julienned yellow bell pepper	60 mL
¼ cup	julienned beet	60 mL
¼ cup	finely chopped Belgian endive	60 mL

1. In a large saucepan of boiling salted water, boil green beans until tender, about 7 minutes. Drain and rinse immediately in cold water until chilled. Drain well.

2. In a small bowl, whisk together balsamic vinegar and salt to taste until salt is dissolved. Slowly add olive oil, whisking constantly. Add peppercorns to taste.

3. In another bowl, combine beans, onion, red and yellow bell peppers, beet and endive. Add dressing and toss to coat. Serve immediately.

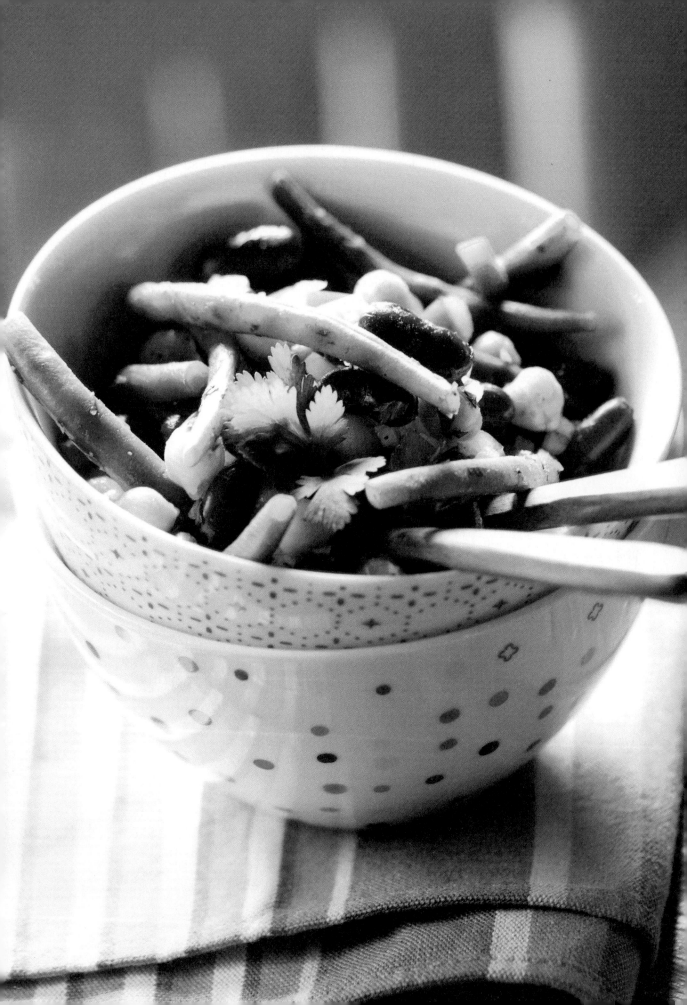

Caprese Salad

See photo, opposite

Serves 4		

Preparation time
10 minutes

2	balls buffalo mozzarella, torn into bite-size pieces	2
2	tomatoes, chopped	2
2	avocados, cut into wedges	2
8	large fresh basil leaves, finely chopped	8
	Fleur de sel or sea salt	
	Freshly ground black pepper	
	Extra virgin olive oil	

1. In four individual dishes, arrange alternating pieces of mozzarella, tomato and avocado, dividing equally among the plates and overlapping as necessary. Sprinkle with chopped basil. Add salt and pepper to taste. Drizzle with olive oil and serve.

Fried Ricotta and Spinach Salad

Serves 4		

Preparation time
15 minutes

Cooking time
25 minutes

Tip

Traditional ricotta is a very firm, dry fresh cheese that can be easily sliced. Look for it at well-stocked supermarkets and specialty cheese shops. If it's not available, omit oil, flour and eggs and skip Step 2, then crumble dry-pressed ricotta cheese, blue cheese or feta cheese on top of salad instead.

• **Preheat broiler**

1	red bell pepper	1
1	yellow bell pepper	1
1 cup	vegetable oil	250 mL
1 lb	traditional ricotta cheese (see Tip, left)	500 g
2 tbsp	all-purpose flour	30 mL
2	eggs, beaten	2
5 oz	baby spinach leaves (about 5 cups/1.25 L)	150 g
1/4 cup	extra virgin olive oil	60 mL
2 tbsp	balsamic vinegar	30 mL
	Salt and freshly ground black pepper	
3 tbsp	toasted pine nuts	45 mL

1. Place bell peppers on a baking sheet and place under preheated broiler and roast, turning often, until skin is blackened all over and peppers are tender, about 20 minutes. Transfer to a bowl, cover and let cool. Remove skin, core and seeds and cut flesh into thin strips.

2. In a large skillet, heat oil over medium heat. Cut ricotta into four slices of equal size. Place flour in a shallow dish and beaten eggs in a bowl. Dip each slice of ricotta in flour, then into egg. In batches as necessary, fry turning once, until golden, 30 to 60 seconds on each side. Transfer to a plate lined with paper towels to drain and set aside.

3. In a bowl, combine spinach, roasted peppers, olive oil, vinegar, and salt and pepper to taste. Arrange in individual dishes and garnish with pine nuts. Place a slice of fried ricotta on top of each portion and serve immediately.

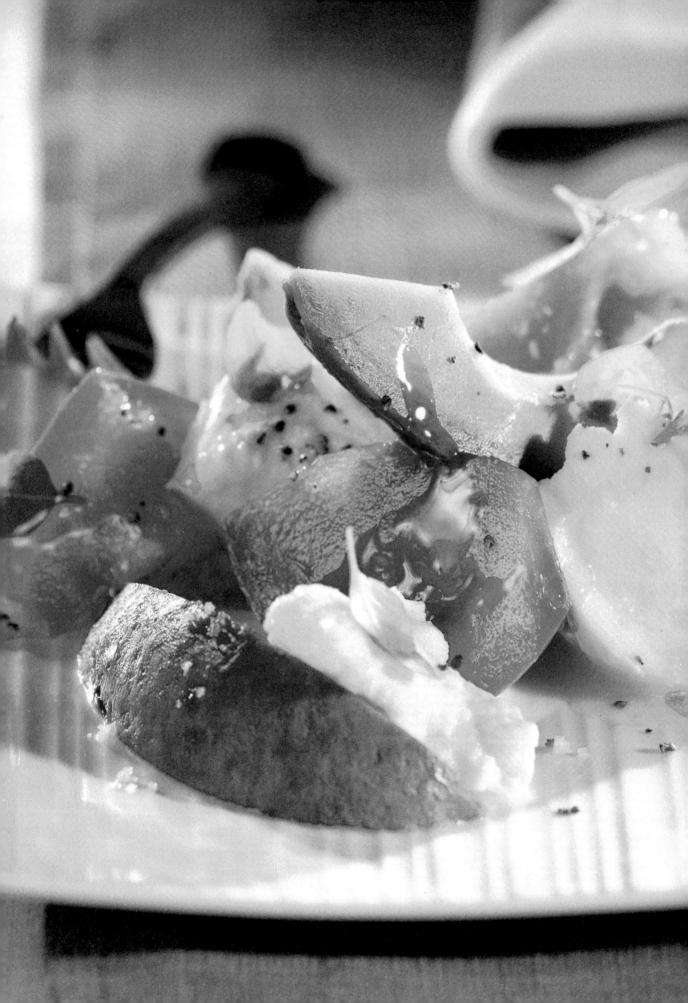

Salade Composée

Serves 4

Preparation time
1 hour

Dressing

7 tbsp	oil	105 mL
4 tsp	vinegar	20 mL
	Juice of 1 lemon, divided	
1 cup	julienned carrots	250 mL
½ tsp	chopped fresh parsley, divided	2 mL
2 tsp	finely chopped French shallots	10 mL
	Salt and freshly ground black pepper	
½ cup	mayonnaise	125 mL
2 tbsp	Dijon mustard	30 mL
1 cup	julienned celeriac	250 mL
	Cayenne pepper	
1 cup	shredded white cabbage	250 mL
1 cup	thinly sliced seeded cucumber	250 mL
½ tsp	chopped fresh chives	2 mL
1	large tomato, cut into wedges	1
½ tsp	finely chopped fresh basil	2 mL
1	head leaf lettuce, leaves separated	1
1	head radicchio, leaves separated	1
1	bunch radishes, leaves trimmed to 1 inch (2.5 cm)	1

1. *Dressing:* In a measuring cup, combine oil, vinegar and half the lemon juice.

2. In a bowl, combine carrots, one-quarter of the dressing, half of the parsley, and shallots. Add remaining lemon juice and salt and pepper to taste.

3. In another bowl, combine mayonnaise and mustard. Add celeriac and season with cayenne to taste.

4. In another bowl, combine cabbage, one-third of the remaining dressing and a little of the carrot mixture to add color. Add salt and pepper to taste.

5. In another bowl, combine cucumber, half of the remaining dressing, chives and salt and pepper to taste.

6. In another bowl, combine tomato, remaining dressing, basil and salt and pepper to taste.

7. On one large platter or 4 individual serving plates, arrange a bed of leaf lettuce and radicchio, then top with carrot, celeriac, cabbage, cucumber and tomato mixtures and garnish with radishes.

Pear and Chicory Salad with Parmesan

Serves 4

Preparation time
10 minutes

Tips

We prefer Packham
pears for this salad
but you can use any
flavorful firm, ripe pear
you prefer.

When buying cheese,
read the label carefully
and make sure to buy
those that are not made
from animal rennet.

1	bunch chicory, trimmed	1
2	pears, thinly sliced (see Tips, left)	2
	Juice of $1/2$ lemon	
	Salt and freshly ground black pepper	
$1/4$ cup	extra virgin olive oil	60 mL
3 oz	vegetarian-friendly Parmesan cheese, shaved (see Tips, left)	90 g

1. Separate chicory leaves from bunch and cut the stems that make up its heart lengthwise into quarters.

2. In a bowl, combine chicory and pears. Season with lemon juice and salt and pepper to taste. Add olive oil. Mix together thoroughly.

3. Arrange salad in individual dishes and generously garnish with Parmesan.

Baby Chicory with Papaya and Green Peppercorns

Serves 4

Preparation time
15 minutes

1	baby chicory, cut into bite-size pieces (see Tip, page 44)	1
1	large very ripe papaya, cut into $3/4$-inch (2 cm) cubes	1
Pinch	brown sugar	Pinch
	Juice of 1 lime	
1 tsp	crushed green peppercorns	5 mL
$1/4$ cup	extra virgin olive oil	60 mL
	Salt	

1. In a large bowl, gently combine chicory and papaya.

2. In a small bowl, dissolve brown sugar in lime juice. Add peppercorns, olive oil, and salt to taste. Add to salad and toss to coat.

Crunchy Vegetable Salad with Raspberry Vinaigrette

1	stalk celery, peeled and julienned	1
4	small fresh artichoke bottoms	4
	Olive oil	
	Salt and freshly ground black pepper	
3 oz	extra fine green beans (haricots verts), cooked	90 g
3 oz	baby yellow and orange carrots, cooked	90 g
⅓ cup	snow peas, cooked	75 mL
⅓ cup	small green peas, cooked	75 mL

Raspberry Vinaigrette

1 tbsp	olive oil	15 mL
1 tsp	raspberry vinegar	5 mL
	Salt and freshly ground black pepper	

1. In a pot of boiling salted water, cook celery until tender-crisp, about 2 minutes. Drain and set aside to cool.

2. Cut artichoke bottoms into quarters. In a skillet, heat oil over high heat. Sauté artichokes until tender-crisp, about 5 minutes. Season with salt and black pepper to taste.

3. In a large bowl, combine cooled salad ingredients.

4. *Raspberry Vinaigrette:* In small bowl, combine oil, raspberry vinegar, and salt and pepper to taste. Stir into salad and serve.

Warm Spinach and Citrus Salad

6	oranges	6
3	grapefruits	3
1 lb	fresh spinach, trimmed	500 g
¾ cup	diced red bell pepper	175 mL
2 tbsp	olive oil	30 mL
2 tsp	balsamic vinegar	10 mL
	Salt and freshly ground black pepper	

1. Peel oranges and grapefruits, then separate into quarters. Cut quarters into fairly large pieces.

2. Place spinach in a round-bottomed stainless steel mixing bowl set over a saucepan of boiling water. Add oranges, grapefruits, bell pepper, olive oil, vinegar, and salt and pepper to taste. Stir gently but quickly, just long enough to warm the salad without cooking it. Serve immediately.

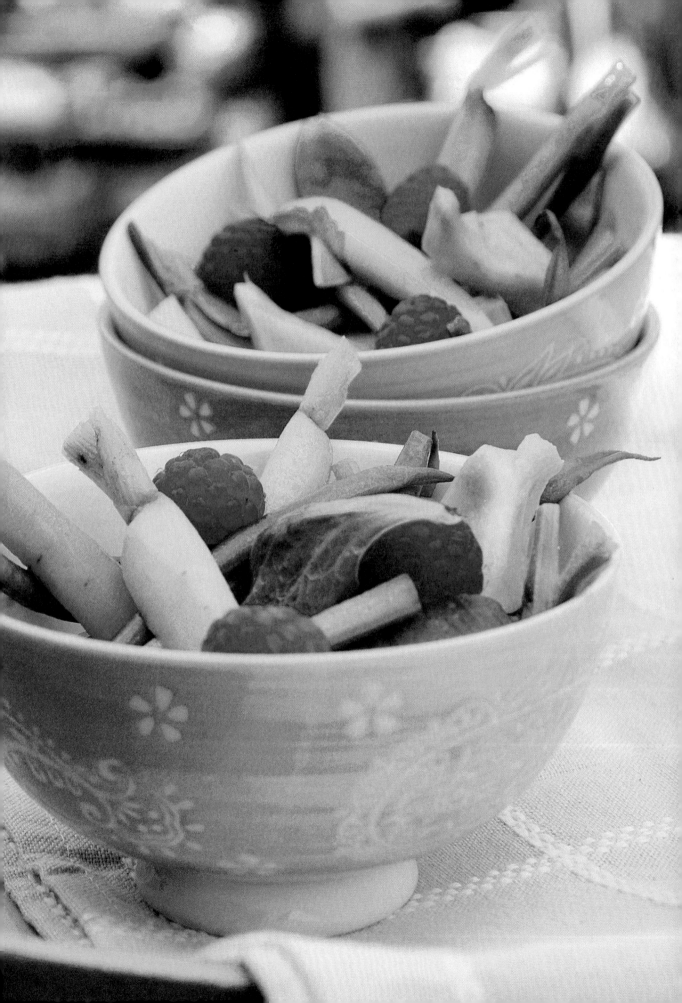

Sicilian Orange Salad

See photo, opposite

Serves 4

Preparation time
15 minutes

Marinating time
30 minutes

4	oranges, peeled and sliced	4
¼ cup	extra virgin olive oil	60 mL
	Salt and freshly ground black pepper	
½ cup	thinly sliced fennel bulb	125 mL
¼ cup	julienned red onion	60 mL
4	large lettuce leaves	4
	Chopped fresh Italian flat-leaf parsley	

1. In a bowl, combine oranges, olive oil, and salt and pepper to taste. Add fennel and red onion. Marinate at room temperature for about 30 minutes.

2. Place a lettuce leaf in the center of each serving plate, fill with salad mixture and garnish with parsley.

Baby Greens and Flowers with Parmesan Tuiles

Serves 4

Preparation time
20 minutes

Cooking time
10 minutes

Tips

Mizuna is a delicate, feathery lettuce green with a peppery mustard flavor.

Make sure you use flowers clearly labeled "not sprayed with pesticides" or use those you've grown yourself, chemical-free. Do not use flowers purchased from florist shops, which are often sprayed with chemicals.

- Preheat oven to 350°F (180°C)
- Ovenproof skillet

Parmesan Tuiles

1½ cups	freshly grated vegetarian-friendly Parmesan cheese (see Tips, page 51)	375 mL
2½ cups	mixed baby greens and sprouts, such as beet shoots, baby Swiss chard leaves, tatsoi, ficoïde glaciale, and/or mizuna lettuce	625 mL
20	nasturtium flowers (see Tips, left)	20
20	borage flowers	20
20	viola (or pansy) flowers	20

Dressing

	Juice of 3 limes	
4 tsp	olive oil	20 mL
	Salt and freshly ground black pepper	

1. *Parmesan Tuiles:* In an ovenproof skillet, in batches, divide Parmesan cheese to form four 5-inch (12 cm) rounds. Press down with a spoon to flatten into disks if necessary. Bake in preheated oven until cheese is melted and golden, 7 to 10 minutes.

2. In a large bowl, combine greens, sprouts, nasturtium, borage and viola flowers.

3. *Dressing:* In a small bowl, combine lime juice, oil, and salt and pepper to taste. Add to salad just before serving, stirring gently to combine.

4. Arrange salad in a dome on individual serving plates and place a Parmesan tuile on top of each.

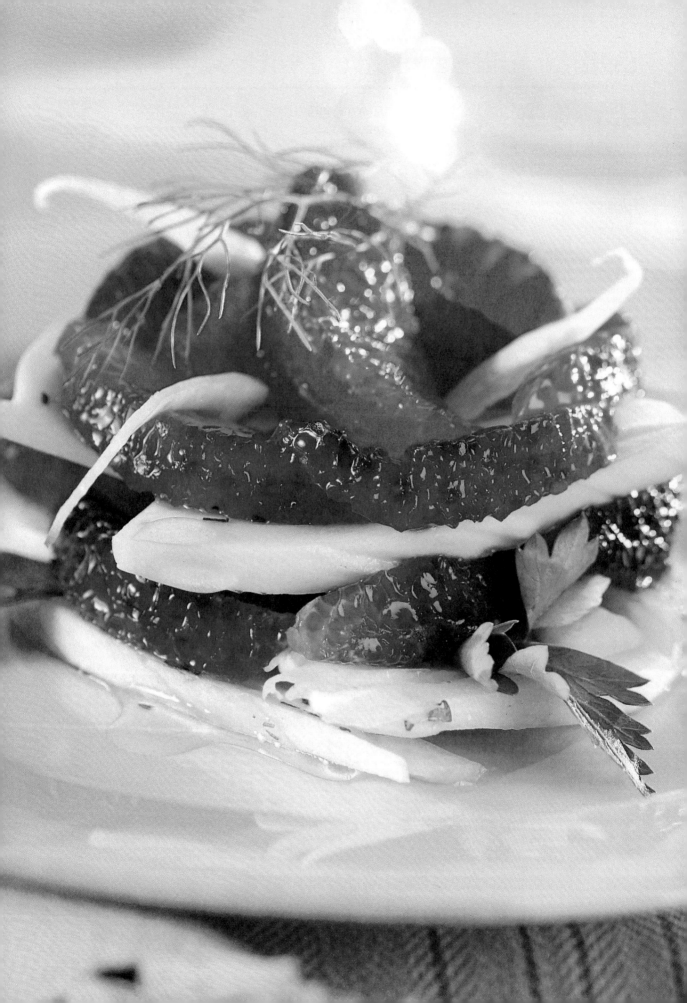

Celeriac and Seeds Salad with Maple Foam

Serves 4

Preparation time
15 minutes

1½ cups	julienned celeriac	375 mL
1½ cups	julienned carrots	375 mL
2 tbsp	pumpkin seeds	30 mL
2 tbsp	sunflower seeds	30 mL
	Salt	
4 tsp	olive oil	20 mL
4 tsp	hazelnut oil	20 mL
	Apple cider vinegar	
½ cup	low-fat (1%) or skim milk	125 mL
2 tsp	pure maple syrup	10 mL

1. In a bowl, combine celeriac, carrots, and pumpkin and sunflower seeds. Add salt to taste, olive oil, hazelnut oil and a few drops of cider vinegar.

2. Warm milk with maple syrup and foam it in the same way you would foam milk for a cappuccino. If you do not have a coffee machine or frother, this can be done using an immersion blender in a container with high sides to prevent splatters.

3. Arrange salad in individual serving bowls and top with maple milk foam.

Chayote Salad

Serves 4

Preparation time
10 minutes

2	chayotes (see Tip, left)	2
2 tbsp	slivered red onion	30 mL
	Finely chopped fresh cilantro leaves	
	Juice of 1 lime	
	Salt	
	Chopped fresh hot chile pepper	
3 tbsp	olive oil	45 mL

Tip

Chayotes are a member of the gourd family. They are referred to by many names, such as mirlitons, chow-chows, cho-chos, vegetable pears or alligator pears. You can find them in specialty produce markets, Asian, South American or Latin American stores and some well-stocked supermarkets.

1. Peel chayotes and cut in half lengthwise. Scoop out seeds, then cut flesh into thin slices.

2. In a bowl, combine chayotes, red onion and cilantro.

3. Season with lime juice and salt and chile pepper to taste. Sprinkle with olive oil and serve immediately.

Garganelli Salad with Artichokes and Squash

Tips

Garganelli pasta is a type of hand-rolled fresh pasta made with eggs. It is similar in shape to penne, but with ridges that run across the width of the tube, not the length. Look for it in specialty Italian food shops or substitute with penne.

Sweet Mama squash is a winter squash with a dark green skin and very sweet yellow flesh. You can use another type of winter squash if you prefer. *To roast squash:* Toss diced, peeled squash with a little olive oil and spread on a baking sheet. Roast in a 425°F (220°C) oven for about 45 minutes or until tender and golden brown.

8	baby artichokes	8
6 tbsp	olive oil, divided	90 mL
	Salt	
8 oz	garganelli pasta (see Tips, left)	250 g
1 cup	roasted diced Sweet Mama squash, chilled (see Tips, left)	250 mL
1	small bunch lemon balm leaves, finely chopped	1
	Juice of 1/2 lemon	
	Freshly ground black pepper	

1. Remove outer leaves of artichokes. Cut off tops of the leaves, trim stems and cut artichokes lengthwise into quarters. Scoop out any fuzzy purple choke.

2. In a heavy saucepan, heat 2 tbsp (30 mL) of the oil over high heat. Sauté artichokes for about 5 minutes or until tender-crisp. Add salt to taste. Transfer to a large bowl.

3. In a large pot of boiling salted water, cook garganelli pasta according to package directions until al dente. Drain and combine with artichokes. Add squash and stir well.

4. Add lemon balm, remaining olive oil and lemon juice. Generously sprinkle with pepper and serve immediately.

Fusilli Salad

Serves 4

Preparation time
30 minutes

Cooking time
10 minutes

Chilling time
2 hours

Tip
The ingredients can be combined while the pasta is still warm.

3 cups	fusilli pasta	750 mL
1 tbsp	olive oil	15 mL
1	tomato, diced	1
1/4 cup	drained capers, chopped	60 mL
1/4 cup	pitted black olives, cut lengthwise into quarters	60 mL
2 tsp	chopped fresh Italian flat-leaf parsley	10 mL
2 tsp	chopped fresh oregano leaves	10 mL
2 tsp	chopped fresh basil leaves	10 mL
2 cups	tomato sauce	500 mL
	Salt and freshly ground black pepper	

1. In a large pot of boiling salted water, cook pasta according to package directions until al dente. Drain and place in a large bowl. Sprinkle with olive oil and toss to coat.

2. Combine pasta, tomato, capers, olives, parsley, oregano, basil and tomato sauce. Season with salt and pepper to taste. Cover and let marinate in the refrigerator for at least 2 hours or for up to 1 day. Serve chilled.

Mediterranean-Style Rice Salad

Serves 4

Preparation time
20 minutes

Cooking time
20 minutes

1 1/4 cups	long-grain parboiled white rice	300 mL
	Olive oil	
4	drained canned artichoke hearts, quartered	4
24	cherry tomatoes, halved	24
24	kalamata olives, pitted or left whole	24
1	yellow bell pepper, finely chopped	1
1	buffalo mozzarella, cut into large cubes	1
	Salt and freshly ground black pepper	
	Juice of 1 lemon	
1/3 cup	olive oil	75 mL
8	leaves fresh basil, chopped	8
8	fresh chives, chopped	8
1	small bunch fresh Italian flat-leaf parsley, chopped	1
2	red endives, leaves separated	2
2 tbsp	drained capers	30 mL

1. Cook rice according to package directions until tender. Drain and let cool on a plate. Drizzle with olive oil.

2. In a bowl, combine rice, artichokes, tomatoes, olives, bell pepper and mozzarella. Add salt and pepper to taste. Add lemon juice and olive oil. Toss with basil, chives and parsley.

3. Arrange salad in a large dish. Decorate with endive leaves and garnish with capers.

Bavarian-Style Warm Potato Salad

1 lb	yellow-fleshed potatoes, unpeeled (about 2)	500 g
2 tbsp	butter	30 mL
½	Vidalia onion, cut into thin slices	½
Pinch	cumin seeds	Pinch
¼ cup	thinly sliced sour pickles	60 mL
1 tbsp	red wine vinegar	15 mL
	Salt and freshly ground black pepper	
1	small bunch fresh Italian flat-leaf parsley, chopped	1
¼ cup	extra virgin olive oil	60 mL

1. Place potatoes in a large pot and add cold, salted water to cover. Bring to a boil over high heat. Reduce heat and boil gently for about 40 minutes or until fork-tender. Drain and let cool just enough to handle.

2. Meanwhile, in a skillet, melt butter over medium heat. Cook onion, stirring occasionally, until lightly golden.

3. Add cumin seeds and pickles. Deglaze with vinegar, scraping up all the browned bits on the bottom of pan. Remove from heat.

4. Peel cooked potatoes while they are still hot. Cut into ½-inch (1 cm) slices and place in a large bowl.

5. Pour warm onion and pickle mixture over potatoes while they are still hot. Add salt and pepper to taste. Add parsley and sprinkle with olive oil. Stir gently and serve.

Potato Salad with Grainy Mustard

1½ lbs	Yukon Gold potatoes, unpeeled (about 6)	750 g
1 cup	finely chopped red onion	250 mL
2 tbsp	chopped fresh Italian flat-leaf parsley	30 mL
2 tbsp	finely chopped fresh chives	30 mL
1 tsp	chopped fresh tarragon leaves	5 mL
½ cup	drained capers, chopped	125 mL
3 tbsp	grainy mustard	45 mL
	Salt and freshly ground black pepper	
¼ cup	olive oil	60 mL
4 tsp	white wine vinegar	20 mL

1. Place potatoes in a large pot and add cold, salted water to cover. Bring to a boil over high heat. Reduce heat and boil gently for about 40 minutes or until fork-tender. Drain and let cool enough to handle. Peel potatoes and cut into small cubes.

2. In a large bowl, carefully combine potatoes, red onion, parsley, chives, tarragon, capers, mustard, and salt and pepper to taste. Add olive oil and vinegar. Cover and refrigerate for at least 2 hours before serving or for up to 1 day.

Lentil Salad

Serves 4

Preparation time
45 minutes

Cooking time
30 minutes

Marinating time
2 hours

Tips

Puy lentils are tiny French green lentils that are often found in specialty stores. If you can't find them, use regular dried green or brown lentils and increase the cooking time by 5 to 10 minutes.

A bouquet garni is a small bundle of aromatic herbs tied together with kitchen string. It is used to add flavor to a simmered or boiled mixture and is generally discarded before the dish is served. It often includes parsley, thyme and bay leaves but can also include any of your favorite herbs that complement the flavors of your dish.

Variation

You can also use a little yogurt in the dressing.

1	onion, cut in half	1
1	whole clove	1
10 oz	Puy lentils (see Tips, left)	300 g
1	carrot, cut into large sticks	1
1	bouquet garni (see Tips, left)	1
1	stalk celery, cut into small sticks	1
1	sprig savory	1
1	onion, finely chopped	1
3	cloves garlic, finely chopped	3
2 tbsp	chopped fresh Italian flat-leaf parsley	30 mL
4 tsp	chopped fresh cilantro leaves	20 mL
1	tomato, cut into large cubes	1
⅔ cup	toasted slivered almonds	150 mL

Dressing

1 tbsp	Dijon mustard	15 mL
¼ cup	olive oil	60 mL
2 tbsp	sherry vinegar	30 mL
	Salt and freshly ground black pepper	

1. Insert clove into one onion half.

2. Place lentils in a large saucepan and cover with water to ¾ inch (2 cm) above lentils. Add carrot, onion halves, bouquet garni, celery and savory and bring to a boil over high heat. Reduce heat to medium-low, cover and simmer gently until lentils are tender but firm, 20 to 30 minutes. Add water if necessary during cooking, but when the lentils are cooked there should not be any liquid left. Transfer lentils to a dish and let cool slightly. Discard carrot, onion halves, bouquet garni, celery and savory sprig.

3. *Dressing:* In a bowl, combine mustard, oil, vinegar, and salt and pepper to taste.

4. While lentils are still warm, add dressing, finely chopped onion, garlic, parsley and cilantro.

5. Cover and marinate salad in the refrigerator for 2 hours. Just before serving, add tomatoes and almonds. Mix thoroughly and adjust seasoning.

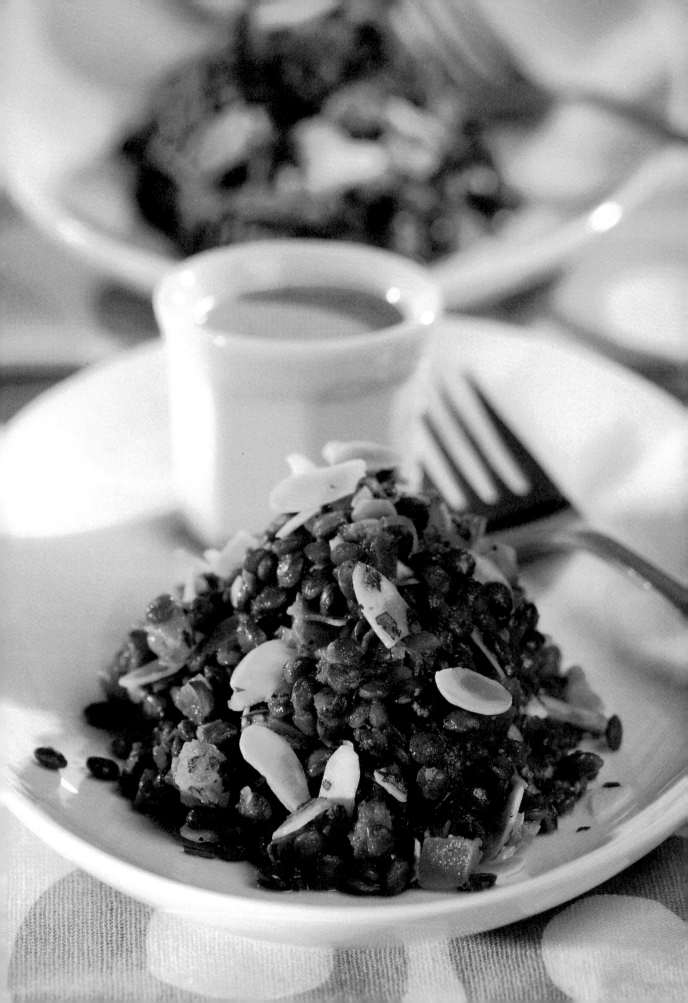

Rice Salad with Almond, Broad Beans and Cilantro

Serves 4

Preparation time
30 minutes

Cooking time
55 minutes

1 cup	long-grain white rice	250 mL
½ cup	wild rice	125 mL
2	tomatoes	2
4 tsp	butter	20 mL
¼ cup	chopped onion	60 mL
3 cups	broad (fava) beans in their pods	750 mL
1	clove garlic, chopped	1
1 cup	slivered almonds, toasted	250 mL
1 tbsp	chopped fresh cilantro	30 mL

Dressing

2 tbsp	olive oil	30 mL
	Juice of 3 lemons	
4 tsp	Dijon mustard	20 mL
	Salt and freshly ground black pepper	
	Ground nutmeg	

1. Cook long-grain rice and wild rice separately according to package directions until tender. Spread out on a baking sheet to cool. Transfer to a large bowl.

2. Meanwhile, in a pot of boiling water, blanch tomatoes, about 30 seconds. Immediately plunge into cold water and let cool. Peel off skins, remove seeds and cut into cubes. Add to rice in bowl.

3. In a saucepan, melt butter over medium heat. Stir in onion. Reduce heat to low, cover and sweat onion until softened, about 5 minutes. Add to rice mixture.

4. In a pot of boiling water, cook beans until pods are tender-crisp. Drain and rinse in cold water until chilled. Remove beans from pods, discarding pods, then add to rice mixture.

5. Add garlic, almonds and cilantro to rice mixture.

6. *Dressing:* In a small bowl, combine olive oil, lemon juice, mustard, and salt, pepper and nutmeg to taste. Add to salad, stir and adjust seasoning.

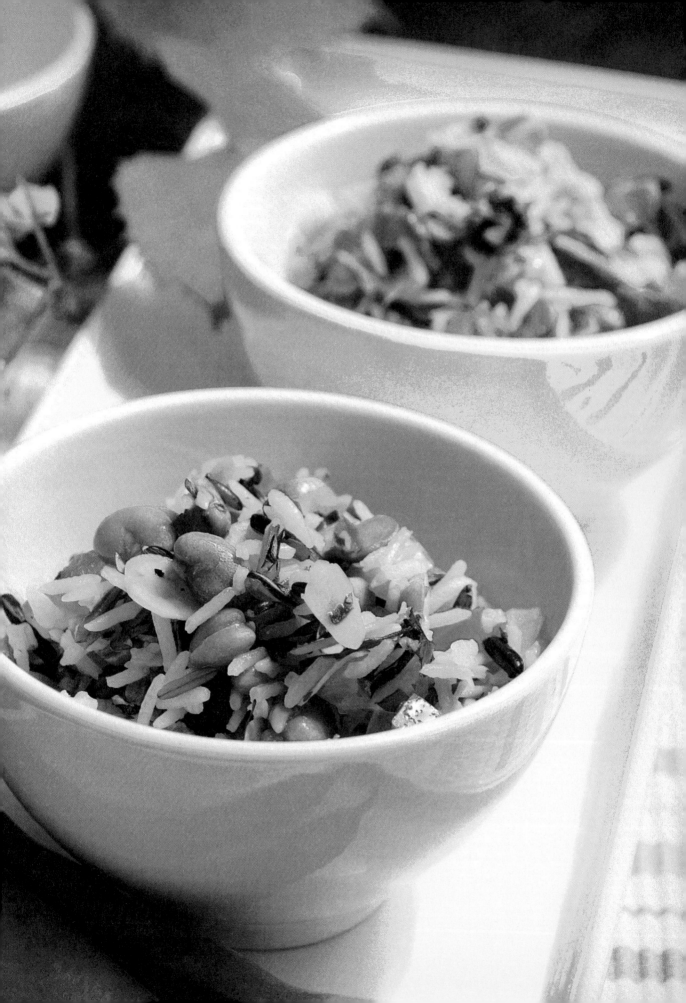

Quinoa Salad

Serves 4

Preparation time
1 hour 15 minutes

Cooking time
1 hour

Tip

Both white and red quinoa are commonly available in health food stores, bulk stores and some well-stocked supermarkets. Using both colors adds a nice look to this salad but you can use 1½ cups (375 mL) of one if you prefer.

Vegetable Stock

2 tbsp	olive oil	30 mL
½ cup	onion trimmings	125 mL
½ cup	chopped carrot	125 mL
¼ cup	chopped celery	60 mL
¼ cup	mushroom trimmings	60 mL
2	cloves garlic	2
10 cups	water	2.5 L
6	sprigs parsley	6
1	sprig thyme	1
1 tbsp	olive oil	15 mL
¾ cup	finely chopped onion	175 mL
1 cup	white quinoa (see Tip, left)	250 mL
½ cup	red quinoa	125 mL
3	star anise	3
	Salt and freshly ground black pepper	
2	ears corn	2
1 cup	small green peas, cooked and cooled	250 mL
1 cup	small cauliflower florets, cooked and cooled	250 mL
1 cup	small broccoli florets, cooked and cooled	250 mL
2 tbsp	chopped fresh Italian flat-leaf parsley	30 mL
1	bird's-eye chile pepper, finely chopped	1
½ cup	olive oil	125 mL
3 tbsp	freshly squeezed lime juice	45 mL

1. *Vegetable Stock:* In a large pot, heat olive oil over medium heat. Stir in onion trimmings, carrot, celery, mushroom trimmings and garlic. Reduce heat to low, cover and sweat vegetables until slightly softened, about 5 minutes. Add water, parsley and thyme and bring to a gentle boil over high heat. Reduce heat and simmer gently until stock is flavorful, about 1 hour. Strain into a clean pot, discarding vegetables. Keep stock hot.

2. In a large saucepan, heat 1 tbsp (15 mL) olive oil over medium heat. Stir in onion. Reduce heat to low, cover and sweat onions until softened, about 5 minutes. Add white and red quinoa, star anise, and salt and pepper to taste. Blend well and add enough hot vegetable stock to cover. Cook slowly, adding more vegetable stock from time to time until quinoa is cooked but still slightly firm. Spread quinoa on a plate to stop the cooking process. Let cool completely. Discard star anise.

3. Meanwhile, in a large pot of boiling water, boil corn for 5 minutes. Remove from heat and let cool slowly in the cooking water. (This will prevent the kernels from shriveling as they cool and allow them to remain juicy.)

4. Place each corn cob vertically in a large bowl and, holding it firmly, use a sharp knife to remove the kernels. Add quinoa, peas, cauliflower, broccoli, parsley, chile pepper, olive oil and lime juice. Mix together carefully and adjust seasoning if necessary.

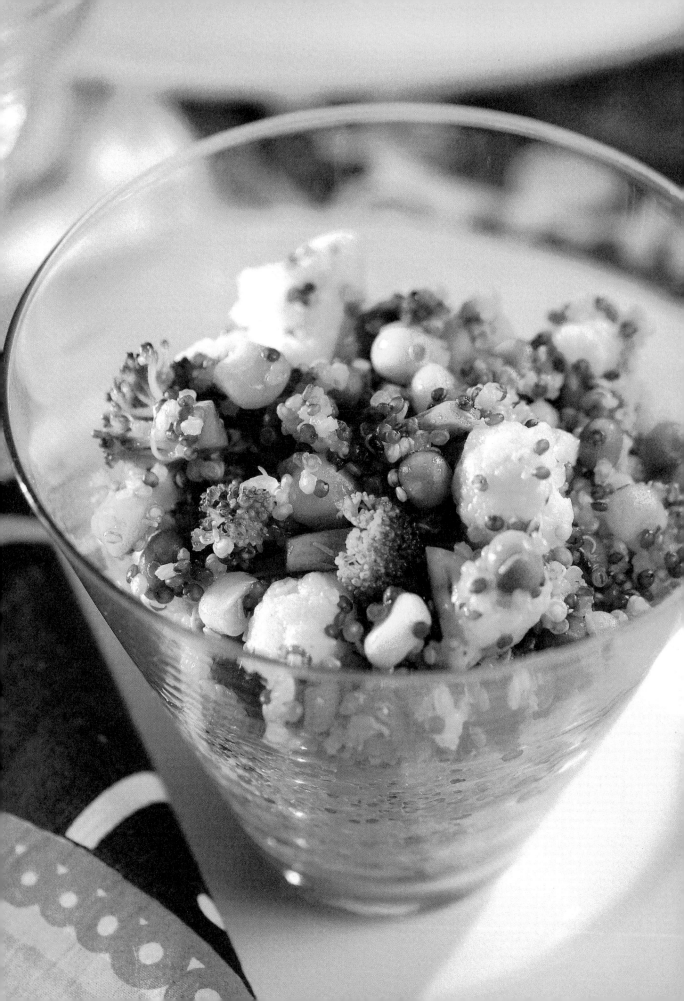

Tabbouleh

Serves 4

Preparation time
15 minutes

Cooking time
1 hour

Chilling time
3 hours

¾ cup	fine bulgur	175 mL
1¼ cups	boiling water	300 mL
3	bunches fresh Italian flat-leaf parsley, chopped	3
½	bunch fresh mint, finely chopped	½
¾ cup	finely chopped onion	175 mL
1	tomato, diced	1
7 tbsp	freshly squeezed lemon juice	105 mL
	Salt and freshly ground black pepper	
4 tbsp	olive oil	60 mL

1. Place bulgur in a bowl. Cover with boiling water and let soften and cool to room temperature. The quantity of water needed may vary according to the quality of the bulgur; add more to moisten, if necessary.

2. Add parsley, mint, onion and tomato to bulgur. Add lemon juice and salt and pepper to taste. Incorporate olive oil, stirring carefully.

3. Cover and refrigerate for at least 3 hours or for up to 8 hours. Serve chilled.

Tabbouleh-Style Quinoa

Serves 4

Preparation time
15 minutes

Cooking time
30 minutes

Chilling time
3 hours

Tip
The color green should dominate in tabbouleh.

¾ cup	white quinoa	175 mL
¾ cup	red quinoa (see Tip, page 64)	175 mL
3	bunches fresh Italian flat-leaf parsley, chopped	3
½	bunch fresh mint, finely chopped	½
¾ cup	finely chopped onion	175 mL
1	tomato, diced	1
7 tbsp	freshly squeezed lemon juice	105 mL
	Salt and freshly ground black pepper	
4 tbsp	olive oil	60 mL

1. In a saucepan, bring 1½ cups (375 mL) water to a boil. Stir in white and red quinoa. Reduce heat to low, cover and simmer until tender, about 15 minutes. Remove from heat and let stand, covered, about 5 minutes. Fluff with a fork. The quantity of water needed may vary according to the quality of the quinoa.

2. Add parsley, mint, onion and tomato to quinoa. Add lemon juice and salt and pepper to taste. Stir carefully and add olive oil.

3. Cover and refrigerate for at least 3 hours or for up to 8 hours. Serve chilled.

Barley and Corn Salad with Macadamia Nuts

Serves 4		
2	ears corn	2
⅔ cup	pearl barley	150 mL
¼ cup	extra virgin olive oil	60 mL
2	large red endives, chopped	2
1 tbsp	red wine vinegar	15 mL
	Salt and freshly ground black pepper	
⅓ cup	chopped toasted macadamia nuts	75 mL

Serves 4

Preparation time
10 minutes

Cooking time
35 minutes

1. In a large pot of boiling water, boil corn for 5 minutes. Remove from heat and let corn cool slowly in the cooking water. (This will prevent the kernels from shriveling as they cool and will allow them to remain juicy.)

2. Meanwhile, in a large saucepan of boiling salted water, gently cook barley until tender, about 35 minutes. Drain and spread out on a plate to let cool. Sprinkle with olive oil and stir from time to time to help barley cool more quickly without drying out.

3. Place each corn cob vertically in a bowl and, holding it firmly, use a sharp knife to remove the kernels. Add barley and endive to kernels in bowl.

4. Add vinegar and season with salt and pepper to taste. Mix together thoroughly and arrange in individual dishes. Sprinkle with macadamia nuts.

Russian Salad

Preparation time
45 minutes

Tips

Dice all the vegetables to the size of small green peas. For the best results, after cooking the vegetables, drain, then run under cold water to stop the cooking process and cool the vegetables quickly, then drain again. Of course, you can also use leftover cooked vegetables from another meal.

Do not mix the beets with the rest of the salad, as they will change its color.

¾ cup	finely diced potatoes, cooked and cooled (see Tips, left)	175 mL
¾ cup	finely diced carrots, cooked and cooled	175 mL
¾ cup	finely diced turnips, cooked and cooled	175 mL
½ cup	diced green beans, cooked and cooled	125 mL
½ cup	frozen small green peas, cooked and cooled	125 mL
⅓ cup	finely diced celery	75 mL
2 tsp	chopped sour pickles	10 mL
4 tsp	drained capers	20 mL
4 tsp	mayonnaise	20 mL
	Salt and freshly ground black pepper	
1	small beet, cooked, cooled and julienned (see Tips, left)	1

1. In a large bowl, combine potatoes, carrots, turnips, green beans, peas and celery. Add pickles and capers.

2. Add mayonnaise and salt and pepper to taste. Mix together carefully.

3. Arrange mixture on a plate in a dome or a circle. Place beets on top of salad.

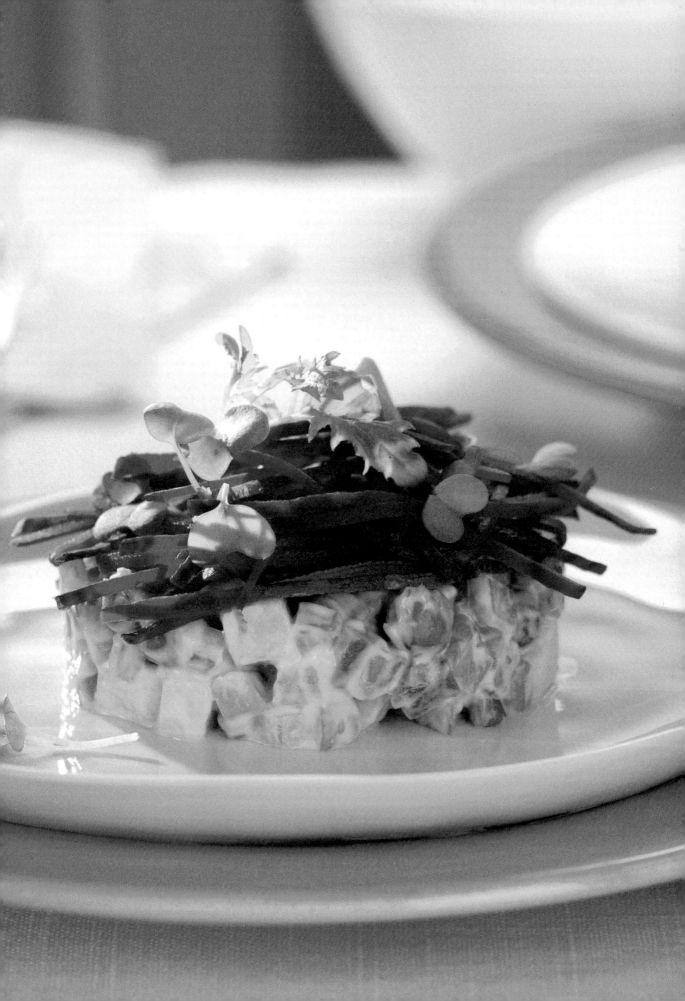

Thai Salad

Preparation time
45 minutes

Cooking time
10 minutes

8 oz	rice vermicelli	250 g
3 oz	fresh coconut meat	90 g
1	stalk lemongrass, very finely chopped	1
	Juice of 4 limes	
3 tbsp	soy sauce	45 mL
2 tbsp	sesame oil	30 mL
2 tbsp	packed brown sugar	30 mL
1 tbsp	vegetable oil	15 mL
6 oz	shiitake mushrooms, stems removed	175 g
6 oz	snow peas, cooked and cooled	175 g
2	bird's-eye chile peppers	2
6 oz	canned water chestnuts, drained	175 g
	Salt	
1 tbsp	black sesame seeds	15 mL
2 tbsp	chopped fresh cilantro leaves	30 mL

1. Cook or soak rice vermicelli according to package directions until tender. Drain well.

2. Using a potato peeler, cut coconut into strips.

3. In a bowl, combine lemongrass, lime juice, soy sauce, sesame oil and brown sugar, stirring to dissolve sugar.

4. In a wok, heat vegetable oil over medium-high heat. Sauté mushrooms until light golden. Add snow peas, chile peppers and water chestnuts. Add vermicelli.

5. Add lemongrass mixture and sauté until noodles are well coated. Add salt to taste.

6. Arrange salad in individual bowls. Sprinkle sesame seeds on top and garnish with coconut shavings and cilantro.

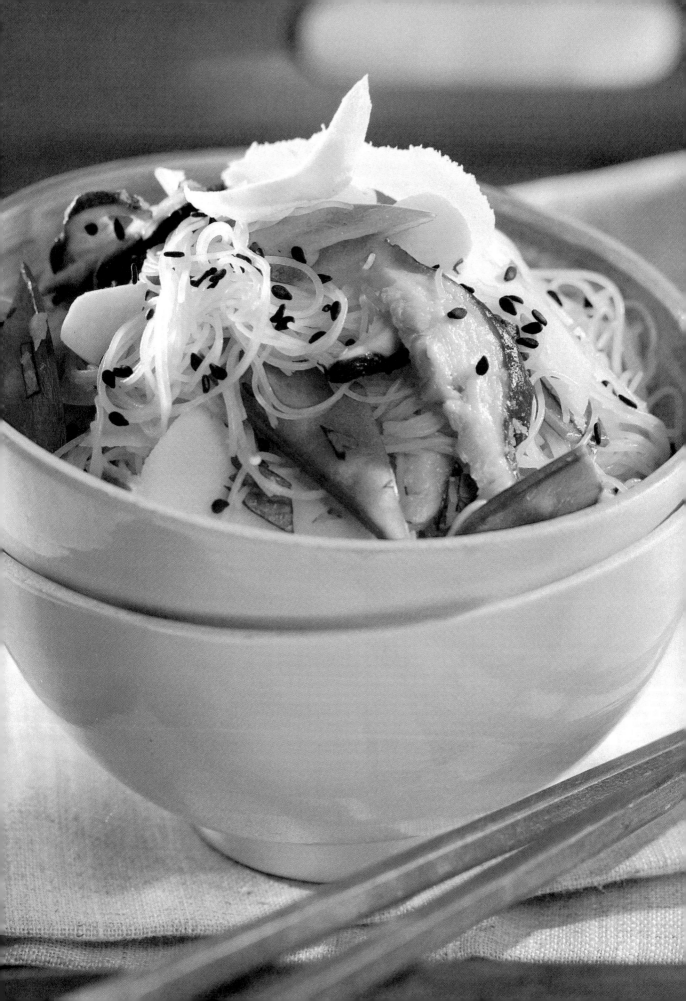

Greek Salad

2	large tomatoes	2
2	cucumbers, peeled	2
8 oz	feta cheese, cut into ¾-inch (2 cm) cubes	250 g
32	kalamata olives	32
	Salt and freshly ground black pepper	
½ cup	extra virgin olive oil	125 mL
	Fresh or dried oregano (see Tip, left)	

1. Remove cores from tomatoes, then cut each into 8 wedges. Cut cucumbers lengthwise into quarters, then cut crosswise into ¾-inch (2 cm) slices.

2. In a bowl, combine tomatoes, cucumbers, feta and olives. Add salt and pepper to taste and olive oil.

3. Arrange salad in individual dishes and sprinkle with oregano to taste.

Japanese Salad

1¼ cups	cooked soybeans	300 mL
1 cup	julienned carrots	250 mL
½ cup	julienned daikon radish	125 mL
2 tbsp	coarsely chopped fresh cilantro leaves	30 mL
2 tbsp	sesame seeds, toasted	30 mL
	Juice of 4 limes	
½	wild lime leaf, cut into small pieces	½
1 cup	roasted peanuts	250 mL
1 tbsp	wakame, chopped if needed (see Tip, left)	15 mL
3 oz	enoki mushrooms	90 g
1 tsp	olive oil	5 mL
½ tsp	sesame oil, optional	2 mL
	Salt and freshly ground black pepper	

1. In a large bowl, combine soybeans, carrots, radish, cilantro, sesame seeds, lime juice, lime leaf, peanuts, wakame and mushrooms. Add olive oil and sesame oil, if using, and carefully blend. Taste and add more sesame oil, if desired. Season with salt and pepper to taste.

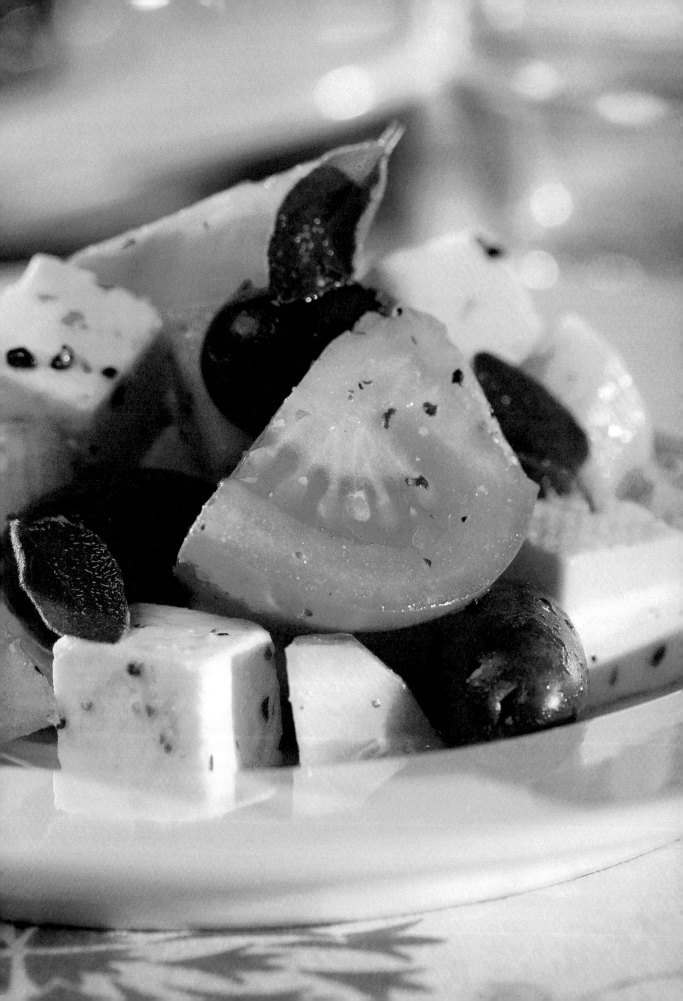

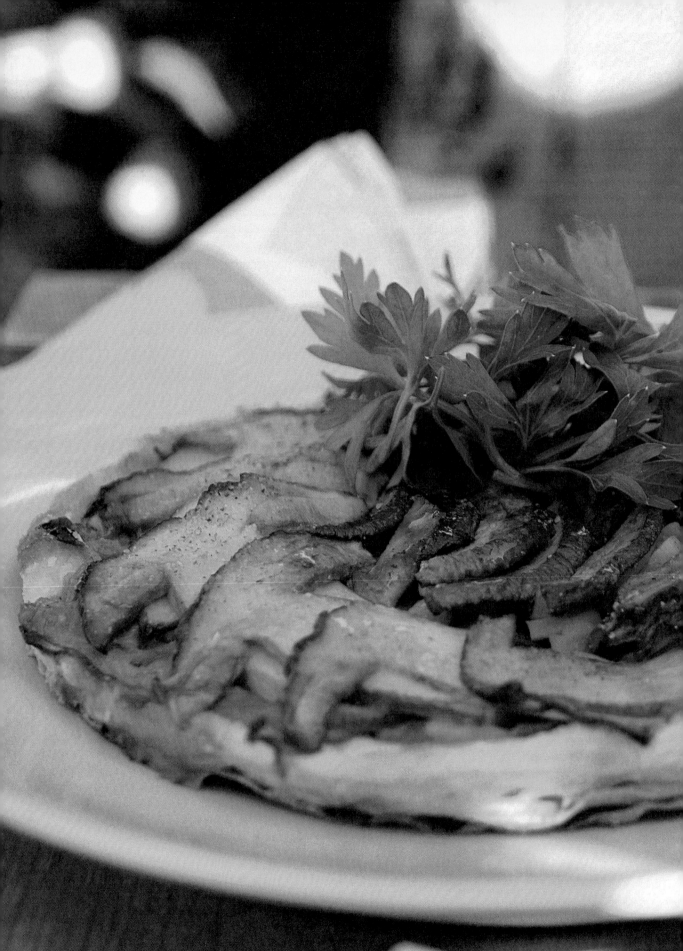

French Mushroom Tart (page 115)

Small Plates and Light Bites

Egg and Spinach–Filled Pastry

Serves 4

Preparation time
20 minutes

Cooking time
5 to 10 minutes

Tips

"Feuilles de Brick" are thin circles of pastry originating in Tunisia. They are available fresh or frozen in some specialty shops or online.

Another type of cheese that melts relatively quickly when cooked can replace the Gruyère, such as provolone, mozzarella or fontina.

When buying cheese, read the label carefully and make sure to buy those that are not made from animal rennet.

The white of the egg should be cooked but the yolk should remain runny. To check while cooking, gently press the pastry bundle with a spatula to feel the texture of the egg.

4 tsp	butter, divided	20 mL
10 oz	spinach, stemmed, divided	300 g
	Salt and black freshly ground pepper	
4	"Feuilles de Brick" pastry sheets (see Tips, left)	4
4	eggs	4
1¼ cups	shredded Gruyère cheese, divided (see Tips, left)	300 mL
1	egg white, beaten	1
	Oil	

1. In a large saucepan, melt half of the butter over medium-high heat. Add half of the spinach and sauté just until wilted. Season with salt and pepper to taste. Using a slotted spoon, transfer to a bowl, let cool, then squeeze dry. Repeat with remaining butter and spinach.

2. Place a pastry sheet on a flat surface. Spoon one-quarter of the spinach into the center. Make a slight depression in the spinach and place one egg on top, without breaking the yolk. Add a quarter of the cheese, then salt and pepper to taste. Fold pastry in half and seal the edges with a little egg white. Repeat with remaining pastry sheets and filling.

3. In a skillet, heat about 1 inch (2.5 cm) oil over medium heat. In batches if necessary, add filled pastry bundles and cook until golden on both sides and egg white is set and yolk is still runny (see Tips, left), about 3 minutes. Transfer to a plate lined with paper towels to drain. Repeat with remaining bundles, adding more oil and adjusting heat as necessary between batches. Serve hot.

Scrambled Eggs with Toasted Baguette

Serves 4

Preparation time
20 minutes

Cooking time
10 minutes

12	diagonal slices baguette	12
4	eggs	4
	Salt and freshly ground black pepper	
1 tbsp	butter (approx.)	15 mL
	Heavy or whipping (35%) cream, optional	

1. Lightly toast baguette slices on both sides.

2. In a bowl, using a fork, whisk eggs until blended, then add salt and pepper to taste.

3. In a skillet, melt a little butter over low heat. Add eggs and cook, stirring constantly with a wooden spatula, until a creamy consistency. If desired, stop the cooking process by drizzling in a little cream or adding some more butter. Serve immediately in small bowls with baguette slices on the side.

Soft-Boiled Eggs and Toast Fingers

Serves 4

Preparation time
15 minutes

Cooking time
8 to 10 minutes

● **Preheat broiler**

4	eggs	4
½	baguette	½
4 tbsp	butter	60 mL

1. Place eggs in a saucepan and add enough cold water to cover. Bring to a boil over high heat. Cover pan, remove from heat and let eggs stand for 4 minutes.

2. Meanwhile, cut baguette into fingers (pieces of bread the width of a finger) and place on a baking sheet. Lightly toast under preheated broiler, turning often, until golden on all sides. Spread one side with butter.

3. Using a slotted spoon, remove eggs from water and place in eggcups. Cut off tops (only the egg white should be coagulated, while the yolk should remain creamy).

4. Place eggcup on a plate and arrange buttered toast fingers next to it.

Omelet and Grilled Vegetable Milles-Feuilles

Serves 4

Preparation time
45 minutes

Cooking time
40 minutes

Tip

This omelet can be served hot or cold. Preheat oven to 350°F (180°C). Remove plastic wrap from dish, cover with foil and heat for 45 minutes or until hot.

Variation

If you like, serve with Red Pepper Coulis (page 260).

- Preheat barbecue grill to medium-high or preheat broiler
- Large rimmed baking sheet
- 10-inch (25 cm) skillet
- 8-inch (20 cm) square glass baking dish, buttered

1	small eggplant (about 8 oz/250 g)	1
1	zucchini	1
¼ cup	olive oil	60 mL
	Salt and freshly ground black pepper	
1	large yellow or red bell pepper	1
2 tbsp	butter, divided	30 mL
10	eggs	10
½ cup	Sun-Dried Tomato Pesto (page 269) or store-bought	125 mL

1. Slice eggplant and zucchini lengthwise. In a bowl, combine olive oil and salt and pepper to taste. Add eggplant and zucchini and marinate for about 30 minutes.

2. Place bell pepper on preheated grill (or place on a baking sheet and place under the broiler) and grill or broil, turning often, until skin is blackened all over and pepper is tender, about 20 minutes. Transfer to a bowl, cover and let cool. Remove skin, core and seeds and cut flesh into strips. Set aside.

3. Arrange eggplant and zucchini in single layers on rimmed baking sheet. Broil, turning once, until tender and lightly golden. Set aside.

4. In skillet, melt 2 tsp (10 mL) of the butter over medium-low heat. In a bowl, beat 2 of the eggs until well blended. Pour into skillet in a very thin layer. Cook, lifting edges with spatula during the first 1 to 2 minutes to allow uncooked eggs to flow underneath, until just set. As completed, transfer to a plate and layer with parchment or waxed paper. Continue with the 8 remaining eggs to prepare 5 very thin omelets, using 2 eggs per omelet and adjusting heat and adding more butter between batches as necessary.

5. Place one layer of omelet in the bottom of prepared baking dish. Add eggplant, then another omelet layer. Add pesto, then another omelet layer. Add zucchini, then another omelet layer. Add bell pepper strips. Top with an omelet layer.

6. Cover with plastic wrap, then place an identical dish on top with a weight inside (such as a can of food) in order to press it down. Refrigerate overnight. Remove from dish and cut into squares.

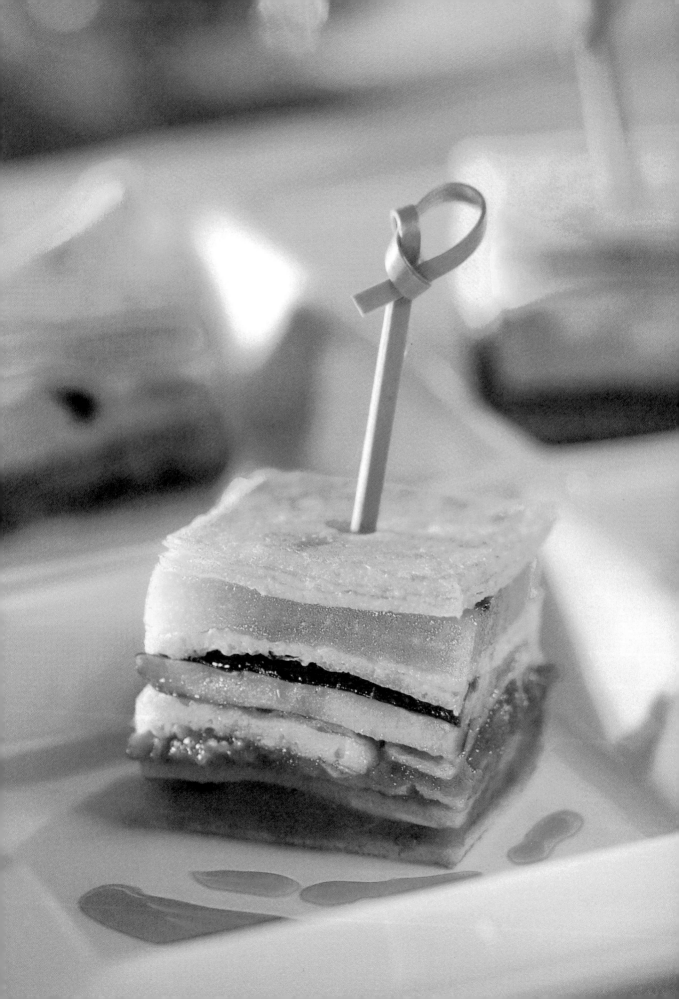

Fried Eggs with Mizuna Salad

Serves 4

Preparation time
20 minutes

Cooking time
8 minutes

Tips

Mizuna is a delicate feathery lettuce green with a peppery mustard flavor.

Make sure you use flowers clearly labeled "not sprayed with pesticides" or use those you've grown yourself, chemical-free. Do not use flowers purchased from florist shops which are often sprayed with chemicals.

Mizuna Salad

2 oz	mizuna lettuce (see Tips, left)	60 g
8	pansies, petals only (see Tips, left)	8
1 tbsp	chopped fresh chervil leaves	15 mL
2 tsp	chopped fresh chives	10 mL
2 tbsp	olive oil	30 mL
2 tsp	freshly squeezed lemon juice	10 mL
	Salt and freshly ground black pepper	
3 tbsp	oil, divided	45 mL
8	diagonal slices baguette	8
8	eggs	8

1. *Mizuna Salad:* In a bowl, combine lettuce, pansies, chervil and chives.

2. In a small bowl, combine olive oil, lemon juice, and salt and pepper to taste. Toss salad with dressing just before serving.

3. In a skillet, heat 1 tbsp (15 mL) of the oil over medium heat. In batches if necessary, add bread slices and fry until toasted on both sides. Transfer to a paper towels to drain.

4. In a large skillet, heat a thin layer of remaining oil over medium heat. One at a time, break eggs into a small bowl, then pour them one at a time into skillet. Fry eggs until white is set, about 30 seconds. Using a slotted spatula, turn eggs over gently and fry just until the white is coagulated and yolk is still creamy, or to desired doneness. Using spatula, place eggs on a plate lined with paper towels to drain. Add more oil to the pan as necessary between eggs.

5. Season eggs with salt and pepper to taste and serve hot on a slice of bread, accompanied by the salad.

Pipérade Omelets

Serves 4

Preparation time
40 minutes

Cooking time
20 minutes

Tips

To easily peel tomatoes, blanch them first, then peel. Then cut in two and remove seeds.

Piment d'Espelette is a mild dried chile pepper from France. If you don't have it, you can substitute with cayenne pepper.

Pipérade

2 tbsp	olive oil	30 mL
1 cup	thinly sliced onion	250 mL
1 cup	large strips green bell pepper	250 mL
2	large tomatoes, peeled, seeded and chopped (see Tips, left)	2
1	clove garlic, chopped	1
1	sprig thyme	1
1	bay leaf	1
Pinch	piment d'Espelette (see Tips, left)	Pinch
	Salt and freshly ground black pepper	

Omelets

12	eggs	12
	Salt and freshly ground black pepper	
4 tbsp	butter, divided	60 mL

1. *Pipérade:* In a skillet, heat oil over high heat. Sauté onion and bell pepper until softened, about 3 minutes.

2. Add tomatoes, garlic, thyme, bay leaf, piment d'Espelette, and salt and pepper to taste. Continue to sauté, stirring frequently, until vegetables are cooked and liquid from tomatoes has evaporated. Set pipérade aside and keep hot.

3. *Omelets:* For each omelet, break 3 of the eggs into a bowl. Add salt and pepper to taste and beat with a fork.

4. In a skillet, melt 1 tbsp (15 mL) of the butter over medium-low heat. Pour in eggs and stir with a fork until they start to set. Cook, without stirring, just until top is no longer shiny. Transfer to a plate. Repeat with remaining eggs and butter to make 3 more omelets.

5. Roll each omelet into a cigar shape and place on a serving plate. Spoon pipérade on top and serve.

Baked Eggs with Mushrooms

Preparation time
25 minutes

Cooking time
6 minutes

Tip

You can use a total of 4½ oz (135 g) of your favorite wild or exotic mushrooms in place of the morels, girolles and chanterelles. Trim off any tough stems from mushrooms and, if they're large, cut into thick slices before cooking.

- Preheat oven to 300°F (150°C)
- Roasting pan
- 4 small ramekins

4 tbsp	butter, divided	60 mL
	Salt	
4	eggs	4
	Boiling water	
½	baguette, cut lengthwise into 4 slices	½
1½ oz	morel mushrooms	45 g
1½ oz	girolle (golden chanterelle) mushrooms (see Tip, left)	45 g
1½ oz	chanterelle mushrooms	45 g
1 tbsp	finely chopped French shallot	15 mL
¼ cup	heavy or whipping (35%) cream	60 mL
½ tsp	finely chopped fresh chives	2 mL
	Freshly ground black pepper	

1. Melt 1 tbsp (15 mL) of the butter and brush inside ramekins. Lightly sprinkle with salt. One at a time, break eggs into a small bowl and pour each carefully into a prepared ramekin without breaking yolks.

2. Place a sheet of parchment paper at the bottom of roasting pan to use as a bain-marie. Place ramekins in bain-marie and pour boiling water around them until water reaches halfway up sides of ramekins.

3. Place bain-marie in preheated oven and bake for about 6 minutes. (The time may vary according to the thickness of the ramekins.) Only the white of the egg should be coagulated, while the yolk should remain creamy.

4. Meanwhile, lightly toast baguette slices.

5. Meanwhile, in a skillet, melt remaining butter over medium-high heat. Sauté mushrooms and shallot until golden and tender, about 5 minutes. Add cream and boil until reduced by about half. Add chives and salt and pepper to taste.

6. Spoon mushroom mixture equally over the eggs in the ramekins. Serve with toasted baguette.

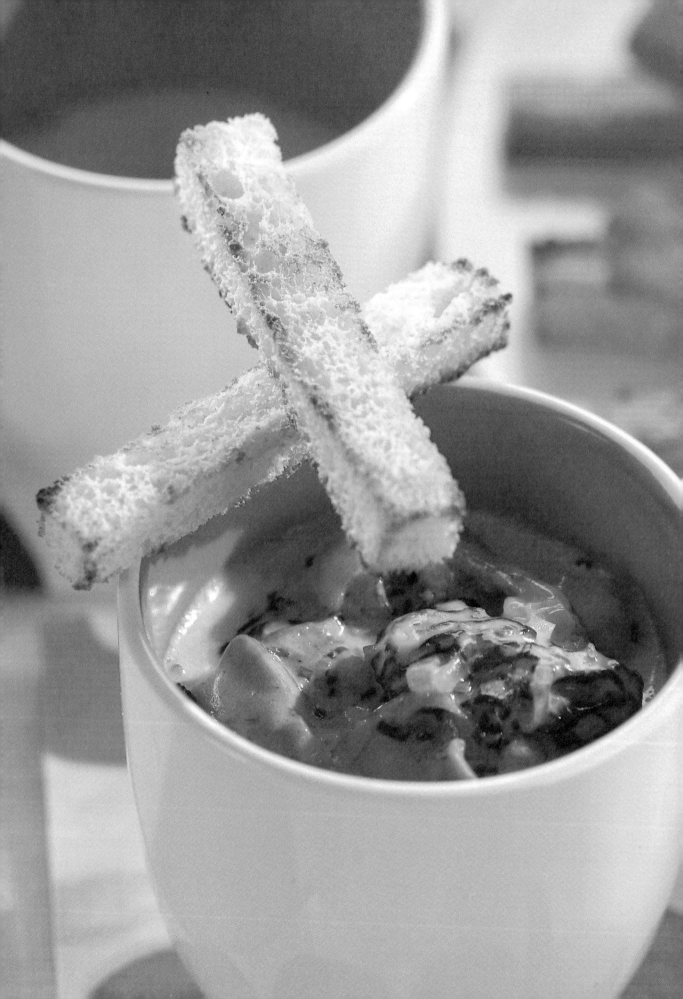

Eggs Florentine

Serves 4

Preparation time
1 hour 15 minutes

Cooking time
55 minutes

● 6- to 8-cup (1.5 to 2 L) baking dish

¼ cup	butter, divided	60 mL
2 lbs	spinach, trimmed	1 kg
	Salt	

Mornay Sauce

1 cup	milk	250 mL
	Salt	
	Cayenne pepper	
	Ground nutmeg	
2 tbsp	butter	30 mL
2 tbsp	all-purpose flour	30 mL
1	egg yolk	1
1 oz	Gruyère cheese, shredded	30 g
4	eggs	4
	Shredded Gruyère cheese	

1. In a skillet, melt 1 tsp (5 mL) of the butter over medium-high heat. Add a few drops of water and one-quarter of the spinach leaves and cook quickly, stirring gently, just until wilted. Transfer to a bowl. Repeat with remaining spinach in 3 batches, adding 1 tsp (5 mL) butter for each batch. Lightly salt and set aside.

2. *Mornay Sauce:* In a saucepan, bring milk almost to a boil over medium heat. Season to taste with salt, cayenne and nutmeg. In another saucepan, melt butter over medium heat. Sprinkle with flour and cook, stirring, about 1 minute to make a roux.

3. Gradually pour hot milk over roux, blending well with a whisk. Bring to a boil and boil, whisking, until thickened, about 3 minutes. Whisk in egg yolk and cheese. Do not boil. Keep sauce hot in a double boiler.

4. In a pot of boiling water, immerse eggs and count 5 minutes from the time the water boils again. Run eggs under cold water and remove shells.

5. Meanwhile, preheat broiler.

6. Chop spinach coarsely. In a skillet, heat 2 tbsp (30 mL) butter over medium-high heat and sauté spinach until hot. Taste and adjust seasoning. Spread spinach over bottom of baking dish.

7. If necessary, reheat eggs by immersing them for a few seconds in boiling salted water, then lay them on top of spinach. Pour Mornay sauce over eggs. Sprinkle Gruyère cheese on top, with a few dabs of remaining butter. Broil until cheese is melted and top is golden. Serve immediately.

Eggs Benedict

Serves 4

Preparation time
45 minutes

Cooking time
20 minutes

Variation

The English muffins can be topped with cooked spinach before the eggs are added.

• **Instant-read thermometer**

1 tsp	white vinegar	5 mL
	Salt	
4	eggs	4
½ cup	butter	125 mL
2	egg yolks	2
1 tbsp	freshly squeezed lemon juice	15 mL
	Cayenne pepper	
2	English muffins, split and toasted	2

1. Fill a saucepan with water about 2 inches (5 cm) deep and add vinegar and a little salt. Bring to a gentle simmer over medium heat.

2. Break 4 eggs into 4 small ramekins or bowls, taking care not to break the yolks. One at a time, pour eggs carefully into water. Simmer gently for 3 minutes (only the white should be coagulated). Using a slotted spoon, carefully remove poached eggs, then immerse them in a bowl of cold water to halt the cooking process. Drain and transfer to a plate. (Keep poaching water hot.)

3. In top of a double boiler over simmering water, melt butter so that it separates to make clarified butter. Pour clear portion into a liquid measuring cup with a spout and discard solids.

4. Place egg yolks in a round-bottomed metal bowl. Add lemon juice and a dash of cold water. Place bowl over a saucepan of boiling water. Using a whisk, beat quickly until temperature reaches 122 to 130°F (50 to 55°C) and eggs have a creamy consistency and after each whisk stroke you see the bottom of the bowl. Remove bowl from heat, then gradually whisk in clarified butter. Season to taste with salt and cayenne pepper. Set sauce aside and keep warm over hot water (temperature should not exceed 104°F/40°C).

5. Reheat poached eggs for a few seconds in boiling water. Drain on paper towels, then place on top of English muffins. Pour sauce overtop and serve.

Eggs in Miniature Pumpkins

Serves 4

Preparation time
30 minutes

Cooking time
45 minutes

Tip

Porcini powder is available from specialty spice shops, online or some well-stocked supermarkets. You can make your own with dried porcini mushrooms. Crumble the dried sliced porcinis and use a spice grinder to grind them to a fine powder.

● **Preheat oven to 350°F (180°C)**

4	miniature pumpkins	4
1 tbsp	butter, cut into 4 pieces	15 mL
	Salt and freshly ground black pepper	
¾ cup	heavy or whipping (35%) cream, divided	175 mL
	Porcini powder (see Tip, left)	
4	eggs	4

1. Make an incision around stem of each pumpkin, remove stem and scoop out seeds. Place on a baking sheet. Bake in preheated oven until tender, about 35 minutes.

2. Once pumpkins are baked, remove from oven and increase temperature to 400°F (200°C).

3. Put a piece of butter in each pumpkin, then add salt and pepper to taste. Pour about ½ cup (125 mL) of the cream into pumpkins, dividing equally. Add a small pinch of porcini powder to each.

4. Add eggs and remaining cream to pumpkins. Sprinkle salt and pepper on top and bake in oven for about 8 minutes for softly set eggs or to desired doneness.

Moroccan Briouats

Serves 4

Preparation time
45 minutes

Cooking time
30 minutes

1 tbsp	olive oil	15 mL
1 cup	finely chopped onions	250 mL
½ tsp	ground cumin	2 mL
½ tsp	ground cinnamon	2 mL
½ tsp	cayenne pepper	2 mL
2 tbsp	chopped fresh cilantro leaves	30 mL
2 tbsp	chopped fresh parsley leaves	30 mL
3½ oz	fresh goat cheese	100 g
4	"Feuilles de Brick" pastry sheets (see Tips, page 76)	4
1	egg, beaten	1
	Vegetable oil	

1. In a skillet, heat oil over low heat. Add onions, cumin, cinnamon and cayenne and cook, stirring occasionally, until onions are very soft, about 15 minutes. Add cilantro and parsley. Let mixture cool completely.

2. Stir in cheese until blended. Spoon one-quarter of mixture onto each pastry sheet. Brush edges with beaten egg and fold one side over filling into a half-moon shape. Brush edges again, then fold in half to make a triangular turnover. Use fingers to pinch edges to seal.

3. In a large skillet, heat a thin layer of oil over medium heat. In batches as necessary, fry briouats, turning once, until golden on both sides, 2 to 3 minutes per side. Transfer to a plate lined with paper towels to drain. Add more oil and adjust heat as necessary between batches to prevent burning. Serve hot.

Cheese Bundles with Arugula Salad

Serves 4

Preparation time
15 minutes

Cooking time
7 minutes

Tips

Curé Nantais is
a French soft
washed-rind cheese,
similar to Saint-Paulin
but with a more
pronounced taste.

It is important that the
spring roll wrapper be
sealed airtight so that
the cheese does not run
while baking.

- **Preheat oven to 450°F (230°C)**

8 oz	soft washed-rind cheese, such as Curé Nantais (see Tips, left)	250 g
4	round spring roll wrappers	4
3 tbsp	basil pesto	45 mL

Arugula Salad

2½ oz	arugula	75 g
2 tbsp	olive oil	30 mL
1 tbsp	balsamic vinegar	15 mL
	Salt and freshly ground black pepper	

1. Cut cheese into 16 equal slices.

2. Place one spring roll wrapper on a work surface. Place one-quarter of the cheese in the center. Add one-quarter of the pesto on top.

3. Brush edges of wrapper with water. Fold wrapper over cheese, pressing out air, and seal edges firmly. Place on a baking sheet. Prepare 3 more bundles in the same way. Bake in preheated oven until wrappers are crispy and golden and cheese is melted, about 7 minutes.

4. *Arugula Salad:* In a bowl, combine arugula, olive oil, vinegar, and salt and pepper to taste. Serve alongside the hot bundles.

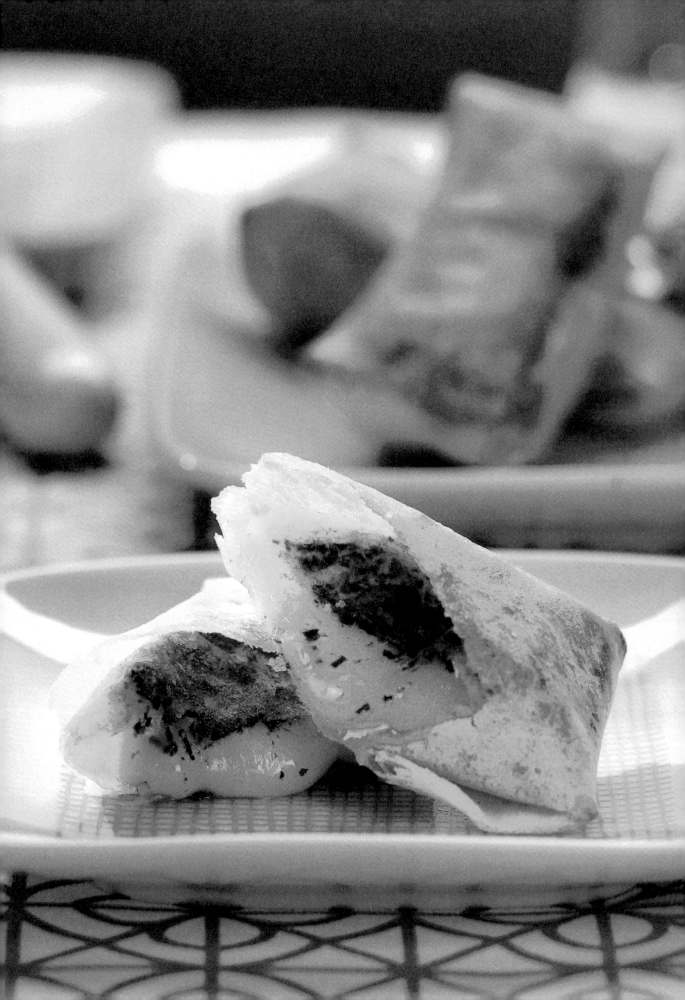

Cheese Soufflés

- Preheat oven to 350°F (180°C)
- Four ¾-cup (175 mL) ramekins, buttered and floured

Béchamel Sauce

1 cup	milk	250 mL
2 tbsp	butter	30 mL
¼ cup	all-purpose flour	60 mL
	Salt	
	Cayenne pepper	
	Ground nutmeg	
3	egg yolks	3
1 cup	shredded Gruyère cheese (see Tip, left)	250 mL
5	egg whites	5

1. *Béchamel Sauce:* In a saucepan, bring milk almost to a boil over medium heat. In another saucepan, melt butter over medium heat. Sprinkle with flour and cook, stirring, about 1 minute to make a roux. Season with salt, cayenne and nutmeg to taste.

2. Gradually pour hot milk over roux, blending well with a whisk. Bring to a boil. Reduce heat and boil gently, whisking, until thick, 5 to 8 minutes.

3. Remove béchamel from heat and whisk in egg yolks and cheese (do not boil). Pour sauce into a bowl and cover with plastic wrap to prevent it from forming a skin.

4. In a bowl, using an electric mixer or whisk, beat egg whites until fairly stiff peaks form. Using a spatula, incorporate a little of the egg whites into the sauce, then add the rest of the egg whites gradually, folding in just until evenly blended.

5. Fill prepared ramekins with egg mixture to about ½ inch (1 cm) below the rims and smooth out the surface. Place ramekins on a baking sheet and bake in preheated oven until golden and puffed and centers are just set, about 20 minutes (the time may vary according to the size and thickness of the ramekins). Serve immediately before the soufflés fall.

Melted Brie on Baguette with Arugula Salad

Serves 4

Preparation time
15 minutes

Cooking time
10 minutes

• **Preheat broiler**

12	large diagonal slices baguette	12
14 oz	Brie cheese, cut into 12 slices	420 g
2 tbsp	olive oil	30 mL
	Freshly ground black pepper	

Arugula Salad

3 oz	arugula	90 g
1/3 cup	olive oil	75 mL
5 tsp	balsamic vinegar	25 mL
	Salt and freshly ground black pepper	
1 tsp	finely chopped fresh chives	5 mL

1. Place baguette slices on a baking sheet and lightly toast on both sides under preheated broiler.

2. Place Brie on top of baguette slices. Drizzle olive oil on top, sprinkle with a little pepper and broil until cheese is slightly melted.

3. *Arugula Salad:* In a bowl, combine arugula, oil, vinegar, and salt and pepper to taste. Sprinkle with chives.

4. Serve baguettes while warm, accompanied by a small portion of arugula salad.

Causa

Serves 4

Preparation time
40 minutes

Cooking time
40 minutes

Chilling time
2 hours

Tip

If the chile pepper is dried, it must be moistened and then crushed with a little oil to make a paste. Aji chile peppers are also sold in paste form. If using aji paste, the quantity should be reduced, as it is very hot.

• 6- to 8-cup (1.5 to 2 L) serving dish

2 lbs	yellow-fleshed potatoes, unpeeled (about 4)	1 kg
1 tsp	crumbled dried aji amarillo chile pepper (see Tip, left)	5 mL
½ cup	olive oil, divided	125 mL
1 cup	mayonnaise	250 mL
1 tsp	chopped garlic	5 mL
3	avocados	3
	Freshly squeezed lime juice	
	Salt and freshly ground black pepper	
3	hard-cooked eggs, thinly sliced	3
	Small green salad	

1. Place potatoes in a large pot and add cold, salted water to cover. Bring to a boil over high heat. Reduce heat and boil gently for about 40 minutes or until fork-tender. Drain and let cool enough to handle.

2. In a small bowl, combine chile pepper and 1 tbsp (15 mL) of the olive oil and mash to a paste.

3. Peel potatoes and, using a potato masher, mash them. Add remainder of olive oil, chile pepper paste, mayonnaise and garlic and mash until blended.

4. Peel avocados and place in a bowl. Using a fork, mash avocados. Add a little lime juice and salt and pepper to taste.

5. Spread half of the potato mixture in a dish. Cover with mashed avocado, then sliced eggs. Top with the rest of the potato mixture. Cover and refrigerate for at least 2 hours, until chilled, or for up to 8 hours. Serve with a small green salad.

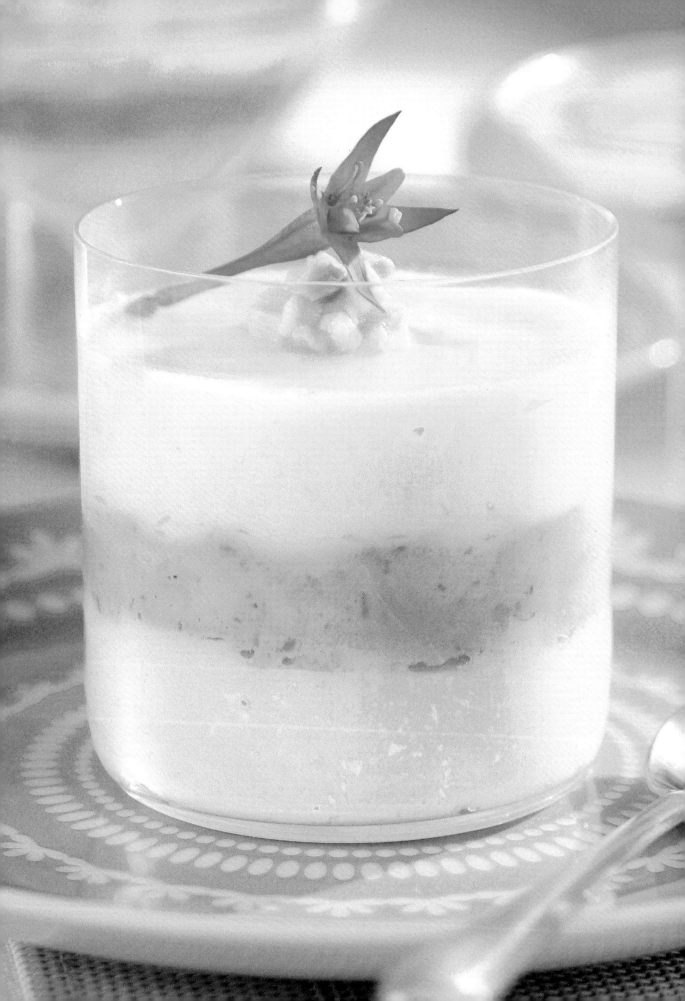

Greek-Style Stuffed Zucchini

Serves 4

Preparation time
20 minutes

Cooking time
20 minutes

● **Preheat oven to 350°F (180°C)**

4	zucchini	4
1/4 cup	extra virgin olive oil	60 mL
	Salt	
4	baby artichokes	4
2	carrots, preferably yellow, thinly sliced	2
8	cipollini onions, quartered	8
8	mushrooms, sliced	8
1	clove garlic, chopped	1
	Salt and freshly ground black pepper	
	Juice of 1/2 lemon	
1 tsp	crushed coriander seeds	5 mL
1	small bunch fresh Italian flat-leaf parsley, chopped	1

1. Cut zucchini in half lengthwise. Scoop out flesh, leaving 1/4-inch (0.5 cm) thick walls and taking care not to break the shells. Discard flesh. Brush cavities lightly with oil and sprinkle with salt. Place on a baking sheet and bake in preheated oven until tender but firm, 20 to 25 minutes. Set aside and let cool.

2. Remove all leaves from the artichokes and scoop out the fuzzy purple chokes. Cut off stems and trim until only the tender bottoms remain. Thinly slice bottoms.

3. In a skillet, heat remaining oil over high heat. Add artichokes, carrots, onions, mushrooms, garlic, and salt and pepper to taste. Sauté until vegetables are brightly colored, carrots are tender-crisp and mushrooms start to brown, about 5 minutes. Sprinkle with lemon juice and coriander.

4. Remove from heat and stir in parsley. Stuff zucchini with vegetable mixture and let cool before serving.

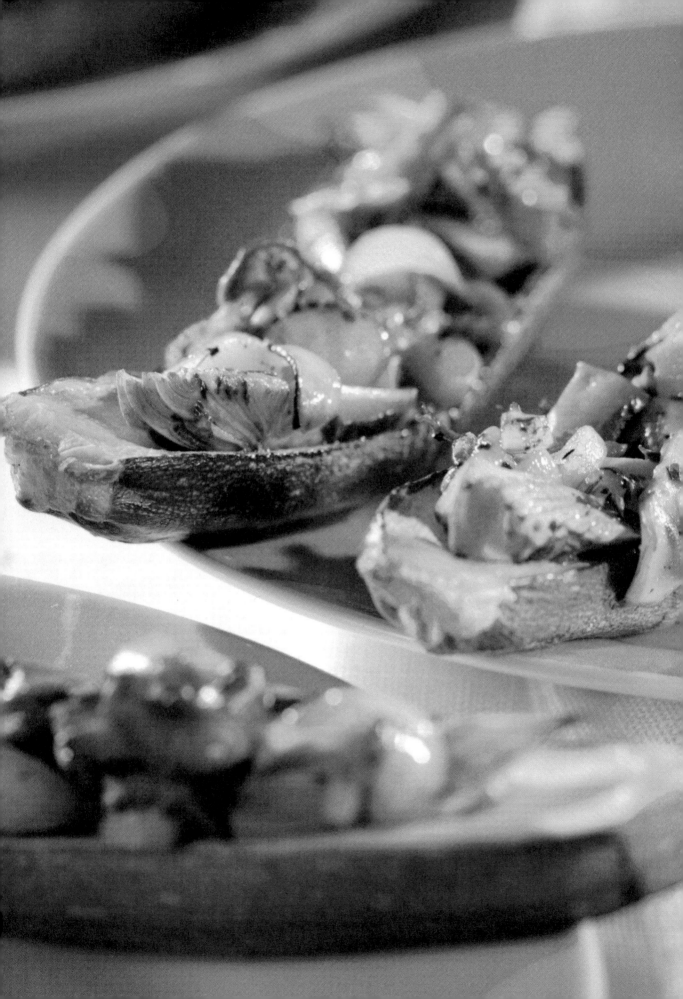

Stuffed Avocados

Serves 4

Preparation time
10 minutes

Tip

All ingredients that make up the stuffing should be prepared before cutting the avocados, as this fruit blackens quickly when it comes into contact with the air. Once it is cut, avocado should be coated with an acidic ingredient as quickly as possible (in this recipe, the lime juice does it) in order to slow down the enzymes that cause this browning.

2	avocados (see Tip, left)	2
1	plum (Roma) tomato, diced	1
2 tbsp	finely sliced Vidalia or other sweet onion	30 mL
	Juice of 1 lime	
2	sprigs cilantro, coarsely chopped, divided	2
1	Belgian endive, thinly sliced, divided	1
	Salt	
	Hot pepper sauce or cayenne pepper	

1. Cut avocados in half lengthwise and remove pits. Using a spoon, scoop out flesh, taking care not to break the shell, which will be used to hold the stuffing. Set aside a few pinches of cilantro and a little endive for the garnish. In a bowl, mash together avocado flesh, tomato, onion, lime juice, cilantro, endive, and salt and pepper sauce to taste.

2. Thoroughly clean avocado shells and fill with mixture. Garnish with reserved cilantro and endive.

Roman-Style Artichokes

Serves 4

Preparation time
20 minutes

Cooking time
1 hour

Variations

This dish can also be simmered on the stovetop, covered, for 20 minutes, then 40 minutes uncovered to allow the sauce to reduce.

This recipe can also be served cold as a first course.

- Preheat oven to 325°F (160°C)
- Deep baking dish

1	small bunch fresh Italian flat-leaf parsley, chopped	1
1	small bunch fresh mint, chopped	1
2	cloves garlic, chopped	2
	Salt and freshly ground black pepper	
3 tbsp	bread crumbs	45 mL
¼ cup	extra virgin olive oil	60 mL
8	artichokes	8

1. In a bowl, combine parsley, mint, garlic, and salt and pepper to taste. Stir in bread crumbs and olive oil until blended.

2. Peel artichoke stems, remove tough outer leaves and cut off points from tips of remaining leaves. Open artichokes gently and, using a spoon, remove the fuzzy purple choke. Fill cavity of each artichoke with herb mixture and pinch upper leaves together to enclose filling. Place artichokes in a deep baking dish with the stems facing up.

3. Add salt and pepper to taste, then cover artichokes completely with warm water and a little olive oil. Bake in preheated oven until tender, about 1 hour. Drain and serve.

Artichoke Bottoms Stuffed with Ratatouille

Serves 4

Preparation time
40 minutes

Cooking time
30 minutes

| 8 | large artichokes | 8 |
| | Juice of ½ lemon | |

Ratatouille

¼ cup	extra virgin olive oil, divided	60 mL
1	clove garlic	1
1	tomato, peeled, seeded and diced	1
½	yellow bell pepper, diced	½
½	red bell pepper, diced	½
1	zucchini, diced	1
1	small eggplant, diced	1
	Salt and freshly ground black pepper	
2	fresh basil leaves, chopped	2

1. Remove all the leaves from the artichokes and scoop out the fuzzy purple chokes. Cut off stems and trim until only the tender bottoms remain. In a large saucepan of boiling salted water, cook artichokes with lemon juice until tender.

2. *Ratatouille:* In a saucepan, heat 1 tbsp (15 mL) of the oil over low heat. Add garlic and cook, stirring, until golden. Remove garlic from saucepan and discard. Add tomato to saucepan and cook, stirring, until very soft, about 5 minutes. Remove from heat.

3. In a skillet, heat 1 tbsp (15 mL) of oil over medium-high heat. Add yellow and red bell peppers and sauté until tender, about 3 minutes. Transfer to a bowl. Add 1 tbsp (15 mL) of oil to skillet and sauté zucchini until tender, about 5 minutes. Add to peppers in bowl. Add remaining 1 tbsp (15 mL) of oil to skillet and sauté eggplant until tender, about 8 minutes. Add to vegetables in bowl, then season with salt and pepper to taste. Gradually stir in tomato, then basil.

4. Garnish artichoke bottoms with ratatouille and serve hot or cold.

Leek and Maroilles Cheese Quiche

Tips

To remove excess water and avoid a soggy crust, pat blanched leeks with paper towels.

We recommend serving a small lamb's lettuce salad with this quiche.

- Preheat oven to 400°F (200°C)
- 9-inch (23 cm) glass pie plate

Pâte Brisée

2 cups	all-purpose flour	500 mL
Pinch	salt	Pinch
½ cup	butter, at room temperature	125 mL
1	egg yolk	1
¼ cup	cold water (approx.)	60 mL

Filling

1 lb	leeks, white part only, thinly sliced	500 g
2	eggs	2
1	egg yolk	1
1 cup	heavy or whipping (35%) or table (18%) cream	250 mL
	Salt	
	Cayenne pepper	
	Ground nutmeg	
4 oz	Maroilles or other pungent washed-rind cheese, thinly sliced (see Tip, page 90)	125 g

1. *Pâte Brisée:* In a bowl, combine flour and salt. Using a pastry blender, cut in butter until crumbs form. Form a well in the center. Add egg yolk and water. Stir together, then gently knead to an even consistency. Squeeze a small amount of dough together; if it is crumbly add more cold water, 1 tbsp (15 mL) at a time. Shape into a disk, wrap in plastic and refrigerate until chilled, about 30 minutes, or for up to 1 day.

2. *Filling:* In a pot of boiling water, blanch leeks until wilted, about 2 minutes. Drain and rinse in cold water to cool, then drain well. Set aside.

3. On a lightly floured surface, roll out pastry and fit into pie plate.

4. In a bowl, whisk together eggs, egg yolk and cream. Stir in salt, cayenne pepper and nutmeg to taste.

5. Arrange leek slices evenly in bottom of pie shell. Pour egg mixture on top.

6. Place cheese slices on top of quiche. Bake in preheated oven until crust is golden and a knife inserted in the center of the filling comes out clean, 30 to 35 minutes. Let cool for 10 minutes before slicing.

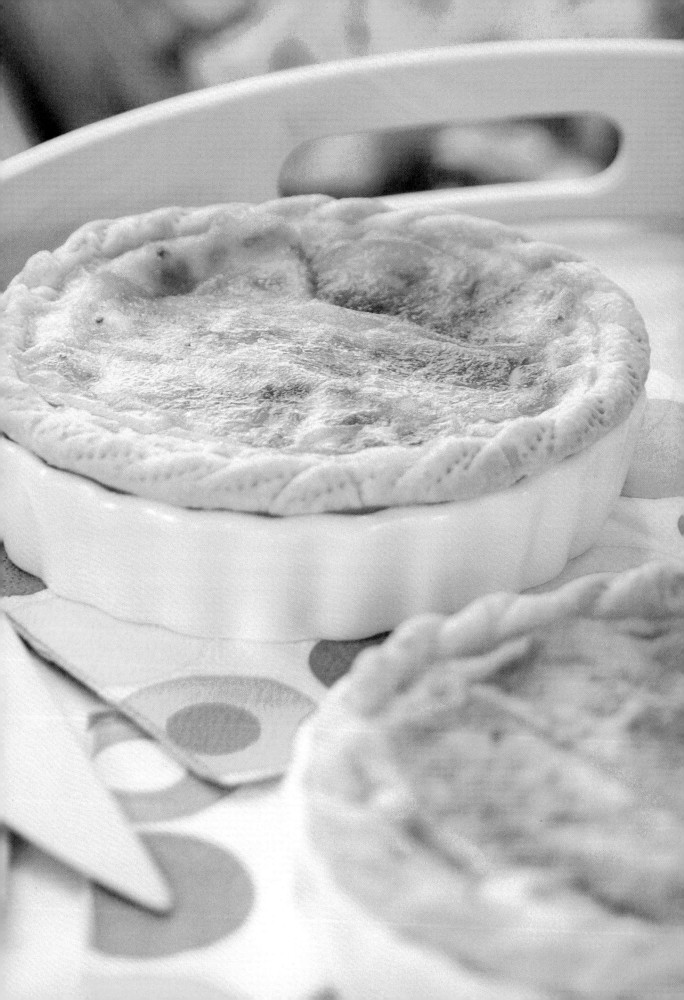

Zucchini, Caramelized Onion and Pine Nut Quiche

Serves 4	

Preparation time
45 minutes

Cooking time
40 minutes

- Preheat oven to 350°F (180°C)
- 9-inch (23 cm) glass pie plate

Pâte Brisée (page 98)

Filling

4 tbsp	extra virgin olive oil, divided	60 mL
2	zucchini, thinly sliced	2
	Salt and freshly ground black pepper	
1	small bunch fresh marjoram	1
½	Vidalia onion, thinly sliced	½
2 tbsp	toasted pine nuts	30 mL
3	eggs	3
6 tbsp	milk	90 mL
6 tbsp	heavy or whipping (35%) cream	90 mL
6	zucchini flowers, optional	6

1. Make Pâte Brisée. Shape into a disk, wrap in plastic and refrigerate until chilled, about 30 minutes, or for up to 1 day.

2. *Filling:* In a skillet, heat 2 tbsp (30 mL) of the olive oil over high heat. Sauté zucchini until browned, about 5 minutes. Add salt and pepper to taste. Sprinkle chopped marjoram on top. Transfer to a bowl and let cool.

3. In same skillet, heat remaining oil over high heat. Sauté onion until well browned, about 3 minutes. Add to zucchini in bowl and let cool.

4. On a lightly floured surface, roll out pastry and fit into pie plate. Spread onions and zucchini evenly over bottom of pie shell. Sprinkle pine nuts on top.

5. In a bowl, whisk together eggs, milk and cream. Stir in salt and pepper to taste. Pour mixture slowly into pie shell, filling to up to ⅛ inch (3 mm) below the rim.

6. Top with zucchini flowers, if using. Bake in preheated oven until crust is golden and a knife inserted in the center of the filling comes out clean, about 35 minutes. Let cool for 10 minutes before slicing.

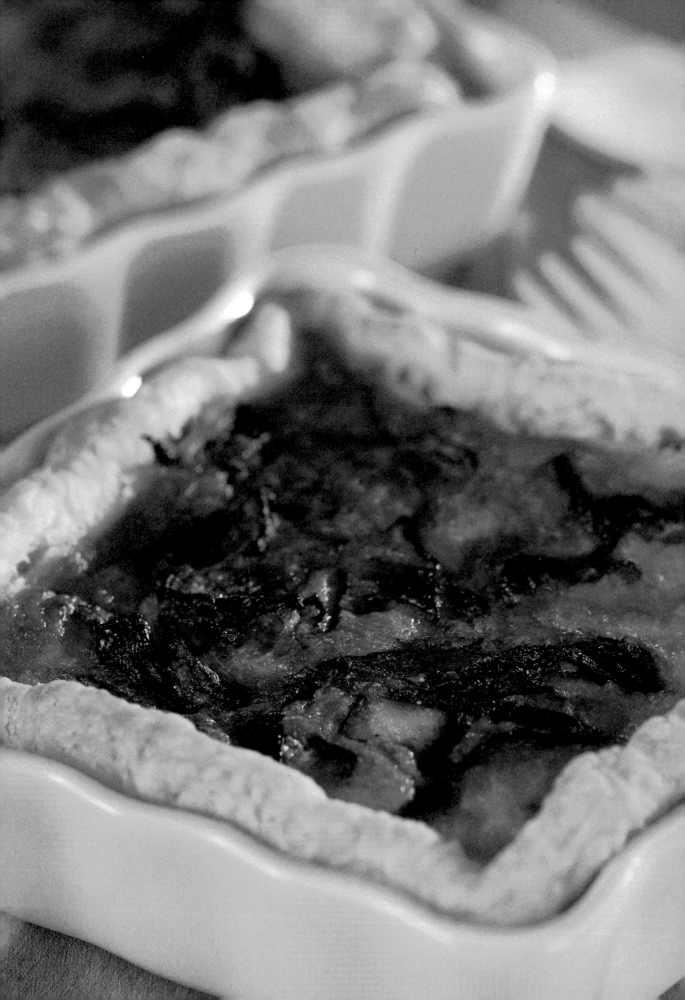

Onion Quiche

Serves 4

Preparation time
55 minutes

Chilling time
30 minutes

Cooking time
30 minutes

- Preheat oven to 400°F (200°C)
- 9-inch (23 cm) pie plate

Pâte Brisée

2 cups	all-purpose flour	500 mL
Pinch	salt	Pinch
½ cup	butter	125 mL
1	egg yolk, beaten	1
¼ cup	water	60 mL

Filling

2	onions	2
2 tbsp	butter	30 mL
2	eggs	2
1	egg yolk	1
1 cup	heavy or whipping (35%) or table (18%) cream	250 mL
	Salt	
	Cayenne pepper	
	Ground nutmeg	

1. *Pâte Brisée:* In a bowl, combine flour and salt. Using a pastry blender, cut in butter until crumbs form. Form a well in the center. Place egg yolk and water in well, stir together, then gently knead to an even consistency. Shape into a disk, wrap in plastic and refrigerate until chilled, about 30 minutes, or for up to 1 day.

2. *Filling:* Cut one of the onions into thin rings and set aside for topping. Cut remaining onion in half lengthwise, then thinly slice crosswise.

3. In a large skillet, melt butter over medium heat. Add lengthwise sliced onion and reduce heat to medium-low. Cook, stirring, until soft and light golden, about 7 minutes. Let cool.

4. On a lightly floured surface, roll out pastry and fit into pie plate.

5. In a bowl, whisk together eggs, egg yolk and cream. Add salt, cayenne pepper and nutmeg to taste.

6. Spread cooked onions on bottom of pie shell, then pour in egg mixture. Arrange reserved onion rings on top.

7. Bake in preheated oven for 10 minutes. Reduce temperature to 375°F (190°C) and bake until crust is golden and a knife inserted in the center of the filling comes out clean, about 20 minutes. Let cool for 10 minutes before slicing.

Caramelized Onion Buns

Serves 4

Preparation time
1 hour 40 minutes

Cooking time
45 minutes

● Large baking sheet, greased or lined with parchment paper

Sponge

Pinch	granulated sugar	Pinch
1 cup	warm water (about 98°F/37°C)	250 mL
2¼ tsp	active dry yeast (¼ oz/8 g package)	12 mL
1 cup	all-purpose flour	250 mL

Dough

2 cups	all-purpose flour (approx.)	500 mL
1½ tsp	salt	7 mL
½ cup	water	125 mL

Caramelized Onions

1 tbsp	extra virgin olive oil	15 mL
1 tbsp	butter	15 mL
1	large Vidalia onion, thinly sliced	1

1. *Sponge:* In a measuring cup or small bowl, combine sugar and water. Sprinkle yeast over top and let stand until frothy, about 10 minutes.

2. Place flour in a bowl and make a well in the center. Pour yeast mixture into the well. Stir together until blended. Cover and let rise in a warm, draft-free place until foamy, about 30 minutes.

3. *Dough:* In a large bowl, combine flour and salt and make a well in the center. Pour water and yeast mixture into well and stir together until a soft dough forms.

4. Transfer dough to a lightly floured work surface and knead, adding more flour as necessary to prevent sticking, until dough is smooth and elastic, about 5 minutes. Place dough in an oiled bowl and turn to coat all over. Cover with a clean tea towel and let rise in a warm, draft-free place until doubled in bulk, about 1 hour.

5. *Caramelized Onions:* Meanwhile, in a skillet, heat oil and butter over medium heat. Add onion and cook, stirring, about 2 minutes. Reduce heat to low and cook, stirring, until onions are very soft and caramelized, about 20 minutes. Let cool.

6. Preheat oven to 425°F (220°C).

7. Cut dough into 12 equal pieces and shape each into a ball. Working with one ball at a time, on a lightly floured surface, roll out to a rectangle about 5 by 3 inches (12 by 7.5 cm) and ½ inch (1 cm) thick. Spoon one-twelfth of the onions in a strip lengthwise along the center of the rectangle. Fold long edges toward center to enclose filling and form a cylinder-shaped bun, pinching edge to seal. Place seam side down on prepared baking sheet, at least 2 inches (5 cm) apart.

8. Bake in preheated oven until buns are golden brown and sound hollow when tapped, about 25 minutes. Serve warm or let cool completely.

Zucchini Flowers with Ricotta Filling and Balsamic Vinegar

Serves 4

Preparation time
25 minutes

Cooking time
25 minutes

Tip

In this recipe we use certified traditional Italian balsamic vinegar. Its authenticity is protected by consortiums in Modena and Reggio Emilia.

- Preheat oven to 350°F (180°C)
- Pastry bag fitted with medium plain tip
- Baking sheet, lined with parchment paper

¼ cup	extra virgin olive oil	60 mL
4	tomatoes, peeled, seeded and diced	4
⅔ cup	ricotta cheese	150 mL
2 tbsp	grated vegetarian-friendly Parmesan cheese (see Tip, page 106)	30 mL
1	egg yolk	1
1	small bunch fresh Italian flat-leaf parsley, chopped	1
Pinch	salt	Pinch
Pinch	freshly ground nutmeg	Pinch
16	zucchini flowers	16
	Traditional balsamic vinegar (see Tip, left)	

1. In a saucepan, heat oil over medium heat. Add tomatoes and cook, stirring, until very soft, about 10 minutes. Set aside.

2. In a bowl, combine ricotta, Parmesan, egg yolk, parsley, salt and nutmeg. Spoon into pastry bag and pipe into zucchini flowers.

3. Place stuffed flowers on prepared baking sheet, at least 1 inch (2.5 cm) apart. Bake in preheated oven until filling is hot, about 15 minutes.

4. Divide tomato sauce equally among four individual serving plates. Serve flowers warm on top of sauce, sprinkled with a few drops of balsamic vinegar to taste.

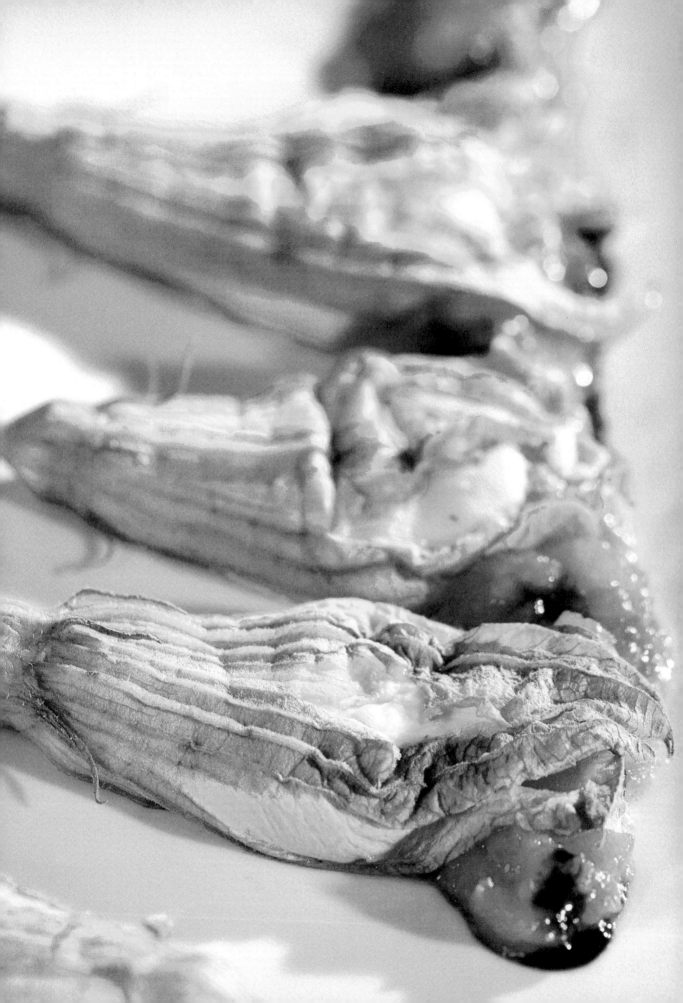

Fried Zucchini Flowers

Serves 4

Preparation time
20 minutes

Cooking time
15 minutes

Tip

When buying cheese, read the label carefully and make sure to buy those that are not made from animal rennet.

• Candy/deep-fry thermometer

16	zucchini flowers	16
16	small cubes (1/16 inch/2 mm) mozzarella cheese	16
3/4 cup	milk	175 mL
1/4 cup	beer	60 mL
2	eggs	2
2/3 cup	sifted all-purpose flour	150 mL
	Salt and freshly ground black pepper	
1 oz	vegetarian-friendly Parmesan cheese, grated (see Tip, left)	30 g
4 cups	vegetable oil	1 L

1. If zucchini flowers have a small zucchini attached, cut off stem end and split zucchini in two to reduce cooking time.

2. Insert a cube of mozzarella in each flower.

3. In a bowl, whisk together milk, beer, eggs and flour. Strain through a fine-mesh sieve into another bowl. Add salt and pepper to taste and Parmesan.

4. In a deep skillet, Dutch oven or deep-fryer, heat oil over medium heat until about 350°F (180°C). Immerse and completely coat zucchini flowers in batter just before frying. Fry, in batches, 4 at a time, turning once, until both sides are golden. Using a slotted spoon, remove from oil and place on a plate lined with paper towels to drain. Serve immediately.

Pressed Grilled Vegetables with Tofu

Serves 4	

Preparation time
1 hour

Cooking time
15 minutes

Refrigerate time
24 hours

- Preheat barbecue grill to high or preheat broiler
- 12- by 3-inch (30 by 7.5 cm) terrine dish or 8- by 4-inch (20 by 10 cm) loaf pan

1	red bell pepper	1
1	yellow bell pepper	1
1	small zucchini, thinly sliced lengthwise	1
1	small eggplant, thinly sliced lengthwise	1
3 tbsp	olive oil	45 mL
4 oz	firm tofu, thinly sliced	125 g
8 oz	cream cheese	250 g
1 tsp	chopped fresh thyme leaves	5 mL
	Salt and freshly ground black pepper	
	Red Pepper Coulis (page 260)	

1. Place bell peppers on grill or under broiler, and grill, turning often, just until skin bubbles (this makes skin easier to remove). Cut in half lengthwise and cut out stem, core and seeds. Cut flesh into long strips about 2 inches (5 cm) wide and peel off skin.

2. Place pepper strips, zucchini and eggplant on grill or on a baking sheet under broiler. Grill or broil, turning once, until tender, about 5 minutes. Let cool.

3. In a skillet, heat oil over high heat. Fry tofu slices, turning once, until golden brown, about 2 minutes per side. Let cool.

4. In a food processor or using an electric mixer, process or beat cream cheese until very soft and smooth. Add thyme and salt and pepper to taste.

5. Line terrine dish with plastic wrap, ensuring that the wrap extends well beyond the rim of the dish.

6. Layer red pepper strips in bottom of dish. Spread with one-quarter of the cream cheese. Arrange zucchini over cream cheese, then spread with one-third of the remaining cream cheese. Arrange tofu on top, then spread with half of the remaining cream cheese. Top with yellow pepper, then remaining cream cheese. Arrange eggplant on top.

7. Using the overhanging plastic wrap, cover terrine well. Cut a piece of cardboard to fit inside the top of the terrine. Place the cardboard on top and weigh it down with food cans or a heavy container. Refrigerate for 24 hours.

8. To serve, unmold terrine onto a cutting board and remove plastic wrap. Cut into slices. Spoon Red Pepper Coulis onto four individual serving plates and top with slices of terrine.

Crêpes with Asparagus

Serves 4

Preparation time
30 minutes

Chilling time
1 hour

Cooking time
20 minutes

• 13- by 9-inch (33 by 23 cm) casserole or baking dish, buttered

Crêpes

2	eggs	2
¾ cup	all-purpose flour	175 mL
Pinch	salt	Pinch
1 cup	milk	250 mL
2 tbsp	butter, melted	30 mL

Béchamel Sauce

4 cups	milk	1 L
¼ cup	butter	60 mL
⅓ cup	all-purpose flour	75 mL
	Salt and freshly ground black pepper	
Pinch	ground nutmeg	Pinch

Filling

8 oz	asparagus, peeled	250 g
2 tbsp	butter	30 mL
¼ cup	finely chopped French shallots	60 mL
1 lb	ricotta cheese	500 g
1	egg yolk	1
	Grated vegetarian-friendly Parmesan cheese (see Tip, page 106)	
2 tbsp	butter, cut into pieces	30 mL

1. *Crêpes:* In a bowl, whisk together eggs, flour and salt to taste. Whisk in milk and melted butter. Cover and refrigerate for at least 1 hour or for up to 8 hours. Strain batter through a sieve before cooking.

2. Heat a nonstick skillet over medium heat. Ladle in a scant ¼ cup (60 mL) batter, swirling pan to coat thinly. Cook until golden on the bottom and top is no longer shiny, about 1 minute. Turn and cook second side for 30 seconds. Transfer to a plate. Repeat to make 8 crêpes in total, adjusting heat as necessary to prevent burning. Let cool on a plate.

3. *Béchamel Sauce:* In a saucepan, bring milk almost to a boil over medium heat. In another saucepan, melt butter over medium heat. Sprinkle with flour and cook, stirring, about 1 minute to make a roux.

4. Gradually pour hot milk over roux, blending well with a whisk. Season with salt and pepper to taste and nutmeg. Bring to a boil. Reduce heat and boil gently, whisking, until thick, about 10 minutes. Cover and set aside.

5. Preheat oven to 350°F (180°C).

6. *Filling:* Cut about 1 inch (2.5 cm) off bottoms of asparagus stalks and discard. Cut off 8 tips, which will be used to garnish the crêpes. Finely chop rest of the asparagus. In a pot of boiling salted water, blanch tips until bright green, about 2 minutes. Drain and run under cold water to stop the cooking. Drain well, cut in half lengthwise and set aside.

7. In a skillet, melt butter over low heat. Add shallots and cook, stirring, until softened, about 5 minutes. Add chopped asparagus and continue cooking and stirring until shallots and asparagus are tender. Transfer to a bowl.

8. Add ricotta, $1/2$ cup (125 mL) of the béchamel sauce and egg yolk to asparagus mixture. Add salt and pepper to taste and mix together thoroughly. Spoon filling onto the center of each crêpe, dividing equally. Fold crêpes over to make half-moon shapes, then in half again to make triangles.

9. Spread half of the remaining béchamel sauce in prepared baking dish and lay folded crêpes on top so they slightly overlap one another. Cover with remaining béchamel and garnish each crêpe with 2 asparagus tip halves laid crosswise. Sprinkle with Parmesan and butter pieces. Bake in preheated oven until hot and bubbly, about 20 minutes. Serve immediately.

Green Pea Flans

Serves 4

Preparation time
40 minutes

Cooking time
30 minutes

- Preheat oven to 350°F (180°C)
- Four $1/2$-cup (125 mL) ramekins, buttered
- Roasting pan

2 cups	small green peas	500 mL
$3/4$ cup	heavy or whipping (35%) cream	175 mL
3	eggs	3
	Salt	
	Cayenne pepper	
	Ground nutmeg	

1. In a saucepan over medium heat, cook peas and cream until peas are very soft. Using a mixer, beat peas and cream together with eggs and salt, cayenne pepper and nutmeg to taste.

2. Strain through a fine-mesh sieve into a measuring cup or other container with a pouring spout, discarding any solids left in strainer.

3. Pour mixture into prepared ramekins. Place a sheet of parchment paper on the bottom of roasting pan to use it as a bain-marie. Place ramekins in bain-marie and pour in boiling water until it reaches halfway up the sides of the ramekins.

4. Place bain-marie in preheated oven and bake until edges of flans are set and center is just slightly jiggly, about 30 minutes. Remove ramekins from water and let cool slightly. Serve hot.

Potato Samosas with Turmeric and Spicy Mango Salad

Makes 72 samosas

Preparation time
1 hour

Cooking time
45 minutes

Tip

Ataulfo mangos are a small variety with golden yellow skin and deep golden yellow, smooth-textured flesh. They have an intense mango flavor and are worth seeking out for this recipe.

- Food mill, ricer or potato masher
- Candy/deep-fry thermometer

1 lb	ratte or fingerling potatoes, unpeeled	500 g

Spicy Mango Salad

1	Ataulfo mango, julienned (see Tip, left)	1
1	bird's-eye chile pepper, chopped	1
	Salt	
	Juice of $1/2$ lime	
1 tbsp	extra virgin olive oil	15 mL
1	small bunch fresh cilantro	1
1 tsp	extra virgin olive oil	5 mL
$1/4$	red bell pepper, diced	$1/4$
1 tbsp	ground turmeric	15 mL
24	large square spring roll wrappers	24
1	egg, beaten	1
4 cups	vegetable oil	1 L

1. Place potatoes in a large pot and add cold, salted water to cover. Bring to a boil over high heat. Reduce heat and boil gently until fork-tender, about 20 minutes. Drain and let cool enough to handle. Peel potatoes while hot and pass through food mill or ricer or mash in a bowl until smooth. Set aside.

2. *Spicy Mango Salad:* Meanwhile, in a bowl, combine mango, chile pepper, salt to taste, lime juice, olive oil and sprigs of cilantro. Set aside.

3. In a skillet, heat oil over medium heat. Add bell pepper and cook, stirring, until softened, about 3 minutes. Add to potato purée. Season with salt to taste and turmeric.

4. Separate spring roll wrappers and cut each one into 3 equal rectangles. Keep wrappers covered with a damp cloth while working.

5. Place 1 tsp (5 mL) of potato mixture about $1/2$ inch (1 cm) from edge on one end of a wrapper rectangle. Fold dough on a 45-degree angle to enclose stuffing in a small triangle. Continue to fold triangle, following its shape, along strip. Once opposite end is reached, moisten last $1/2$ inch (1 cm) of wrapper with beaten egg to seal the triangle. Place on a baking sheet and cover with a damp towel. Repeat procedure with remaining filling and wrappers.

6. In a deep skillet, Dutch oven or deep fryer, heat oil to 350°F (180°C). In batches to avoid crowding, fry samosas, turning once, until deep golden and hot inside. Using a slotted spoon, remove from oil and place on a baking sheet lined with paper towels to drain. Serve warm with mango salad.

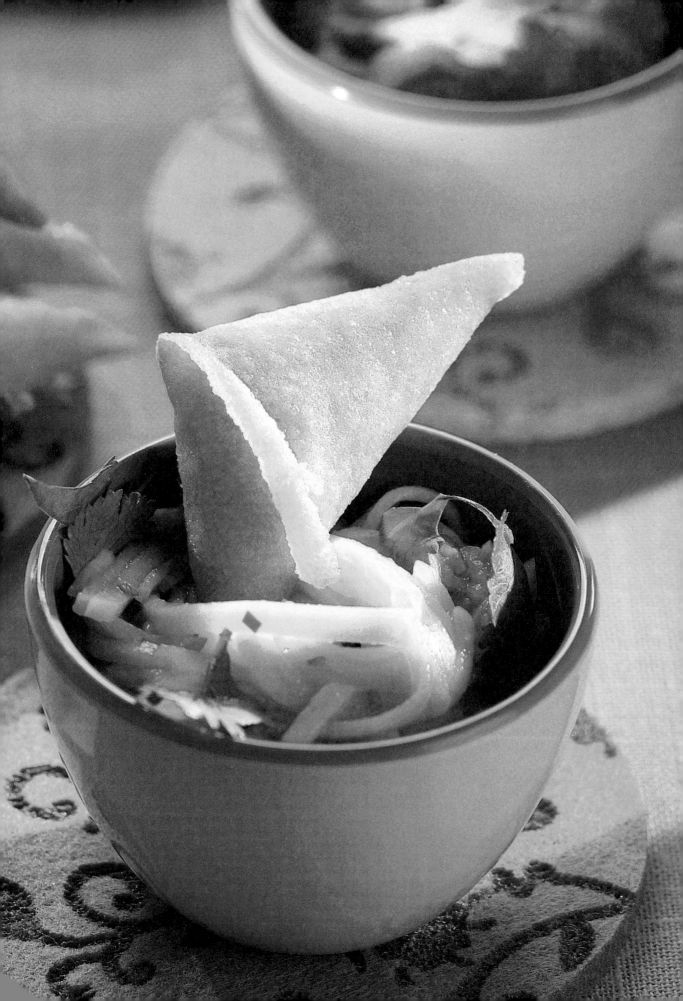

Potato and Spinach Roulade

Serves 4

Preparation time
1 hour 15 minutes

Cooking time
1 hour 30 minutes

Tip

When rolling out the dough, the length of the rectangle is not so important, but the roulade should be able to fit into a large pot of boiling water. If it will not, make two smaller roulades.

- Food mill, ricer or potato masher
- Cheesecloth
- Kitchen string
- Large pot, at least 10 inches (25 cm) wide

2 lbs	potatoes, unpeeled (about 4)	1 kg
3	egg yolks	3
	Salt and freshly ground black pepper	
Pinch	ground nutmeg	Pinch
2½ cups	all-purpose flour	625 mL
½ cup	butter, divided	125 mL
½	onion, finely chopped	½
1	clove garlic, minced	1
1 lb	baby spinach leaves	500 g
1 cup	freshly grated Grana Padano cheese, divided	250 mL

1. Place potatoes in a large pot and add cold, salted water to cover. Bring to a boil over high heat. Reduce heat and boil gently until fork-tender, about 40 minutes. Drain and let cool enough to handle. Peel while still hot and pass through food mill or ricer, or mash in a bowl until smooth. Immediately spread mashed potatoes on a work surface to allow steam to escape. Let cool for 5 minutes.

2. Mound the potatoes and make a well in the center. Place egg yolks, salt and pepper to taste, and nutmeg in the well. Mix together well, then add flour. Knead quickly to make a smooth dough. Cover loosely with plastic wrap and set aside.

3. In a large pot, melt 3 tbsp (45 mL) of the butter over medium-low heat. Add onion and garlic and cook, stirring, until softened and translucent but not browned, about 5 minutes. Increase heat to high. Add spinach, one handful at a time, and cook, stirring, just until spinach is wilted. Transfer to a colander and drain off excess liquid. Return to pot and add half of the cheese and salt and pepper to taste.

4. Using a rolling pin, on a floured work surface, roll out dough into a rectangle less than a ½ inch (1 cm) thick and about 10 inches (25 cm) wide (see Tip, left).

5. Cut a large rectangle of double-layer cheesecloth that is larger than the dough. Carefully transfer dough to on top of the cheesecloth. Spread spinach mixture uniformly on dough, leaving a 1-inch (2.5 cm) border of dough all around the edge.

6. Starting at one 10-inch (25 cm) wide end, roll up dough very tightly jelly-roll style, lifting it with the cheesecloth and wrapping the cheesecloth around the outside of the roll. Tie the ends closed with string and tie string every 2 inches (5 cm) along the roll to keep it held firmly together.

7. Bring a large pot of salted water to a gentle boil over high heat. Add roulade, reduce heat and boil gently until roulade is firm and hot in the center, about 40 minutes, adding more hot water and adjusting heat as necessary to keep at a gentle boil.

8. Meanwhile, to make beurre noisette, in a small saucepan, cook remaining butter over medium heat until a hazelnut-brown color, reducing heat as necessary to prevent burning. Remove from heat and keep warm.

9. Using two large slotted spatulas or tongs, carefully remove roulade from water and drain well. Transfer to a cutting board and remove cheesecloth. Cut into slices and top with beurre noisette. Sprinkle with remaining cheese. Serve immediately.

Huancayo-Style Potatoes

Serves 4

Preparation time
40 minutes

Cooking time
25 minutes

Tip

Fromage frais is a name for any type of soft, fresh cultured cheese. It is very perishable, so it must be used soon after it is made. You can often find it at specialty cheese shops — Neufchâtel is an example. If you can't find it, use the mildest feta cheese you can find.

1 lb	potatoes, unpeeled (about 4 small)	500 g
6 oz	fromage frais or mild feta cheese (see Tip, left)	175 g
¾ cup	milk	175 mL
¼ cup	aji amarillo paste	60 mL
4 tsp	cooking vegetable oil	20 mL
	Salt and freshly ground black pepper	
4	eggs, hard-cooked and cooled	4
4	lettuce leaves	4
¼ cup	small black olives	60 mL

1. Place potatoes in a large pot and add cold, salted water to cover. Bring to a boil over high heat. Reduce heat and boil gently until fork-tender, about 25 minutes. Drain and let cool.

2. Using an electric mixer, beat cheese, milk, aji amarillo paste, oil, and salt and pepper to taste until texture is smooth. Cover and refrigerate sauce until serving, for up to 1 day.

3. Peel potatoes and cut into round slices about ½ inch (1 cm) thick. Cut eggs into quarters.

4. Arrange lettuce leaves on individual serving plates. Cover with slices of potato and pour a generous amount of cheese sauce on top. Arrange quartered eggs and olives around the edge of the dish.

Eggplant Rolls with Buffalo Mozzarella

Serves 4

Preparation time
30 minutes

Cooking time
30 minutes

Tips

To easily peel tomatoes, blanch them first, then peel. Then cut in two and remove seeds.

If buffalo mozzarella isn't available, you can use four bocconcini 1½ inches (4 cm) in diameter, cut in half.

- Preheat barbecue grill to medium or preheat broiler
- Preheat oven to 300°F (150°C)
- Rimmed baking sheet

1	small eggplant	1
	Salt and finely crushed black peppercorns	
1 tbsp	balsamic vinegar	15 mL
3 tbsp	extra virgin olive oil, divided	45 mL
2	very ripe plum (Roma) tomatoes, peeled (see Tips, left)	2
1	ball buffalo mozzarella (see Tips, left)	1
8	leaves fresh basil	8

1. Remove stem of eggplant. Slice eggplant lengthwise into at least 8 slices. Place on preheated barbecue grill or on a baking sheet under broiler, and grill or broil, turning once, until eggplant is tender and browned, about 5 minutes per side. Transfer to a dish or leave on baking sheet and sprinkle with salt and pepper to taste, balsamic vinegar and 2 tbsp (30 mL) of the oil. Set aside.

2. Cut tomatoes in quarters lengthwise and remove seeds. Place tomato pieces skin side down on rimmed baking sheet. Salt to taste and sprinkle with remaining olive oil. Bake in preheated oven until softened, about 20 minutes. Let cool slightly.

3. Cut mozzarella into 8 slices. Place a baked tomato quarter on each slice, followed by a basil leaf. Wrap a slice of eggplant around the stack and secure with a toothpick, if necessary. Serve immediately.

French Mushroom Tart

Preparation time
35 minutes

Cooking time
20 minutes

Tip

Serve this tarte very hot with a small green salad.

• **Preheat oven to 400°F (200°C)**

3 tbsp	butter, divided	45 mL
2 tbsp	olive oil	30 mL
2	onions, thinly sliced	2
1	clove garlic, minced	1
	Salt and freshly ground black pepper	
	Chopped fresh savory leaves	
10 oz	puff pastry	300 g
5 oz	wild or exotic mushrooms, thinly sliced	150 g

1. In a skillet, heat 1 tbsp (15 mL) of the butter and olive oil over medium heat. Stir in onions and garlic. Reduce heat to low, cover and cook, stirring occasionally, until very soft and light golden, about 20 minutes. Add salt and pepper to taste, then add savory. Let cool.

2. Cut puff pastry dough into 4 equal pieces and roll each out to a circle about $1/8$ inch (3 mm) thick and 4 inches (10 cm) in diameter. Place circles on a baking sheet, at least 1 inch (2.5 cm) apart, and prick dough lightly with a fork. Spread cooled onion mixture over dough.

3. Arrange mushrooms on top of dough in a rosette pattern, slightly overlapping. Melt remaining 2 tbsp (30 mL) of butter and lightly brush over mushrooms.

4. Bake in preheated oven for 5 minutes. Reduce temperature to 350°F (180°C) and bake until pastry is crisp and golden brown, 10 to 15 minutes.

French-Style Tomato Tart

Serves 4

Preparation time
35 minutes

Cooking time
20 minutes

See photo, opposite

• **Preheat oven to 400°F (200°C)**

10 oz	puff pastry	300 g
4 tsp	olive oil, divided	20 mL
2 oz	Emmenthal cheese, shredded	60 g
	Chopped fresh thyme leaves	
10	small tomatoes, sliced into thin rounds	10
	Fleur de sel or sea salt	
	Freshly ground black pepper	

1. Cut puff pastry dough into 4 equal pieces and roll each out to a circle about $1/8$ inch (3 mm) thick and 4 inches (10 cm) in diameter. Place on a baking sheet, at least 1 inch (2.5 cm) apart, and prick with a fork. Drizzle half of the olive oil over the dough, then sprinkle Emmenthal and thyme on top.

2. Arrange tomatoes evenly on top of cheese, overlapping slices as necessary. Season lightly with salt. Drizzle with remaining olive oil and add pepper to taste.

3. Bake in preheated oven for 5 minutes. Reduce temperature to 350°F (180°C) and bake until pastry is crisp and golden brown, 10 to 15 minutes.

French-Style Zucchini and Blue Cheese Tart

Serves 4

Preparation time
30 minutes

Cooking time
30 minutes

Tip
We suggest sautéing the zucchini quickly at high heat to avoid cooking it too much. This eliminates some of the water and prevents the tart from being too moist.

• **Preheat oven to 400°F (200°C)**

8 oz	puff pastry	250 g
4	zucchini	4
3 tbsp	olive oil	45 mL
	Salt	
7 oz	Gorgonzola or other blue cheese	210 g
	Freshly ground black pepper	
$1/4$ cup	chopped walnuts	60 mL

1. Roll out pastry dough into a circle about $1/16$ inch (2 mm) in thickness. Place on a baking sheet and prick with a fork.

2. Cut zucchini in half lengthwise, then thinly slice crosswise into half moons. In a large skillet, heat oil over high heat. Sauté zucchini just until liquid is released but zucchini is still firm, about 5 minutes (see Tip, left). Transfer to a bowl and salt lightly. Let cool.

3. Using a spatula, spread half the Gorgonzola over dough. (If the cheese you use is less creamy, cut it into little pieces and distribute over entire surface of dough.) Arrange zucchini slices evenly on top, overlapping slightly. Add pepper to taste, then spread remaining Gorgonzola on top.

4. Bake in preheated oven until pastry is crisp and golden brown, about 25 minutes. Sprinkle walnuts on top, cut into pieces and serve.

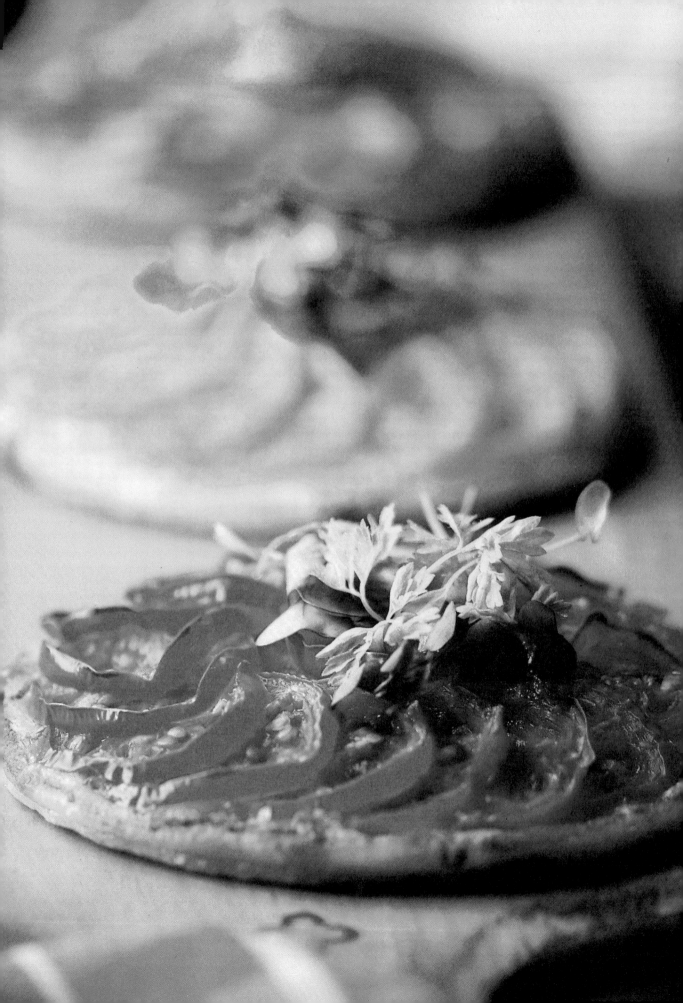

Tarte Flambée

Serves 4

Preparation time
25 minutes

Cooking time
10 minutes

Tip

Fromage frais is a name for any type of soft, fresh cultured cheese. It is very perishable, so it must be used soon after it is made. You can often find it at specialty cheese shops — Neufchâtel is an example. If you can't find it, use the mildest feta cheese you can find.

Variation

You can add pieces of Muenster cheese on top of the tart just before putting it in the oven.

- Preheat oven to 475°F (240°C)

2 tbsp	butter	30 mL
1	onion, finely chopped	1
¾ cup	crème fraîche	175 mL
¾ cup	fromage frais (see Tip, left)	175 mL
	Salt and freshly ground black pepper	
	Ground nutmeg	
1 lb	pizza dough	500 g
1 tbsp	olive oil	15 mL

1. In a skillet, melt butter over medium heat. Add onion and cook, stirring, until softened but not browned, about 5 minutes. Let cool slightly.

2. In a bowl, combine crème fraîche and fromage frais. Season with salt, pepper and nutmeg to taste.

3. Roll out dough very thinly on a baking sheet.

4. Spread crème fraîche mixture over dough. Distribute onion evenly over top, then drizzle with olive oil.

5. Bake in preheated oven until crust is crisp and golden, about 10 minutes. Cut into pieces and serve.

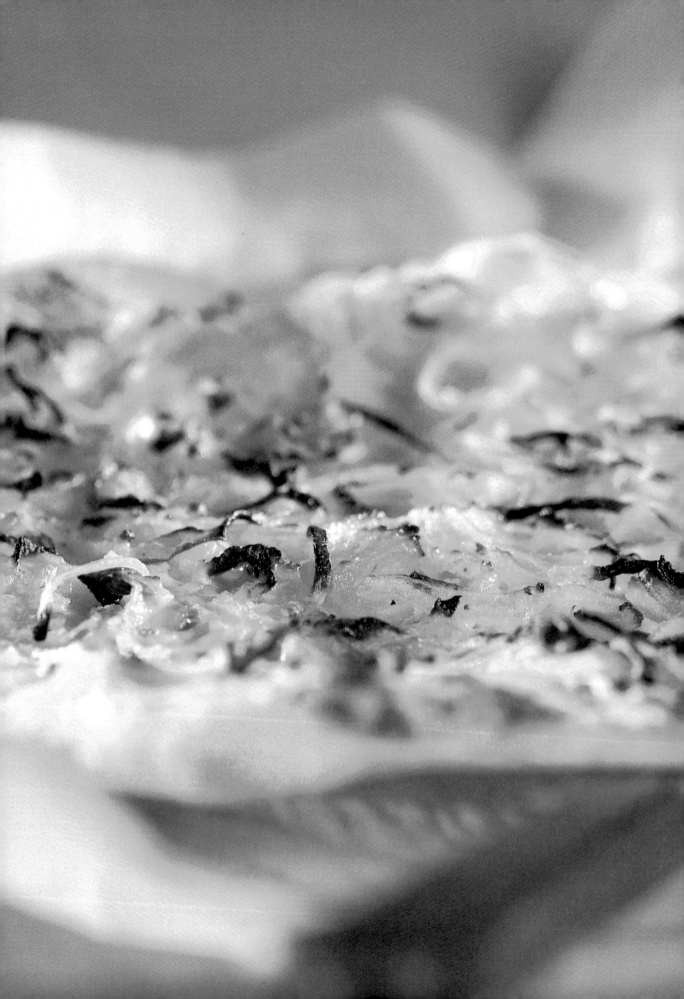

Onion Tomato Tarte Tatin

Serves 4

Preparation time
50 minutes

Cooking time
30 minutes

Variation

You can put a small quenelle of goat cheese on each tart before serving.

- Preheat oven to 400°F (200°C)
- Four 3-inch (7.5 cm) tart pans, oiled

2 tbsp	butter	30 mL
1 lb	onions, thinly sliced	500 g
½ tsp	chopped fresh savory leaves	2 mL
	Salt and freshly ground black pepper	
½ cup	sun-dried tomatoes	125 mL
5 oz	puff pastry	150 g
1	egg, beaten	1
	Mixed salad greens	

1. In a deep skillet, melt butter over medium heat. Add onions and cook, stirring, about 2 minutes. Reduce heat to medium-low, add savory and cook, stirring occasionally, until onions are very soft and golden brown, about 20 minutes. Season with salt and pepper to taste. Let cool slightly.

2. Meanwhile, in a heatproof bowl, cover sun-dried tomatoes with boiling water and let stand until softened. Drain well and pat dry.

3. Cut pastry into 4 equal pieces. On a lightly floured surface, roll out each piece into a circle that is slightly larger than the tops of the tart pans.

4. Arrange rehydrated tomatoes evenly over bottoms of tart pans, then top with onion mixture. Fit pastry circles overtop, tucking in edges between pan and vegetables. Prick tops with a fork and brush with egg.

5. Place pans on a baking sheet and bake in preheated oven until pastry is crisp and golden brown, about 25 minutes. Let cool slightly. Run a knife around edge of pastry, then flip over onto serving plates. Serve with a green salad on the side.

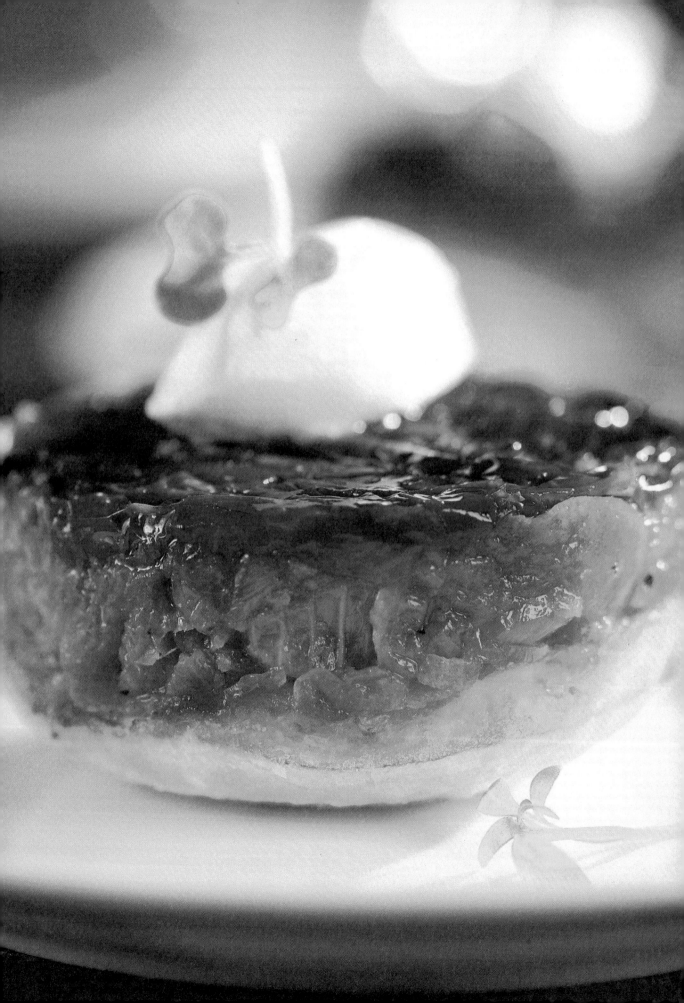

Vegetable Tian

Serves 4

Preparation time
55 minutes

Cooking time
35 minutes

Tip

Slice all the vegetables to the same thickness, as a uniform appearance will make the dish look more attractive.

- Candy/deep-fry thermometer
- Preheat oven to 400°F (200°C)
- 6- to 8-cup (1.5 to 2 L) gratin or baking dish

4 cups	vegetable oil	1 L
1	small eggplant	1
3 tbsp	olive oil, divided	45 mL
1 cup	thinly sliced onions	250 mL
	Sprig thyme, chopped	1
1	zucchini, thinly sliced crosswise	1
1	large tomato, thinly sliced	1
	Salt and freshly ground black pepper	
½ cup	bread crumbs	125 mL

1. In a deep skillet, heat vegetable oil over medium heat to 350°F (180°C). Cut eggplant crosswise into slices $\frac{1}{6}$ inch (4 mm) thick and pat dry. In batches to avoid crowding, fry, turning once, until golden and tender, 2 to 3 minutes. Using a slotted spoon, remove from pan and place on a baking sheet lined with paper towels to drain. Set aside.

2. In a skillet, heat 1 tbsp (15 mL) of the olive oil over medium-low heat. Add onions and thyme and cook, stirring, until soft but not browned, about 5 minutes. Spread in bottom of gratin dish.

3. Layer zucchini, tomato slices and eggplant, alternating and overlapping, on top of onions. Season with salt and pepper to taste between layers. Sprinkle bread crumbs on top, then drizzle with remaining olive oil.

4. Bake in preheated oven until vegetables are tender and topping is browned, about 20 minutes. Cut into pieces and serve hot.

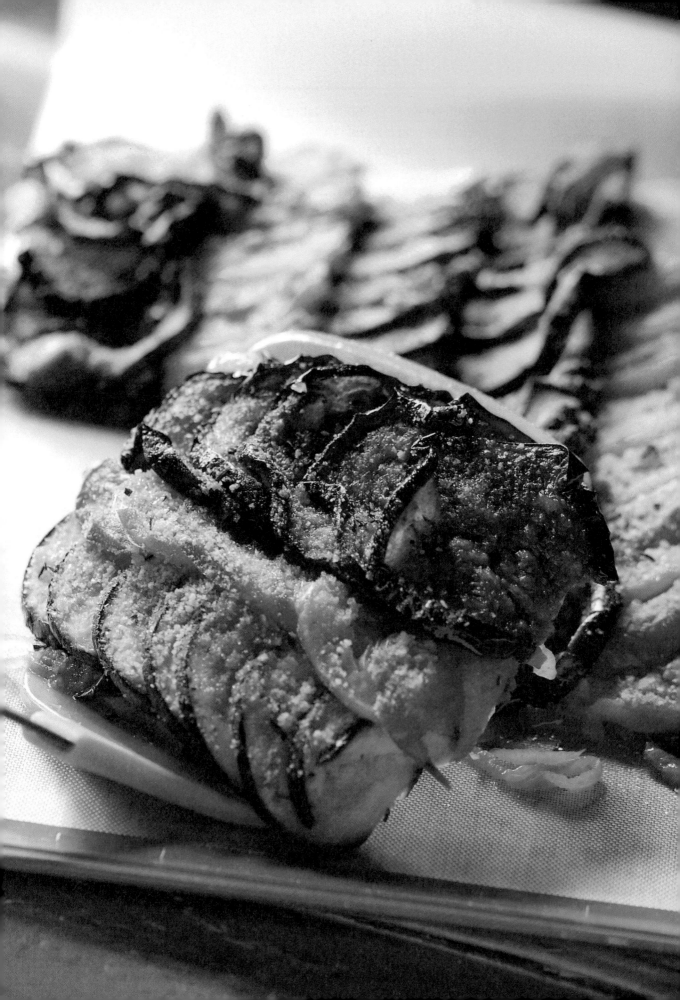

Vegetable Timbales

Serves 4

Preparation time
1 hour 15 minutes

Cooking time
30 minutes

- Preheat oven to 350°F (180°C)
- Four ¾-cup (175 mL) ramekins, bottoms lined with parchment paper, sides greased

¼ cup	extra virgin olive oil, divided	60 mL
½ cup	diced red bell pepper	125 mL
	Salt and freshly ground black pepper	
½ cup	diced yellow bell pepper	125 mL
½ cup	diced carrots	125 mL
¾ cup	diced eggplant	175 mL
1	medium zucchini, cut in half lengthwise and thinly sliced	1
2	small blue potatoes, unpeeled	2
¼ cup	thinly sliced red onion	60 mL

1. In a skillet, heat 1 tbsp (15 mL) of the oil over high heat. Add red pepper and sauté until slightly tender, about 2 minutes. Transfer to a bowl and add salt and pepper to taste. Repeat with yellow pepper, carrots, eggplant and zucchini, cooking them one at a time and adding more oil as necessary between each. Transfer to separate bowls.

2. Cut potatoes in half, then cut crosswise into very thin slices. Add 1 tbsp (15 mL) of oil to skillet and sauté potatoes until starting to soften. Transfer to a bowl and add salt and pepper to taste.

3. Reduce heat to medium and add 1 tsp (5 mL) of oil to skillet. Add red onion and cook, stirring, until softened, about 4 minutes. Transfer to another bowl.

4. Divide red onion among prepared ramekins, then cover completely with a row of slightly overlapping potato slices.

5. Line the sides of the ramekins with zucchini slices, standing them on one end and slightly overlapping, with the skin toward the outside.

6. Spoon red bell pepper on top and level with back of spoon. Repeat in turn with yellow bell pepper, eggplant and carrot to make individual colored layers. Top with another layer of potato.

7. Bake in preheated oven until potatoes are tender and timbales are hot inside, about 25 minutes. Run a knife carefully around inside edge of ramekins. Invert a serving plate on top of ramekin, then flip both over to unmold timbale onto plate. Remove parchment paper. Serve hot.

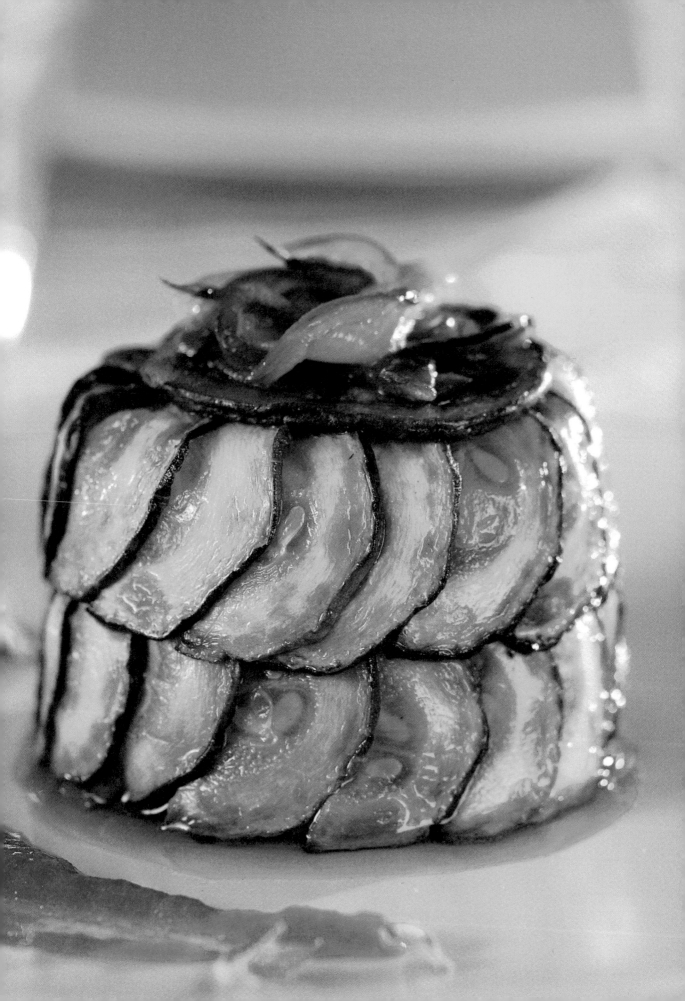

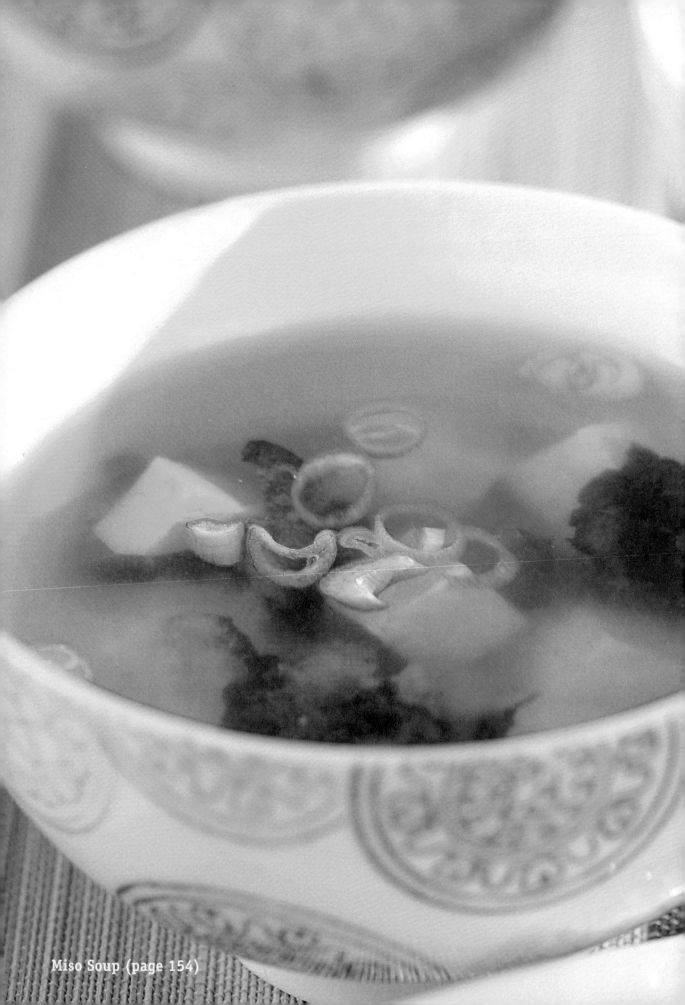

Miso Soup (page 154)

Soups

Vegetable Stock

Makes about 6 cups (1.5 L)

Preparation time
5 minutes

Cooking time
1 hour

Tip

This vegetable stock can be used in all the recipes where it is listed as an ingredient, and it is obviously of higher quality than what you find at the supermarket. It is not really made to be consumed as is.

2	stalks celery, cut into chunks	2
3	carrots, cut into chunks	3
2	onions, cut in half	2
1	leek, green part only	1
6	sprigs parsley	6
2	cloves garlic	2
4	bay leaves	4
1 tsp	whole black peppercorns	5 mL
4	whole cloves	4
2	sprigs thyme	2
9 cups	cold water	2.25 L

1. In a large pot, combine celery, carrots, onions, leek, parsley sprigs, garlic, bay leaves, peppercorns, cloves and thyme sprigs. Add cold water. Bring to a boil over high heat. Reduce heat and boil gently until stock is flavorful, about 45 minutes. In batches as necessary, strain through a fine-mesh sieve, discarding solids.

Rapini, Barley and Corn Soup

Serves 4

Preparation time
20 minutes

Cooking time
40 minutes

Tip

Cut off and discard the toughest part of the rapini stalks. Cut the other parts into pieces no longer than $\frac{1}{2}$ inch (1 cm).

3 tbsp	pot barley	45 mL
2 tbsp	extra virgin olive oil	30 mL
2 tbsp	diced celery	30 mL
2 tbsp	diced carrot	30 mL
2 tbsp	finely chopped onion	30 mL
1	bunch rapini, cut into $\frac{1}{2}$-inch (1 cm) pieces (see Tip, left)	1
5 cups	Vegetable Stock (above) or ready-to-use broth	1.25 L
1 cup	corn kernels	250 mL

1. In a saucepan of boiling salted water, cook barley until tender, about 40 minutes. Drain.

2. Meanwhile, in a pot, heat oil over medium-high heat. Sauté celery, carrot and onion until softened, about 3 minutes.

3. Add rapini and stock and bring to a boil. Stir in corn. Reduce heat and simmer until rapini is soft, about 15 minutes. Stir in barley. Ladle into warmed bowls.

Cream of Eggplant Soup

Serves 4

Preparation time
45 minutes

Cooking time
1 hour

- • Preheat oven to 400°F (200°C)
- • Blender, food processor or immersion blender

1 lb	eggplant	500 g
2 tsp	olive oil	10 mL
2 tbsp	butter, divided	30 mL
½ cup	thinly sliced onion	125 mL
½ cup	thinly sliced leeks, white parts only	125 mL
5 tsp	all-purpose flour	25 mL
2 cups	Vegetable Stock (page 128) or ready-to-use broth (approx.)	500 mL
1 cup	heavy or whipping (35%) cream (approx.)	250 mL
	Salt and freshly ground black pepper	
2	hard-cooked eggs	2
3 oz	wild mushrooms, sliced	90 g
2 tsp	chopped fresh cilantro leaves	10 mL

1. Cut eggplant lengthwise in half, brush with olive oil and place on a baking sheet, cut side up. Bake in preheated oven until very soft, about 45 minutes. Using a spoon, scoop out flesh and set aside. Discard skin.

2. In a pot, melt 1 tbsp (15 mL) of the butter over medium heat. Add onion and leek, reduce heat to low and cook, stirring, until softened but not browned, about 8 minutes. Add flour and cook, stirring, about 3 minutes. Stir in eggplant.

3. Increase heat to medium-high. Stir in vegetable stock and cream and bring to a simmer. Reduce heat and simmer gently, stirring often, until flavors have blended, about 15 minutes. Add salt and pepper to taste.

4. Meanwhile, separate egg whites from yolks and chop separately. Set aside.

5. In a skillet, melt remaining butter over high heat. Sauté mushrooms until tender and browned, about 4 minutes. Set aside.

6. In batches as necessary, transfer soup to blender (or use immersion blender in the pot) and purée until smooth. Return to pot, if necessary. Reheat over medium heat, stirring often, until steaming. Check seasoning. Adjust consistency as needed by adding a little cream or vegetable stock.

7. Ladle hot soup into warmed bowls. Garnish with mushrooms, chopped egg yolks and whites and cilantro.

Squash Soup with Ginger and Goat Cheese

Tip

A quenelle is an oblong shape with tapered ends, like a football. You can shape the cheese into a quenelle using two spoons for a fancy presentation, or just dollop or crumble the cheese on top of the soup.

Variation

This soup can be garnished with mild, creamy blue cheese instead of goat cheese. It's truly delicious.

• Blender, food processor or immersion blender

3 tbsp	butter	45 mL
3 tbsp	thinly sliced French shallots	45 mL
2 cups	chopped pepper (acorn) squash	500 mL
1 tbsp	grated fresh gingerroot	15 mL
2½ cups	Vegetable Stock (page 128) or ready-to-use broth	625 mL
	Salt and freshly ground black pepper	
4 tbsp	fresh goat cheese	60 mL
	Finely chopped fresh chives	

1. In a pot, melt butter over medium heat. Add shallots and cook, stirring, until softened but not browned, about 3 minutes. Add squash, ginger and vegetable stock. Season with salt and pepper to taste. Bring to a boil. Reduce heat and boil gently until squash is soft, about 20 minutes.

2. In batches as necessary, transfer soup to blender (or use immersion blender in the pot) and purée until smooth. Return to pot, if necessary. Reheat over medium heat until steaming. Check seasoning.

3. In a bowl, combine cheese and chives to taste. Ladle soup into warm bowls and garnish each with a quenelle of cheese (see Tip, left).

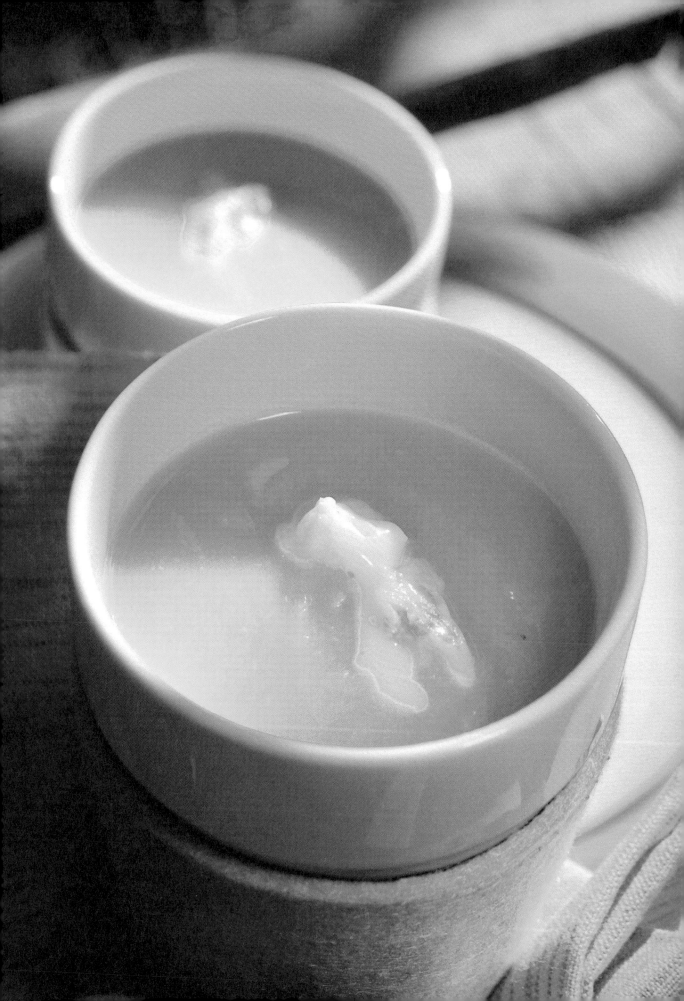

Gazpacho

Serves 4

Preparation time
40 minutes

Chilling time
6 hours

Tip

Piment d'Espelette is a dried mild chile pepper from the Basque region of France.

- Preheat broiler or barbecue grill to high
- Food processor

2	red bell peppers	2
4	tomatoes, peeled and diced	4
1	cucumber, coarsely chopped	1
½	red onion, diced	½
1 cup	tomato juice	250 mL
1 cup	cubed day-old bread, crusts removed	250 mL
2 tbsp	sherry vinegar	30 mL
2 tbsp	extra virgin olive oil	30 mL
	Salt	
	Piment d'Espelette (see Tip, left)	
2	hard-cooked eggs	2

1. Place bell peppers on a baking sheet and broil, or place on preheated grill and roast, turning often, until skin is slightly blackened and blistered. Transfer to a bowl, cover and let cool.

2. Peel roasted peppers and discard cores and seeds. Cut flesh into chunks.

3. In a food processor, purée roasted peppers, tomatoes, cucumber, red onion, tomato juice, bread, vinegar and olive oil until smooth. Transfer to a bowl. Season with salt and piment d'Espelette to taste. Cover and chill in refrigerator for 6 hours.

4. Separate egg whites from yolks and chop separately.

5. Ladle gazpacho into chilled bowls and topped with chopped egg yolks and whites.

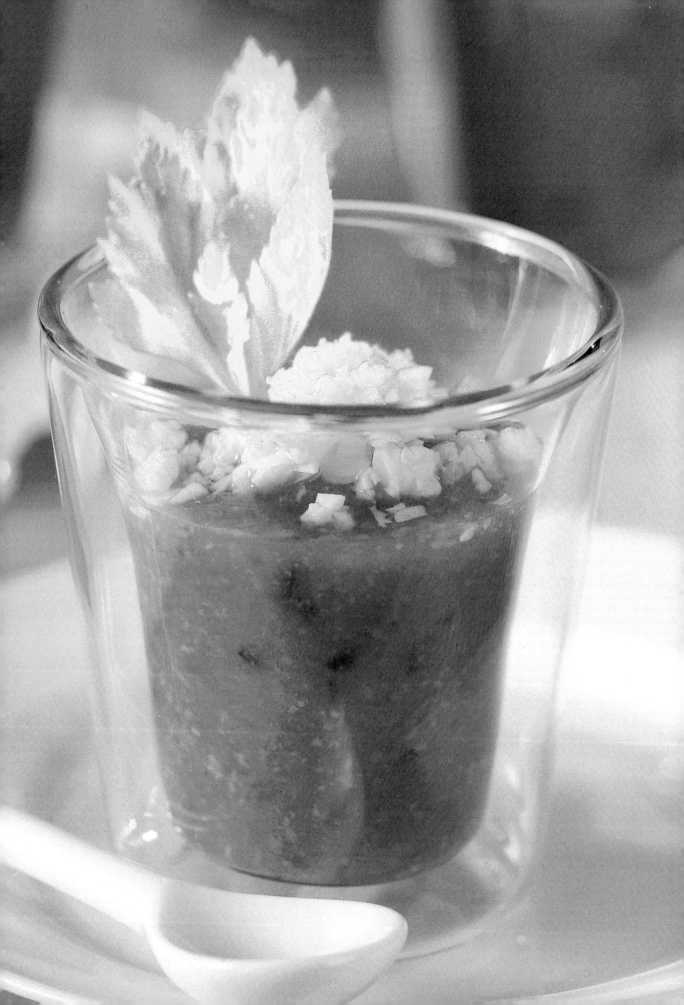

Hearty South American–Style Fava Bean Soup

Serves 4

Preparation time
1 hour

Cooking time
35 minutes

Tips

Fava beans, also known as broad beans, are native to North Africa. Once the beans have been removed from their inedible pods, steam or blanch them for 1 minute, then remove the outer skins before using in recipes. Two cups (500 mL) canned, frozen or soaked and cooked dried fava beans can be used in this soup.

Aji panca are mild dark red peppers with a fruity, slightly smoky flavor. The paste is available in jars at Latin food stores. If you can't find it, use 2 tsp (10 mL) minced canned chipotle peppers in adobo sauce.

Fromage frais is a name for any type of soft, fresh cultured cheese. It is very perishable, so it must be used soon after it is made. You can often find it at specialty cheese shops — Neufchâtel is an example.

1 lb	shelled fava beans (see Tips, left)	500 g
1 lb	potatoes, unpeeled (about 4 small)	500 g
2	ears corn	2
3 tbsp	vegetable oil, divided	45 mL
1	large onion, finely chopped	1
4 tsp	aji panca paste (see Tips, left)	20 mL
2 tsp	chopped garlic	10 mL
2/3 cup	jasmine rice	150 mL
	Salt	
1	bunch fresh oregano, chopped	1
8	eggs	8
8 oz	fromage frais, cut into cubes (see Tips, left)	250 g
1/2 cup	evaporated milk	125 mL

1. In a pot of boiling water, blanch fava beans until almost tender, about 5 minutes. Drain and set aside.

2. Place potatoes in a pot and add cold, salted water to cover. Bring to a boil over high heat. Reduce heat and boil gently until fork-tender, about 30 minutes. Drain until cool enough to handle. Cut into quarters and set aside.

3. In another large pot, bring 8 cups (2 L) salted water to a boil over high heat. Add corn and boil until tender, about 5 minutes. Using tongs, transfer corn to a bowl and reserve cooking water. When cool enough to handle, cut cobs of corn in half crosswise. Set aside.

4. In a large pot, heat 2 tbsp (30 mL) of the oil over medium heat. Add onion and cook, stirring, until softened but not browned, about 5 minutes. Add aji panca paste and garlic and cook, stirring, for 1 minute. Add rice and stir to coat well.

5. Add reserved corn cooking water and salt to taste and bring to a boil. Reduce heat and simmer for 15 minutes. Stir in oregano and potatoes and simmer for 10 minutes.

6. In a bowl, whisk 4 of the eggs until blended. Gradually pour into soup while stirring constantly. Stir in cheese, corn and fava beans. Simmer, stirring, until heated through (do not let boil).

7. Just before serving, in a large skillet, heat remaining oil over medium-high heat. Fry remaining 4 eggs sunny-side up.

8. Stir evaporated milk into soup and ladle into warmed bowls. Place a fried egg on top of each serving.

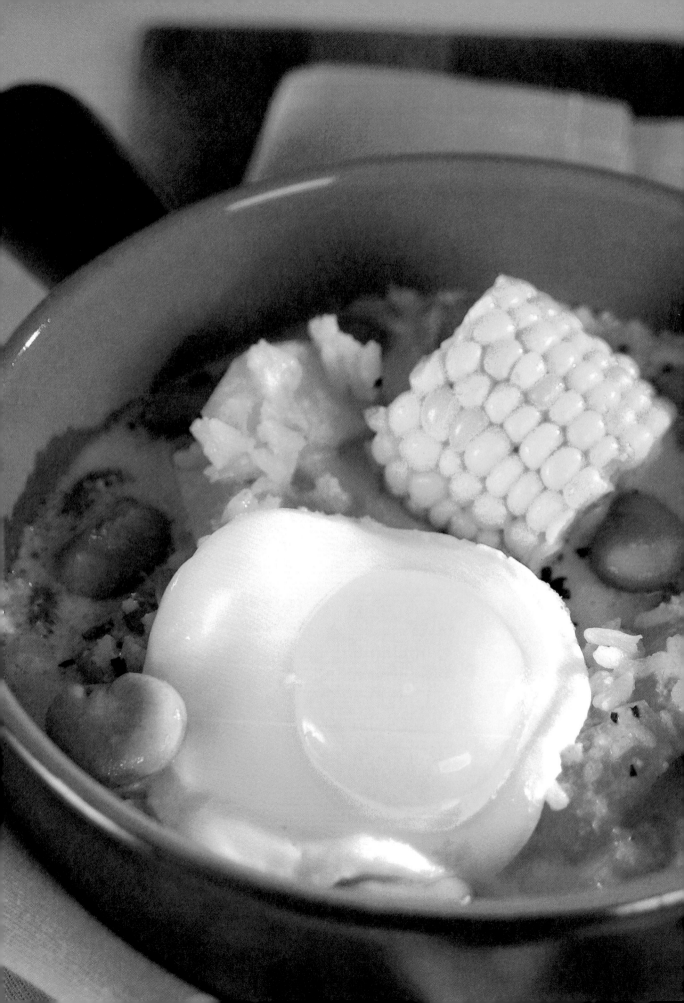

Parsley Root Soup

Tip

Parsley root comes from a variety of parsley grown specifically for its roots. The taste is similar to a blend of celery and carrot. To use, trim off the greens and use them for stock or some other use and peel the root as you would a carrot.

Variation

You can drizzle a little nut oil or truffle oil into each bowl.

• Blender, food processor or immersion blender

1 lb	parsley roots, peeled and thinly sliced (see Tip, left)	500 g
¼ cup	butter	60 mL
½ cup	chopped French shallots	125 mL

Béchamel Sauce

3 cups	milk (approx.)	750 mL
2½ tbsp	butter	37 mL
¼ cup	all-purpose flour	60 mL
	Salt	
	Cayenne pepper	
1¼ cups	heavy or whipping (35%) cream	300 mL

1. In a pot of boiling water, blanch parsley roots for 2 minutes. Drain well.

2. In a clean pot, melt butter over medium heat. Add shallots and cook, stirring, until softened but not browned, about 5 minutes. Add parsley roots, cover and reduce heat to low. Cook until parsley roots are very soft but not browned, about 10 minutes.

3. *Béchamel Sauce:* Meanwhile, in a saucepan, bring milk almost to a boil over medium heat. In another saucepan, melt butter over medium heat. Sprinkle with flour and cook, stirring, for 1 minute to make a roux.

4. Gradually pour hot milk over roux, blending well with a whisk. Season with salt and cayenne pepper to taste. Bring to a boil. Reduce heat and boil gently, whisking, until slightly thickened, about 5 minutes.

5. Add béchamel to parsley root mixture. Salt lightly and cook over low heat, stirring often, until flavors are blended, about 15 minutes.

6. In batches as necessary, transfer to blender (or use an immersion blender in the pot) and purée until smooth. Strain through a sieve back into the pot.

7. Return soup to medium heat, add cream and adjust seasoning. Add a little milk if mixture is too thick.

Spinach and Potato Soup au Gratin

Serves 4

Preparation time
20 minutes

Cooking time
30 minutes

Tip

When buying cheese, read the label carefully and make sure to buy those that are not made from animal rennet.

• Preheat oven to 500°F (260°C)
• 4 ovenproof onion soup or other soup bowls

2 tbsp	butter	30 mL
3 tbsp	finely chopped French shallots	45 mL
1	large potato, cut into ½-inch (1 cm) cubes	1
3⅓ cups	water	825 mL
	Salt and freshly ground black pepper	
Pinch	freshly grated nutmeg	Pinch
6 oz	spinach, trimmed and chopped	175 g
4 tbsp	shredded Gruyère cheese (see Tip, left)	60 mL
4	quail eggs, optional	4

1. In a pot, melt butter over medium heat. Add shallots and cook, stirring, until softened but not browned, about 3 minutes. Add potatoes and water, increase heat to high and bring to a boil. Add salt and pepper to taste and nutmeg. Reduce heat and boil gently until potato is tender.

2. Stir in spinach and simmer for 2 minutes.

3. Ladle soup into bowls and place on a baking sheet. Sprinkle each with Gruyère cheese and gently place a quail egg, if using, in the center of each bowl. Bake in preheated oven until cheese is browned and egg is just set, about 3 minutes.

Classic Leek and Potato Soup

Serves 4

Preparation time
45 minutes

Cooking time
30 minutes

Variation

This soup is a base that can be garnished in many ways, for example, with julienned vegetables, a poached egg, sautéed mushrooms or a quenelle of goat cheese.

• Blender, food processor or immersion blender

2 tbsp	butter	30 mL
6	leeks, white parts only, thinly sliced	6
4 cups	water	1 L
1 lb	potatoes, peeled and cut into cubes	500 g
	Salt	
2 tsp	heavy or whipping (35%) cream	10 mL
	Sprigs chervil	

1. In a pot, melt butter over medium heat. Add leeks, reduce heat to low and cook, stirring, until softened but not browned, about 10 minutes.

2. Add water, potatoes and salt to taste. Increase heat to high and bring to a boil. Reduce heat to low, cover and simmer until potatoes are very soft and soup is flavorful, 20 to 25 minutes.

3. In batches as necessary, transfer to blender (or use immersion blender in the pot) and purée until smooth. Return to pot, if necessary. Stir in cream and reheat over medium heat, stirring often, until steaming. Adjust seasoning.

4. Ladle into warm bowls and garnish with chervil sprigs.

Lentil Soup

● **Blender, food processor or immersion blender**

2 tbsp	butter	30 mL
½ cup	finely chopped onion	125 mL
½ cup	thinly sliced leek, green part only	125 mL
1 cup	Puy lentils, sorted and rinsed	250 mL
4 cups	cold water	1 L
1	sprig thyme	1
1	bay leaf	1
	Salt	
2 tsp	white vinegar	10 mL
4	eggs	4

1. In a pot, melt butter over medium heat. Add onion and leek and cook, stirring, until softened but not browned, about 5 minutes.

2. Add lentils, water, thyme and bay leaf, increase heat to high and bring to a boil. Reduce heat and simmer until lentils are tender, about 20 minutes. Discard thyme sprig and bay leaf.

3. In batches as necessary, transfer to blender (or use immersion blender in the pot) and purée until smooth. Strain through a sieve back into the pot. Reheat over medium heat until steaming.

4. Meanwhile, fill a saucepan with 3 inches (7.5 cm) of water and bring to a simmer over medium-high heat. Add vinegar. Reduce heat to a gentle simmer. One at a time, crack each egg into a small dish and carefully drop into simmering water. Poach until white is set and yolk is the desired consistency, 3 to 5 minutes.

5. Ladle soup into warmed bowls. Using a slotted spoon, remove poached eggs from water, draining well, and place one in each bowl of soup.

Cream of Corn and Pepper Soup with Potato Croquettes

Serves 4

Preparation time
55 minutes

Cooking time
45 minutes

• Blender, food processor or immersion blender

¼ cup	butter	60 mL
1	onion, finely chopped	1
	Piment d'Espelette (see Tip, page 132)	
6 cups	corn kernels	1.5 L
2½ cups	milk (approx.)	625 mL
	Salt	
	Cayenne pepper	
	Hot Fingerling Potato Croquettes (page 22)	

1. In a pot, melt butter over medium heat. Add onion and piment d'Espelette to taste and cook, stirring, until softened but not browned, about 5 minutes. Add corn and milk (adding more if necessary to cover the vegetables). Season with salt and cayenne pepper to taste.

2. Cover and cook over low heat until corn is very soft and soup is flavorful, about 40 minutes.

3. In batches as necessary, transfer to blender (or use immersion blender in the pot) and purée until smooth. Strain through a sieve back into the pot. Adjust seasoning as needed. Reheat over medium heat, stirring, until steaming.

4. Ladle soup into warm bowls and sprinkle potato croquettes on top.

Minestrone

Preparation time
30 minutes

Cooking time
35 minutes

Variation

This soup is excellent topped with basil pesto.

2 tbsp	extra virgin olive oil	30 mL
¼ cup	finely chopped onion	60 mL
1	clove garlic, chopped	1
2	large savoy cabbage leaves, chopped	2
1	stalk celery, diced	1
1	carrot, diced	1
1	leek, white part only, chopped	1
8 cups	water	2 L
	Salt and freshly ground black pepper	
2	plum (Roma) tomatoes, chopped	2
1	small potato, diced	1
1	zucchini, diced	1
⅓ cup	small tube pasta, such as tubettini	75 mL
¾ cup	cooked white beans	175 mL
1 cup	spinach leaves	250 mL

1. In a pot, heat oil over medium heat. Add onion and garlic and cook, stirring, until softened, about 5 minutes. Add cabbage, celery, carrot and leek. Reduce heat to low and cook, stirring, until softened but not browned, about 8 minutes.

2. Add water, increase heat to medium-high and bring to a boil. Reduce heat and simmer until vegetables are slightly tender, about 5 minutes. Season with salt and pepper to taste.

3. Add tomatoes, potato and zucchini. Simmer until vegetables are soft, about 15 minutes.

4. Meanwhile, in a saucepan of boiling salted water, cook pasta according to package directions until al dente. Drain well.

5. Stir beans and spinach into soup and cook for 1 minute. Divide pasta among warm bowls and ladle soup overtop.

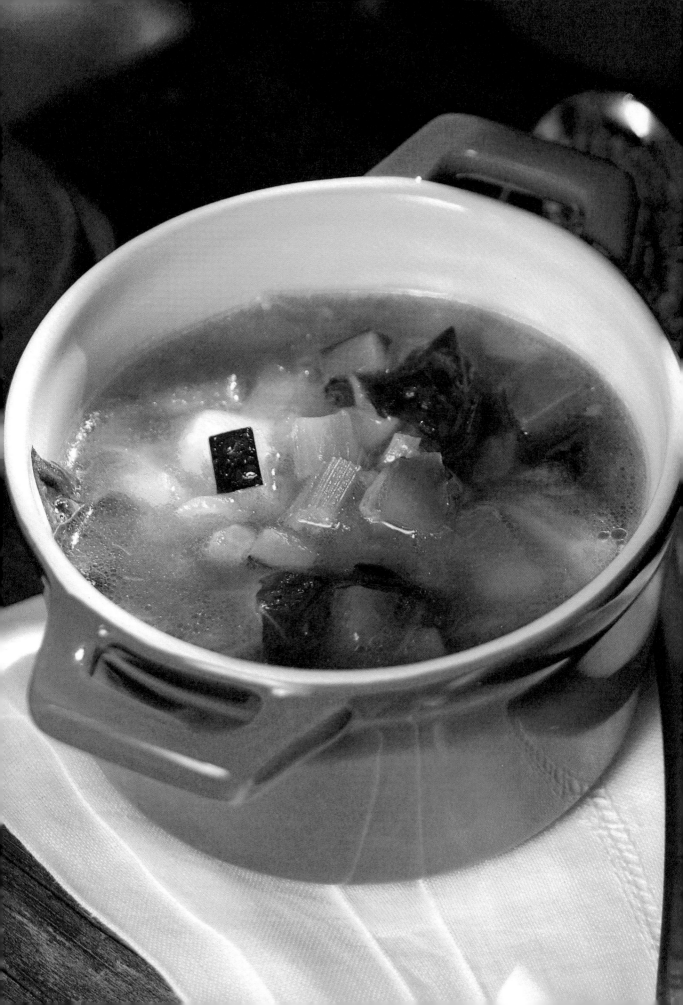

Pasta Fagioli Soup

Serves 4

Preparation time
20 minutes

Cooking time
1 hour

• Food mill, blender or food processor

2	cloves garlic	2
1	sprig rosemary	1
2	leaves fresh sage	2
5 tbsp	extra virgin olive oil, divided	75 mL
½ cup	diced celery	125 mL
½ cup	diced carrot	125 mL
½ cup	diced onion	125 mL
¼ cup	chopped peeled tomato	60 mL
2½ cups	cooked white beans (cannellini or borlotti)	625 mL
6 cups	Vegetable Stock (page 128) or ready-to-use broth	1.5 L
	Salt and freshly ground black pepper	
½ cup	small pasta, such as tubettini	125 mL

1. Chop garlic, rosemary and sage together.

2. In a pot, heat ¼ cup (60 mL) of the oil over medium-high heat. Sauté celery, carrot and onion until lightly browned, about 5 minutes. Add garlic mixture and sauté until lightly browned, about 2 minutes.

3. Add tomato, beans, stock, and salt and pepper to taste and bring to a boil. Reduce heat and simmer until vegetables are soft and beans start to break apart, about 45 minutes.

4. Meanwhile, in a pot of boiling salted water, cook pasta according to package directions until al dente. Drain well and set aside.

5. Using a slotted spoon, transfer about half of the vegetable solids to food mill, blender or food processor and press or purée until smooth, adding some of the liquid to blender if necessary. Return to pot and stir in pasta.

6. Ladle soup into warm bowls and drizzle with remaining olive oil.

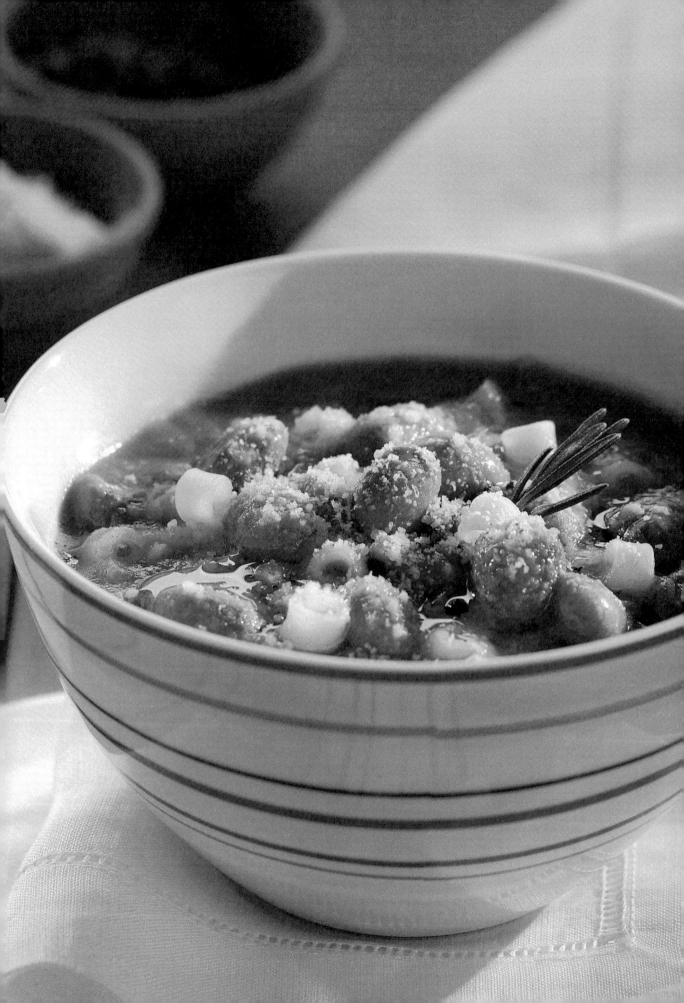

Potage Saint-Germain

Preparation time
15 minutes

Cooking time
1 hour

Tip

A bouquet garni is a small bundle of aromatic herbs tied together with kitchen string. It is used to add flavor to a simmered or boiled mixture and is generally discarded before the dish is served. It often includes parsley, thyme and bay leaves but can also include any of your favorite herbs that complement the flavors of your dish.

• Blender, food processor or immersion blender

2 tbsp	butter	30 mL
1	leek, green part only, thinly sliced	1
¼ cup	thinly sliced onion	60 mL
1	clove garlic, chopped	1
1 cup	dried split peas, sorted and rinsed	250 mL
4 cups	cold water	1 L
1	bouquet garni (see Tip, left)	1
4	slices bread	4
1 tsp	vegetable oil or clarified butter (ghee)	5 mL
	Salt	
3 tbsp	heavy or whipping (35%) cream, optional	45 mL
	Sprigs chervil	

1. In a pot, melt butter over medium heat. Add leek and onion and cook, stirring, until softened but not browned. Add garlic, split peas, water and bouquet garni and bring to a boil. Reduce heat to medium-low, cover and boil gently until peas are tender, about 45 minutes.

2. Meanwhile, cut bread into cubes. In a skillet, heat oil over medium-high heat. Add bread cubes and brown gently in oil. Place on a plate lined with paper towels to drain.

3. Discard bouquet garni from soup and season with salt to taste.

4. In batches as necessary, transfer soup to blender (or use immersion blender in the pot) and purée until smooth. Strain through a sieve back into the pot. Stir in cream, if desired, to thin the soup. Reheat over medium heat, stirring often, until steaming. Adjust seasoning.

5. Ladle soup into warm bowls and garnish with chervil sprigs. Serve croutons in a separate bowl on the side.

Onion Soup

Serves 4

Preparation time
45 minutes

Cooking time
30 minutes

Variation

Serve this soup topped with a toasted baguette slice and shredded Gruyère and broil until browned.

2 tbsp	butter	30 mL
2	large onions, thinly sliced (about 12 oz/375 g)	2
3 cups	water	750 mL
1	bottle (12 oz/341 mL) lager beer	1
	Salt and freshly ground black pepper	

1. In a pot, melt butter over medium heat. Stir in onions. Reduce heat to medium-low and cook, stirring, until very soft and golden, about 15 minutes.

2. Add water, beer, and salt and pepper to taste. Increase heat to high and bring to a boil. Reduce heat to low, cover and simmer until flavors are blended, about 15 minutes.

3. Adjust seasoning. Ladle into warm bowls.

Rice and White Quinoa Soup with Lemon

Serves 4

Preparation time
5 minutes

Cooking time
30 minutes

● **Blender**

¼ cup	white quinoa	60 mL
4 cups	Vegetable Stock (page 128) or ready-to-use broth	1 L
⅓ cup	Arborio rice	75 mL
2	eggs	2
3 tbsp	grated vegetarian-friendly Parmesan cheese (see Tip, page 137)	45 mL
	Freshly ground black pepper	
	Grated zest and juice of ½ lemon	
	Chopped fresh Italian flat-leaf parsley	

1. In a saucepan of boiling salted water, cook quinoa until tender, about 13 minutes. Drain and set aside.

2. Meanwhile, in a pot, bring vegetable stock to a boil over high heat. Add rice, reduce heat and boil gently until tender, about 20 minutes.

3. In a bowl, beat eggs with cheese. Season with pepper to taste and add lemon zest and juice. Gradually pour mixture into pot, stirring gently.

4. Transfer half of the soup to blender and purée until smooth. Return to pot and stir well.

5. Stir in quinoa and parsley. Ladle into warm bowls.

Cold Cucumber and Tomato Soup

Serves 4

Preparation time
30 minutes

Chilling time
6 hours

● **Food processor**

1	cucumber	1
2	tomatoes, peeled and seeded	2
2 tsp	chopped white onion	10 mL
3 tbsp	plain yogurt	45 mL
½ cup	Vegetable Stock (page 128) or ready-to-use broth	125 mL
	Salt	
	Hot pepper sauce	
	Finely chopped fresh chives	
2	radishes, chopped	2

1. Cut cucumbers in half lengthwise and scoop out seeds, then cut into chunks.

2. In a food processor, purée cucumber, tomatoes and onion.

3. Transfer to a bowl and stir in yogurt and vegetable stock, then add salt and hot pepper sauce to taste.

4. Cover and refrigerate until chilled, about 6 hours. Ladle into chilled bowls and garnish with chives and chopped radish.

Savoy Cabbage, Bean and Squash Minestrone

Tips

Borlotti beans are known by several other names, including romano beans, cranberry beans and rosecoco beans.

To soak and cook dried beans: In a bowl, cover dried beans with at least 4 inches (10 cm) of cold water. Cover and let soak for 24 hours. Drain beans and transfer to a large pot. Add fresh cold water to cover by at least 3 inches (7.5 cm). Bring to a boil over high heat. Reduce heat and boil gently until beans are tender, about 1 hour. Drain well.

1 cup	fresh shelled borlotti (romano or cranberry) beans (see Tips, left)	250 mL
5 tbsp	extra virgin olive oil, divided	75 mL
3 tbsp	finely diced celery	45 mL
3 tbsp	finely diced carrot	45 mL
3 tbsp	finely diced onion	45 mL
1	clove garlic, chopped	1
	Chopped fresh rosemary leaves	
	Chopped fresh sage leaves	
2 cups	cubed ($\frac{1}{2}$ inch/1 cm) winter squash	500 mL
1 cup	chopped savoy cabbage	250 mL
	Salt and freshly ground black pepper	
4 cups	Vegetable Stock (page 128) or ready-to-use broth	1 L
4	slices baguette	4

1. In a saucepan, cover beans with cold salted water and bring to a boil over high heat. Reduce heat and boil gently until tender, about 20 minutes. Drain, reserving cooking water.

2. Meanwhile, in a pot, heat $\frac{1}{4}$ cup (60 mL) of the olive oil over medium-high heat. Sauté celery, carrot, onion, garlic, rosemary and sage until softened and lightly browned, about 5 minutes.

3. Add squash, reduce heat to low and cook, stirring, for 3 minutes. Add cabbage and cook, stirring, for 3 minutes. Season with salt and pepper to taste.

4. Add stock, increase heat to high and bring to a boil. Reduce heat and simmer until squash is almost tender, about 10 minutes. Stir in beans and as much cooking water as needed to thin soup to desired consistency. Adjust seasoning.

5. Just before serving, in a skillet, heat remaining oil over medium-high heat. Fry baguette slices, turning once, until golden brown, about 2 minutes per side.

6. Ladle soup into warm bowls and top with a toasted baguette slice.

Cold Yellow Tomato and Orange Soup with Thai Basil

Serves 4		
Preparation time 15 minutes		
Chilling time 6 hours		

- Food processor

1¼ lbs	yellow tomatoes, peeled (about 4 medium)	625 g
1 cup	freshly squeezed orange juice	250 mL
2 tbsp	extra virgin olive oil	30 mL
	Salt	
Pinch	cayenne pepper	Pinch
2 tbsp	sour cream	30 mL
8	leaves fresh Thai basil, finely chopped	8

1. In a food processor, purée tomatoes, orange juice, olive oil, salt to taste and cayenne pepper.

2. Transfer to a bowl, cover and refrigerate until chilled, about 6 hours. Ladle into chilled bowls and garnish with sour cream and basil.

Barley Soup with Mushroom Fumet

Serves 4		
Preparation time 20 minutes		
Cooking time 1 hour 15 minutes		

3 oz	dried mushrooms	90 g
6 cups	water	1.5 L
2 tbsp	olive oil	30 mL
⅔ cup	chopped celery	150 mL
½ cup	chopped onion	125 mL
½ cup	chopped carrot	125 mL
1 cup	pearl barley	250 mL
	Salt and freshly ground black pepper	
1	small bunch fresh Italian flat-leaf parsley, chopped	1
4	leaves fresh basil	4

1. In a saucepan, combine mushrooms and water. Bring to a boil over high heat. Remove from heat and let steep for 30 minutes. Drain well, reserving liquid and mushrooms separately. Strain liquid through a fine-mesh sieve or coffee filter to remove any grit.

2. In a pot, heat oil over medium-high heat. Sauté celery, onion and carrot until softened and browned, about 5 minutes. Stir in barley until well coated. Stir in reserved mushroom liquid and salt and pepper to taste and bring to a boil. Reduce heat and simmer for 20 minutes.

3. Chop reserved mushrooms and stir into soup. Simmer until barley is tender, about 20 minutes.

4. Stir in parsley. Adjust seasoning. Ladle into warm bowls and garnish with basil.

Hot and Sour Soup

See photo, opposite

Serves 4		
Preparation time 15 minutes		
Cooking time 20 minutes		

3 cups	Vegetable Stock (page 128) or ready-to-use broth	750 mL
2 tbsp	soy sauce	30 mL
1 lb	firm tofu, cut into strips	500 g
½ cup	thinly sliced bamboo shoots	125 mL
⅔ cup	thinly sliced shiitake mushroom caps	150 mL
1 tbsp	rice vinegar	15 mL
	Sambal oelek	
2 tbsp	tapioca starch	30 mL
2 tbsp	cold water	30 mL

1. In a saucepan, bring vegetable stock to a boil over high heat. Add soy sauce, tofu, bamboo shoots and mushrooms. Reduce heat and simmer until mushrooms are tender, about 5 minutes.

2. Add rice vinegar and sambal oelek to taste. In a small bowl, combine tapioca starch and cold water. Stir into soup. Cook, stirring, until slightly thickened and clear, about 2 minutes. Ladle into warmed bowls.

Cream of Cauliflower Soup with Hazelnut Oil

Serves 4		
Preparation time 20 minutes		
Cooking time 50 minutes		

- Blender or food processor

1	small cauliflower, cut into large pieces (about 12 oz/375 g trimmed)	1
3 cups	milk	750 mL
1 tbsp	vegetable oil	15 mL
1	small potato, diced	1
	Salt	
	Hazelnut oil	

1. In a saucepan, combine cauliflower and milk and bring to a simmer over medium heat, stirring occasionally. Reduce heat to low, cover with lid slightly ajar and simmer until cauliflower is soft, 30 to 40 minutes.

2. Meanwhile, in a skillet, heat vegetable oil over low heat. Add potato and cook, stirring often, until lightly browned, about 10 minutes. Transfer to a plate lined with paper towels and sprinkle with salt. Set aside.

3. In batches as necessary, transfer cauliflower mixture to blender and purée until smooth. Return to pot and reheat over medium heat, stirring, until steaming. Add salt to taste.

4. Ladle soup into warmed bowls. Garnish with fried potato and drizzle with a little hazelnut oil.

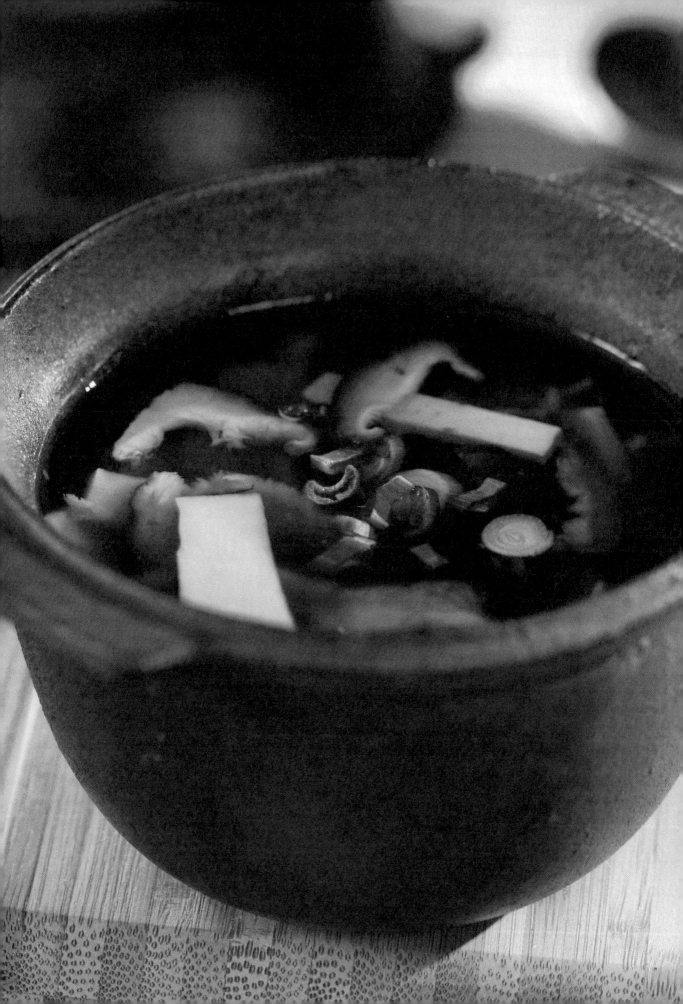

Hearty Wheat, Fromage Frais and Wild Mushroom Soup

Serves 4

Preparation time
40 minutes

Cooking time
50 minutes

Tip

We prefer a deeply flavored wild mushroom such as black trumpet (also called black chanterelle), but your favorite wild mushroom will work in this soup.

1 tsp	vegetable oil	5 mL
1 cup	finely chopped onions	250 mL
1	clove garlic, chopped	1
1½ tsp	aji amarillo paste	7 mL
	Salt and freshly ground black pepper	
	Ground cumin	
1 cup	wheat berries, rinsed	250 mL
8 cups	water	2 L
2	medium potatoes, diced	2
2 tbsp	butter	30 mL
¾ cup	sliced wild mushrooms (see Tip, left)	175 mL
8 oz	fromage frais, diced (see Tip, page 118)	250 g
1 tsp	chopped fresh Italian flat-leaf parsley	5 mL

1. In a pot, heat oil over medium heat. Add onions and cook, stirring, until softened but not browned, about 5 minutes. Stir in garlic, aji amarillo paste, and salt, pepper and cumin to taste. Add wheat berries and stir to coat well.

2. Add water, increase heat to high and bring to a boil. Reduce heat to low, cover and simmer until wheat berries are slightly tender, about 30 minutes. Add potatoes, cover and simmer until wheat berries and potatoes are tender, about 15 minutes.

3. Meanwhile, in a small skillet, melt butter over high heat. Sauté mushrooms until tender and browned, about 5 minutes.

4. Stir cheese, mushrooms and parsley into soup. Adjust seasoning. Ladle into warmed bowls.

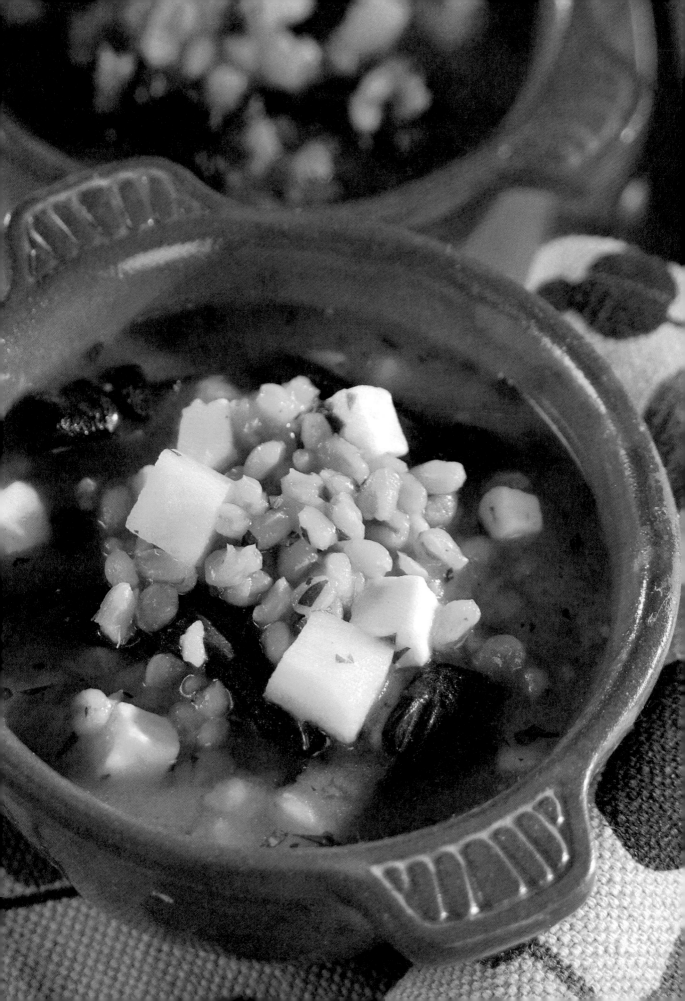

Cabbage and Bean Soup

Tip

If you can't find fresh beans, soak and cook ⅔ cup (150 mL) dried beans (see Tips, page 146).

1¼ cups	fresh shelled borlotti (romano or cranberry) beans (see Tip, left)	300 mL
6 cups	cold water	1.5 L
	Salt	
¼ cup	extra virgin olive oil, divided	60 mL
⅔ cup	diced celery	150 mL
½ cup	diced carrot	125 mL
½ cup	diced onion	125 mL
1	clove garlic, chopped	1
2	leaves fresh sage, chopped	2
	Chopped fresh rosemary leaves	
	Chopped fresh oregano leaves	
2 cups	chopped savoy cabbage	500 mL
	Freshly ground black pepper	
¼ cup	grated vegetarian-friendly Parmesan cheese (see Tip, page 187)	60 mL

1. In a saucepan, cover beans with cold water and add salt to taste. Bring to a boil over high heat. Reduce heat and boil gently until slightly tender, about 10 minutes. Set aside.

2. Meanwhile, in a pot, heat half of the olive oil over medium-high heat. Sauté celery, carrot, onion, garlic, sage, rosemary and oregano until softened, about 5 minutes. Add cabbage, reduce heat to low and cook, stirring, until cabbage is wilted but not browned, about 5 minutes.

3. Add beans along with all the cooking water, increase heat to high and bring to a boil. Reduce heat and simmer until beans and vegetables are soft, about 15 minutes. Season with salt and pepper to taste.

4. Ladle into warm bowls, sprinkle with Parmesan and drizzle with remaining olive oil.

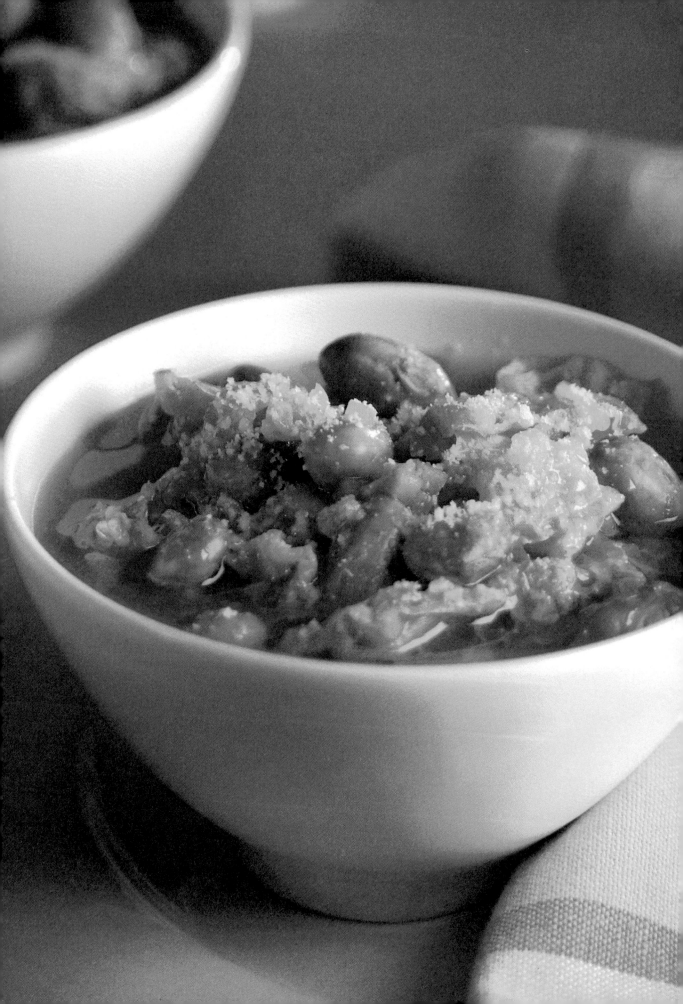

Wonton Soup

8 oz	firm tofu, finely chopped	250 g
2	shiitake mushroom caps, chopped	2
1½ tbsp	chopped drained canned water chestnuts	22 mL
½ tsp	finely chopped fresh gingerroot	2 mL
1	egg, beaten	1
1 tsp	soy sauce	5 mL
20	wonton wrappers	20
4 cups	Vegetable Stock (page 128) or ready-to-use broth	1 L
	Finely chopped fresh chives	
	Soy sauce	

1. In a bowl, combine tofu, mushrooms, water chestnuts, ginger, egg and soy sauce.

2. Place about 1 tbsp (15 mL) of the tofu mixture in center of each wonton wrapper. Moisten the edges of the wrapper and bring up the sides around the filling to form a purse shape, pinching firmly at the top, or fold into a triangle, pressing out any air pockets. Cover with a clean tea towel while preparing remaining wontons.

3. In a saucepan, bring vegetable stock to a boil over high heat. Reduce heat to low, cover and keep hot.

4. Meanwhile, in a pot of boiling salted water, in batches as necessary, cook wontons until tender, about 8 minutes, adjusting heat as necessary to maintain a gentle boil. Using a slotted spoon, remove from water and drain well.

5. Ladle hot stock into warm bowls, add wontons and garnish with chives. Season with soy sauce to taste.

Miso Soup

Tip

To preserve the nutritional value of miso, it is important not to boil it.

⅓ oz	wakame seaweed	10 g
	Warm water	
3 cups	Vegetable Stock (page 128) or ready-to-use broth	750 mL
2 tbsp	miso	30 mL
4 oz	semi-firm tofu, cut into cubes	125 g
	Tamari sauce	
2	green onions, finely chopped	2

1. In a bowl, cover wakame with warm water and let soak for 5 minutes. Drain.

2. Meanwhile, in a saucepan, bring vegetable stock to a boil over high heat. Reduce heat to keep stock simmering. Stir in miso until blended, then stir in drained wakame and tofu. Season with tamari sauce to taste. Reduce heat and simmer to blend flavors, about 10 minutes (do not let it boil).

3. Ladle into warm bowls and garnish with green onions.

Pea Soup

Serves 4

Soaking time
24 hours

Preparation time
30 minutes

Cooking time
2 hours

Tip

Herbes salées is a paste, similar to pesto, made with herbs and sometimes vegetables and seasoned with salt. You can make your own or purchase it in jars at specialty food stores. If you don't have it, you can add other chopped fresh herbs or your favorite pesto.

6 oz	dried yellow split peas, sorted and rinsed	175 g
1	whole clove	1
½	onion	½
1	carrot, cut in half lengthwise	1
1	bouquet garni (see Tip, page 144)	1
2 tbsp	butter	30 mL
¼ cup	diced carrot	60 mL
¼ cup	diced celery	60 mL
¼ cup	diced turnip	60 mL
	Salt and cayenne pepper	
	Chopped fresh parsley or herbes salées (see Tip, left)	

1. In a pot, cover dried peas with at least 4 inches (10 cm) cold water. Cover and let soak for 24 hours.

2. Bring pot of soaked peas to a boil over high heat. Drain well, clean pot and return peas to pot.

3. Stick clove into onion and add to pot. Add halved carrot, bouquet garni and 8 cups (2 L) water. Bring to a simmer over high heat. Reduce heat to low, cover and simmer until peas are very soft, 1½ to 2 hours.

4. Meanwhile, in a small skillet, melt butter over medium heat. Add diced carrot, celery and turnip and cook, stirring, until slightly softened but not browned, about 3 minutes. Stir into soup and season with salt and cayenne pepper to taste. Simmer until turnip is tender, about 15 minutes.

5. Discard onion, clove, carrot halves and bouquet garni. Stir in parsley or herbes salées and adjust seasoning. Ladle into warm bowls.

Stracciatella

Serves 4

Preparation time
5 minutes

Cooking time
12 minutes

Tip

Depending on the stock or broth you use, you may need to add salt to taste at the end of cooking to brighten the flavors of this soup.

4 cups	Vegetable Stock (page 128) or ready-to-use broth	1 L
4	eggs	4
½ cup	grated vegetarian-friendly Parmesan cheese (see Tip, page 137)	125 mL
	Freshly ground black pepper	
Pinch	freshly grated nutmeg	Pinch

1. In a saucepan, bring vegetable stock to a boil over high heat.

2. Meanwhile, in a bowl, whisk eggs until blended. Whisk in Parmesan, pepper to taste and nutmeg.

3. Stir the boiling stock as you pour in the egg mixture. Cook, stirring occasionally with a fork, until egg is opaque and soup is slightly thickened, about 2 minutes. Adjust seasoning and ladle into warm bowls.

Cold Green Asparagus Soup

Serves 4

Preparation time
20 minutes

Cooking time
20 minutes

Chilling time
6 hours

Tip

Use only the tender green parts of the asparagus stems. Save the tips for another recipe.

Variation

You can garnish the soup with asparagus tips cooked in boiling salted water.

● **Blender, food processor or immersion blender**

3 tbsp	butter	45 mL
¾ cup	very finely chopped onion	175 mL
1 lb	green asparagus stalks, thinly sliced (see Tip, left)	500 g
1½ cups	cold water	375 mL
½ cup	heavy or whipping (35%) cream	125 mL
	Salt	

1. In a pot, melt butter over medium heat. Add onion and cook, stirring, until softened but not browned, about 5 minutes. Add asparagus and cook, stirring, until liquid is released, about 5 minutes.

2. Add water, increase heat to medium-high and bring to a gentle boil. Reduce heat and simmer until asparagus is tender, about 10 minutes.

3. In batches as necessary, transfer to blender (or use immersion blender in the pot) and purée until smooth, adding cream. Transfer to a bowl and season with salt to taste. Cover and refrigerate until chilled, about 6 hours.

4. Adjust seasoning. Ladle into chilled bowls.

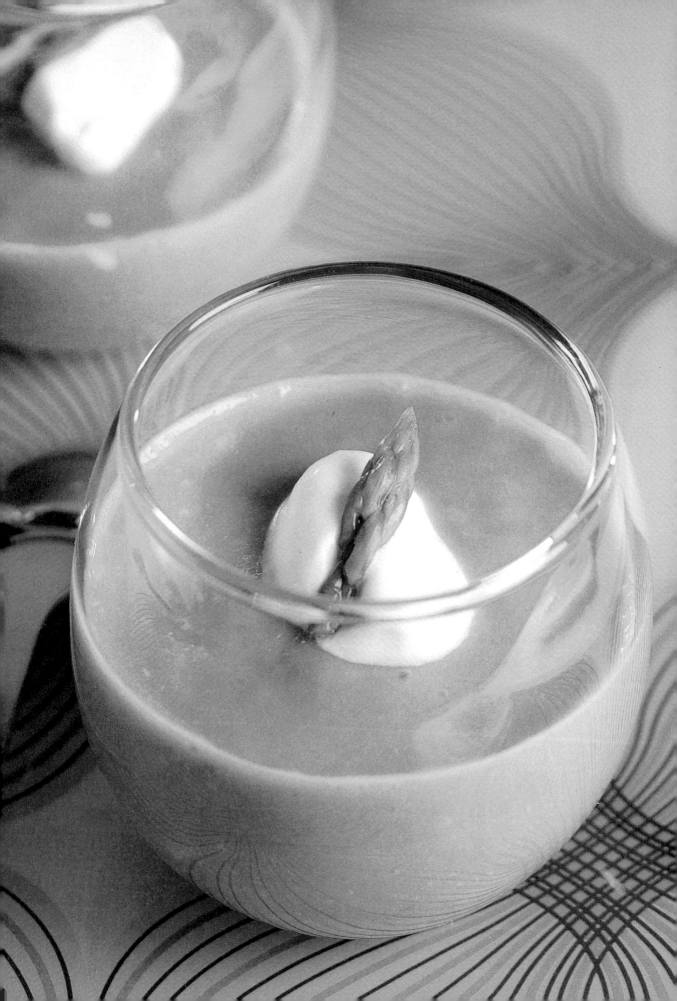

Saffron Vegetable Soup

Tip

When chopping the carrots, celery, onion, leeks and potato, cut them into small, uniformly sized pieces just under ½ inch (1 cm), so that a few pieces at once will fit on a spoon. Cut the green beans to about the size of the peas.

3 tbsp	butter	45 mL
3	leeks, white parts only, finely chopped	3
1 cup	diced carrots	250 mL
1 cup	diced celery	250 mL
¾ cup	diced onion	175 mL
1	medium potato, diced	1
1	clove garlic, chopped	1
4 cups	Vegetable Stock (page 128) or ready-to-use broth	1 L
¼ tsp	saffron threads	1 mL
	Salt and freshly ground black pepper	
½ cup	chopped green beans	125 mL
½ cup	fresh or frozen green peas	125 mL
½ cup	heavy or whipping (35%) cream	125 mL

1. In a pot, melt butter over medium heat. Add leeks, carrots, celery and onion and cook, stirring, until softened but not browned, about 8 minutes. Add potato, garlic, vegetable stock, saffron, and salt and pepper to taste and bring to a boil. Reduce heat and simmer until potato is almost tender, about 15 minutes.

2. Stir in beans and peas. Simmer until potato is tender and beans and peas are tender-crisp, about 5 minutes.

3. Stir in cream and adjust seasoning. Simmer, stirring, until steaming, about 1 minute. Ladle into warm bowls.

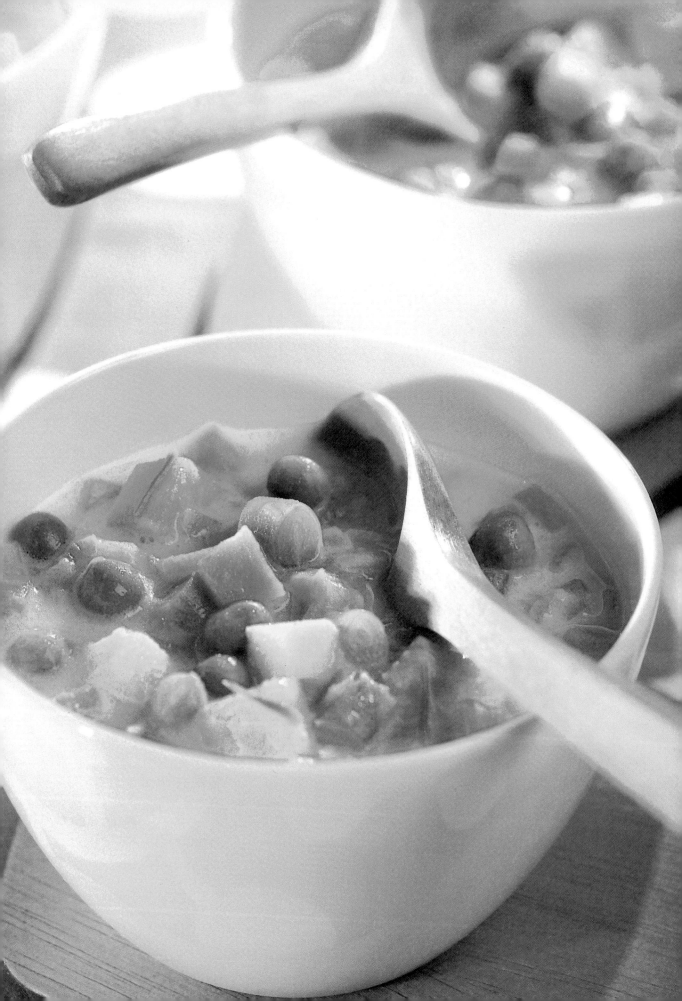

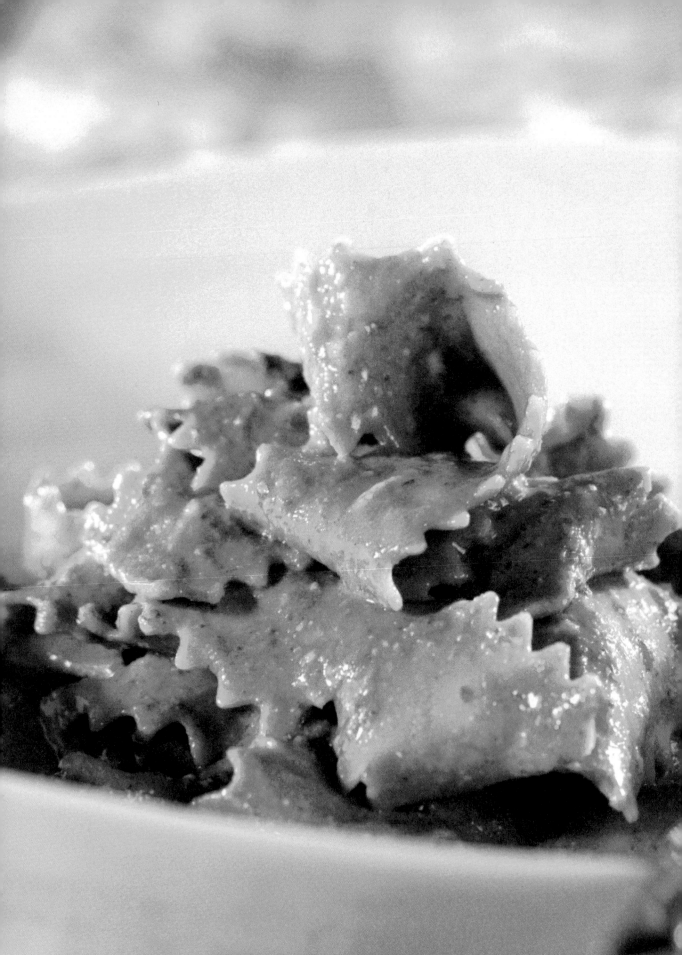

Chestnut Pappardelle with Pesto (page 202)

Mains

Red Curry Tofu with Shiitake Mushrooms and Bamboo Shoots

Serves 4

Preparation time
15 minutes

Cooking time
20 minutes

¼ cup	butter, divided	60 mL
¼ cup	vegetable oil, divided	60 mL
1 lb	firm tofu, cut into thin strips	500 g
½	onion, thinly sliced	½
1	yellow bell pepper, thinly sliced	1
12	shiitake mushroom caps, thinly sliced	12
4	cloves garlic, chopped	4
2 tbsp	chopped fresh gingerroot	30 mL
1	can (8 oz/227 mL) sliced bamboo shoots, drained	1
2 tbsp	Thai red curry paste	30 mL
1½ cups	coconut milk	375 mL
	Salt	

1. In a large skillet or wok, heat 2 tbsp (30 mL) each of the butter and vegetable oil over medium-high heat. Sauté tofu until lightly golden, about 5 minutes. Transfer to a bowl and set aside.

2. Add remaining butter and oil to pan and swirl to coat. Sauté onion, bell pepper and mushrooms until onion is softened and mushrooms start to brown, about 5 minutes. Add garlic and ginger and sauté until golden, about 1 minute.

3. Add reserved tofu, bamboo shoots, red curry paste, coconut milk and salt to taste. Bring to a simmer, stirring. Reduce heat and simmer until sauce is slightly thickened and flavors are blended, about 5 minutes.

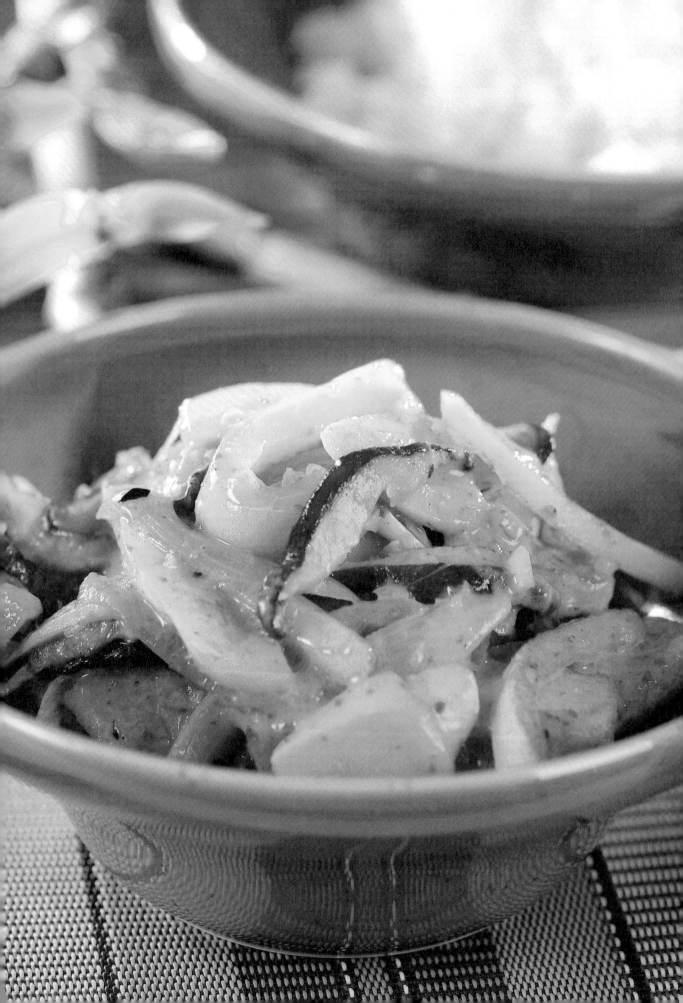

Green Curry Vegetables and Jasmine Rice

Serves 4

Preparation time
30 minutes

Cooking time
25 minutes

²⁄₃ cup	jasmine rice, rinsed	150 mL
1 cup	water	250 mL
4 oz	extra fine green beans (haricots verts), trimmed	125 g
¼ cup	vegetable oil	60 mL
½	red onion, thinly sliced	½
1	carrot, thinly sliced	1
6	cloves garlic, minced	6
1	red bell pepper, thinly sliced	1
1	yellow zucchini, thinly sliced	1
3 cups	chopped napa cabbage	750 mL
1 cup	coconut milk	250 mL
½ cup	Vegetable Stock (page 128) or ready-to-use broth	125 mL
2 tbsp	Thai green curry paste	30 mL
	Soy sauce	
1	tomato, chopped	1
2 tsp	tapioca starch	10 mL
1 tbsp	cold water	15 mL

1. In a saucepan with a tight-fitting lid, combine rice and water and bring to a boil over high heat. Reduce heat to low, cover and simmer until rice is tender and liquid is absorbed, about 20 minutes.

2. Meanwhile, in a pot of boiling salted water, blanch beans until bright green, about 2 minutes. Drain and rinse under cold water to stop the cooking. Drain and set aside.

3. In a large skillet, heat oil over medium-high heat. Sauté red onion and carrot until browned, about 7 minutes. Add garlic and sauté for 1 minute. Add bell pepper, zucchini and cabbage and sauté until tender, about 5 minutes.

4. Stir in coconut milk, vegetable stock and curry paste. Season with soy sauce to taste and bring to a simmer. Reduce heat and simmer until slightly thickened and flavors are blended, about 5 minutes. Stir in tomato and beans.

5. In a small bowl, stir together tapioca starch with 1 tbsp (15 mL) cold water. Stir into pan and simmer, stirring, until sauce thickens slightly and beans are heated through, about 2 minutes.

6. Fluff rice with a fork and divide among serving bowls. Spoon curry overtop.

Tofu Spring Vegetable Stew

12	carrots, cut into chunks	12
12	turnips, cut into wedges	12
12	pearl onions	12
12	small yellow-fleshed potatoes, cut into chunks	12
20	green beans, cut in half	20
¾ cup	green peas	175 mL
2 tbsp	butter	30 mL
2 tbsp	granulated sugar	30 mL
	Salt and freshly cracked black peppercorns	
3 tbsp	olive oil	45 mL
2	cloves garlic	2
1 lb	semi-firm tofu, cut into ¾-inch (2 cm) cubes	500 g
	Zest and juice of 1 orange	
¾ cup	Vegetable Stock (page 128) or ready-to-use broth	175 mL
¼ cup	hoisin sauce	60 mL
¼ cup	chopped fresh Italian flat-leaf parsley	60 mL

1. Place carrots and turnips in a large pot and add cold salted water to cover by 3 inches (7.5 cm). Bring to a boil over high heat. Reduce heat and boil gently until slightly tender, about 15 minutes. Add onions and boil until vegetables are tender, about 10 minutes. Drain well and return to pot.

2. Meanwhile, place potatoes in another pot and add cold salted water to cover by 2 inches (5 cm). Bring to a boil over high heat. Reduce heat and boil gently until almost tender, about 15 minutes. Add green beans and peas and boil until tender, about 3 minutes. Drain well.

3. Add butter, sugar, a little salt and a generous amount of pepper to carrot mixture. Cook over high heat, stirring until browned. (This will caramelize the sugar on the vegetables, giving them a brown glaze.) Remove from heat.

4. In a large skillet, heat oil over medium-high heat. Add garlic cloves and cook, stirring, until golden, about 5 minutes. Using a slotted spoon, remove garlic and discard, leaving oil in the pan. Add tofu to pan and cook, stirring, until nicely browned, about 5 minutes.

5. Add potato mixture and cook, stirring, until hot. Stir in orange zest and juice, vegetable stock and hoisin sauce and bring to a boil, stirring to coat vegetables. Stir in glazed carrot mixture and parsley. Adjust seasoning and serve.

Vegetarian Cassoulet

Serves 4

Soaking time
24 hours

Preparation time
50 minutes

Cooking time
about 2 hours

Tip

A bouquet garni is a small bundle of aromatic herbs tied together with kitchen string. It is used to add flavor to a simmered or boiled mixture and is generally discarded before the dish is served. It often includes parsley, thyme and bay leaves but can also include any of your favorite herbs that complement the flavors of your dish.

- 10-cup (2.5 L) shallow baking dish

Beans

1¼ cups	dried white beans	300 mL
1	whole clove	1
1	onion	1
1	carrot, cut into large pieces	1
4	cloves garlic	4
1	bouquet garni (see Tip, left)	1
	Salt	
2 tbsp	butter	30 mL
1 tbsp	oil	15 mL
2	onions, finely chopped	2
2	cloves garlic	2
1	tomato, peeled, seeded and finely chopped	1
1	bouquet garni (see Tip, left)	1
	Salt and freshly ground pepper	
4	seitan or tofu vegetable sausages	4
8 oz	smoked tofu, cut into 4 pieces	250 g
⅓ cup	bread crumbs	75 mL

1. In a bowl, cover dried beans with at least 4 inches (10 cm) of cold water. Cover and let soak for 24 hours. Drain beans and transfer to a large pot.

2. Stick clove into onion and add to beans in pot with carrot, garlic, bouquet garni and 6 cups (1.5 L) water. Bring to a boil over high heat. Reduce heat and boil gently until beans are tender, about 1 hour, adding more water if necessary to prevent drying out. Drain, reserving 1 cup (250 mL) cooking liquid. Discard onion with clove, carrots, garlic and bouquet garni. Season beans to taste with salt.

3. Meanwhile, preheat oven to 425°F (220°C).

4. In a large skillet, melt butter and heat oil over medium heat. Add onions and cook, stirring occasionally, until softened but not browned, about 8 minutes. Add garlic, tomato and bouquet garni. Season with salt and pepper to taste. Cook, stirring occasionally, until liquid has evaporated from tomatoes and mixture is thick, about 10 minutes. Remove from heat. Discard garlic and bouquet garni.

5. Stir beans into tomato mixture and stir in enough of the reserved cooking liquid to moisten to a slightly loose consistency. Transfer to baking dish and nestle seitan and tofu into bean mixture. Sprinkle with bread crumbs.

6. Bake in preheated oven until mixture is bubbling, seitan and tofu are hot and topping is golden, about 25 minutes.

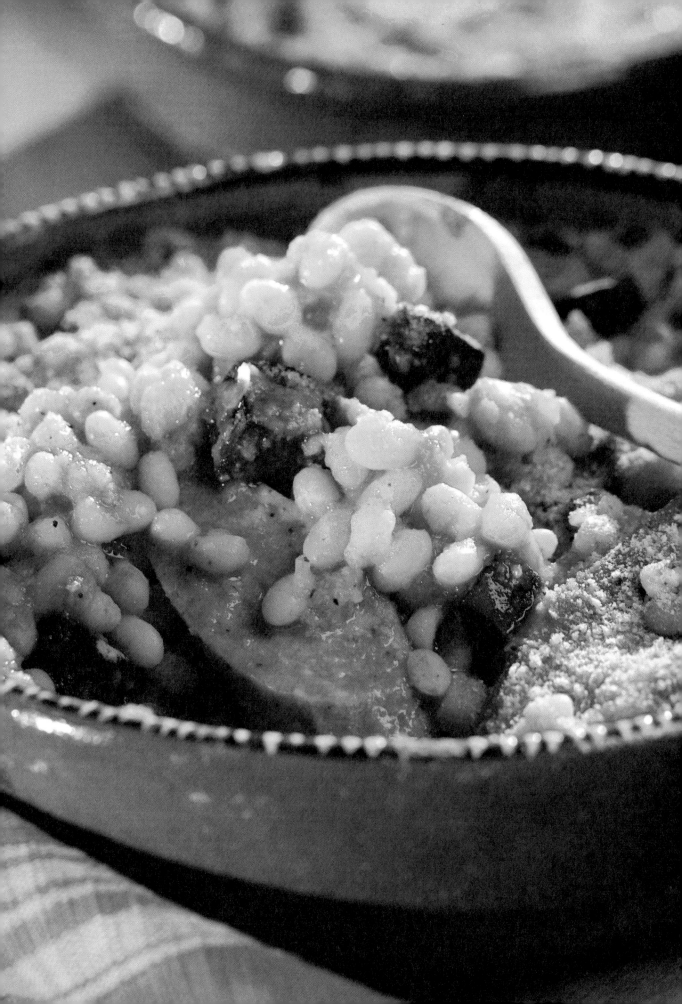

Vegetarian Chili

Serves 4

Soaking time
24 hours

Preparation time
50 minutes

Cooking time
2 hours

Tip

In place of dried beans, you can use two 14 to 19 oz (398 to 540 mL) cans kidney beans, drained and rinsed (or 3½ cups/825 mL), and skip Steps 1 and 2.

Beans

1¾ cups	dried kidney beans (see Tip, left)	425 mL
1	carrot, cut into chunks	1
½	onion	½
1	clove garlic	1
1	bouquet garni (see Tip, page 166)	1
¼ cup	olive oil	60 mL
1 cup	finely chopped onions	250 mL
1	small red bell pepper, cut into 1-inch (2.5 cm) strips	1
1	small green bell pepper, cut into 1-inch (2.5 cm) strips	1
2	cloves garlic, chopped	2
2	hot chile peppers, chopped	2
½ tsp	ground cumin	2 mL
1	can (28 oz/796 mL) diced tomatoes, drained, juice reserved	1
1 cup	Vegetable Stock (page 128) or ready-to-use broth	250 mL
	Salt and freshly ground black pepper	
	Chopped fresh cilantro	
	Tortilla chips	
	Lime wedges	

1. In a bowl, cover dried beans with at least 4 inches (10 cm) of cold water. Cover and let soak for 24 hours. Drain beans and transfer to a large pot.

2. Add carrot, ½ onion, garlic, bouquet garni and water to cover by at least 3 inches (7.5 cm). Bring to a boil over high heat. Reduce heat and boil gently until beans are almost tender, about 50 minutes. Drain well. Discard carrot, onion, garlic and bouquet garni.

3. In a pot, heat oil over medium heat. Add finely chopped onions and cook, stirring, until softened but not browned, about 5 minutes. Add red bell pepper, green bell pepper, garlic, chile peppers and cumin and cook, stirring, until peppers are softened, about 5 minutes.

4. Stir in tomatoes, vegetable stock and beans. Add enough of the reserved tomato juice to thin, as necessary. Season with salt and pepper to taste. Bring to a boil, stirring. Reduce heat to low, cover and simmer for 15 minutes. Stir in cilantro to taste, cover and simmer until beans are tender and flavors are blended, about 5 minutes.

5. Serve with tortilla chips and lime wedges to squeeze overtop.

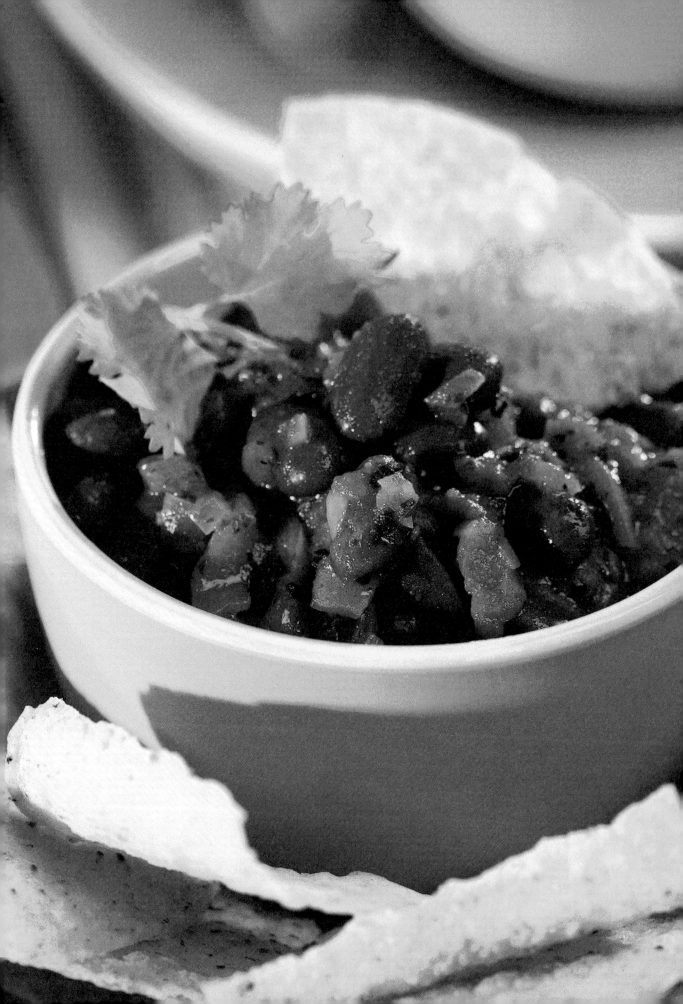

Cabbage Rolls

Tip

To separate cabbage leaves, using a sharp knife, remove and discard core from cabbage. Pull off and discard outer leaves of cabbage. Gently separate remaining leaves from head, keeping them intact.

- Preheat oven to 400°F (200°C)
- 8-inch (20 cm) baking dish, buttered

6 tbsp	long-grain white rice	90 mL
¾ cup	Vegetable Stock (page 128) or ready-to-use broth	175 mL
8	large green cabbage leaves (see Tip, left)	8
3 tbsp	butter, divided	45 mL
1	large onion, finely chopped	1
1 tbsp	olive oil	15 mL
6 oz	shiitake mushrooms, stems removed, caps sliced	175 g
3	cloves garlic, chopped	3
5 oz	smoked or extra-firm tofu, cut into ½-inch (1 cm) cubes	150 g
	Salt and freshly ground black pepper	

1. In a small saucepan, combine rice and vegetable stock and bring to a boil over high heat. Cover, reduce heat to low and simmer until rice is tender and most of liquid is absorbed, about 20 minutes. Remove from heat and let stand, covered, for 5 minutes. Fluff with a fork.

2. Meanwhile, in a large pot of boiling salted water, in batches as necessary, blanch cabbage leaves until slightly softened, about 4 minutes. Using tongs, transfer to a colander and rinse with cold water until cool. Drain well. Cut away protruding part of the thick mid-ribs. (This will make it easier to roll up the cabbage rolls.)

3. In a skillet, melt 2 tbsp (30 mL) of the butter over medium heat. Add onion and cook, stirring, until softened but not browned, about 5 minutes. Transfer to a bowl.

4. Add remaining butter and the oil to same skillet and heat over medium-high heat. Add mushrooms and cook, stirring, until browned, about 5 minutes. Add to onions in bowl. Stir in rice, garlic and tofu. Season with salt and pepper to taste.

5. Place cabbage leaves on a work surface with smooth side up. Spoon about ½ cup (125 mL) filling in the center of each leaf. Fold in sides of leaf over filling, then roll up to enclose filling. Place seam side down in prepared baking dish and cover with foil.

6. Bake in preheated oven until cabbage is tender and filling is hot, about 30 minutes.

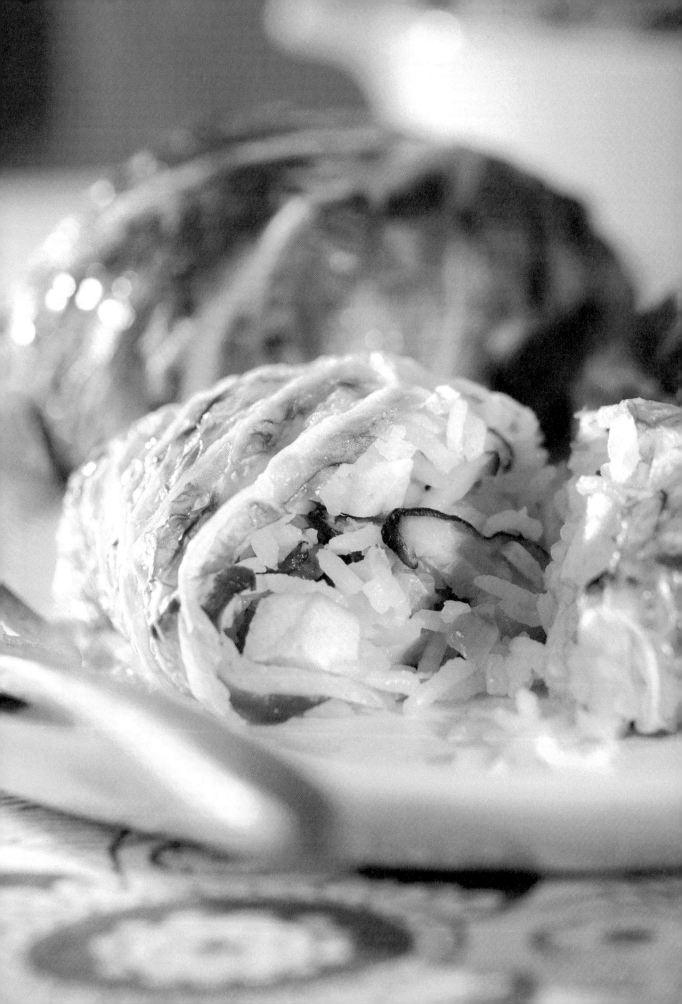

Cabbage Cooked in Butter with Braised Lentils

Serves 4

Preparation time
40 minutes

Cooking time
1 hour 15 minutes

- Preheat oven to 350°F (180°C)
- 6- to 8-cup (1.5 to 2 L) ovenproof saucepan with lid

1 cup	Puy lentils, sorted and rinsed	250 mL
1	carrot	1
1	onion, halved	1
2	cloves garlic	2
1	bouquet garni (see Tip, page 166)	1
	Salt and freshly ground black pepper	
1 lb	savoy cabbage (about ⅓ medium), cut into strips	500 g
6 tbsp	butter	90 mL
1	carrot, diced	1
1	onion, finely chopped	1

1. In ovenproof saucepan, combine lentils, carrot, two onion halves, garlic and bouquet garni. Add enough cold water to cover by $1\frac{1}{2}$ inches (4 cm) and bring to a boil over high heat.

2. Cover and bake in preheated oven until lentils are tender, adding water as needed to prevent lentils from drying out, for about 1 hour. (When lentils are cooked, there should no longer be any liquid.) Season with salt and pepper to taste. Discard carrot, onion halves, garlic and bouquet garni. Spread lentils on a large plate to stop them cooking.

3. In a large pot of boiling water, blanch strips of cabbage until slightly wilted, about 2 minutes. Drain and rinse with cold water until chilled. Drain well.

4. In a large skillet, melt butter over low heat. Add diced carrot and finely chopped onion and cook, stirring, until softened, about 10 minutes. Add cabbage and cook, stirring gently, just until cabbage is warmed and remains very firm. Stir in lentils and season to taste with salt and pepper.

Tartiflette

Serves 4

Preparation time
40 minutes

Cooking time
45 minutes

Tips

Reblochon cheese is a French soft cheese with a washed-rind. It has a creamy texture and mild flavor. If it's not available, you can substitute Port Salut or fontina cheese.

When buying cheese, read the label carefully and make sure to buy those that are not made from animal rennet.

- Preheat oven to 350°F (180°C)
- 8-cup (2 L) baking dish, buttered

2½ lbs	round waxy potatoes, peeled (about 8)	1.25 kg
¼ cup	butter, divided	60 mL
2 tbsp	vegetable oil, divided	30 mL
1	onion, thinly sliced	1
1	clove garlic, cut in half	1
	Salt and freshly ground black pepper	
1	round (1 lb/450 g) Reblochon cheese (see Tips, left)	1

1. Place potatoes in a pot and add enough cold salted water to cover. Bring to a boil over high heat. Reduce heat and boil gently until potatoes are fork-tender, about 20 minutes. Drain and cut into thick slices. Set aside.

2. Meanwhile, in a large skillet, melt half each of the butter and oil over medium-high heat. Sauté onion until slightly golden, about 5 minutes. Transfer to a bowl.

3. Add 1 tbsp (15 mL) of the remaining butter and half the remaining oil to skillet and heat over medium-high heat. In batches as necessary, fry potato slices, turning once, until lightly golden on both sides, about 3 minutes per side. Transfer to a plate. Add more butter and oil and adjust heat between batches as necessary.

4. Rub the insides of the buttered baking dish with cut sides of garlic. Arrange alternating layers of potatoes and onions in dish, seasoning with salt and pepper to taste between the layers and ending with a potato layer.

5. Cut Reblochon cheese in half horizontally and place, cut sides up, on top of potato layer.

6. Bake in preheated oven until hot in the center and cheese is golden, about 20 minutes.

Squash and Cortland Apples with Cheese

Tip

Clarified butter, also known as drawn butter, is made by slowly melting unsalted butter, allowing the water to evaporate and the milk solids to settle. *To make clarified butter:* In a small heavy saucepan, heat unsalted butter over low heat until melted. Skim foam from top and carefully strain out milk solids. It keeps indefinitely in the refrigerator.

- Preheat oven to 400°F (200°C)
- Pastry bag fitted with plain tip, optional

4	sheets phyllo pastry	4
2 tbsp	clarified butter (see Tip, left)	30 mL
1	small buttercup squash (about 1 lb/500 g)	1
¼ cup	butter, divided	60 mL
	Salt and freshly ground black pepper	
4	Cortland or other tart cooking apples	4
4 oz	Brie cheese, thinly sliced	125 g
4 tsp	toasted pine nuts	20 mL

1. Place one sheet of phyllo on a cutting board and brush lightly with clarified butter. Place a second sheet on top and brush lightly. Stack remaining two sheets on top, brushing each. Cut into 8 rectangles. Place on a large baking sheet. Bake in preheated oven until pastry is golden and crispy, 3 to 4 minutes. Let cool.

2. Reduce oven to 350°F (180°C). Cut squash in half and scrape out seeds. Place on another baking sheet, cut side down. Bake until tender, about 30 minutes. Let cool slightly. Leave oven on.

3. Scoop out squash pulp with a spoon, discarding skins. While it is still hot, pass through a food mill or purée in a food processor. Transfer to a bowl, if necessary. Stir in half of the butter and salt and pepper to taste.

4. Cut apples into quarters and cut out cores. Cut each quarter into thin wedges. In a large skillet, melt remaining butter over medium-high heat. Add apples and sauté until tender but not soft, about 5 minutes. Remove from heat.

5. Place 4 pastry rectangles on baking sheet. Place half the apples on rectangles in a uniform pattern so they are slightly overlapping. Spoon squash into pastry bag and pipe evenly over apples (or spread with a spatula).

6. Place remaining pastry rectangles on top to form the second layer. Arrange remaining apples on top. Place slices of Brie on top and garnish with pine nuts. Bake until hot and cheese is melted, about 10 minutes.

Ciabattas with Grilled Vegetables, Goat Cheese and Alfalfa Sprouts

Serves 4

Preparation time
20 minutes

Cooking time
20 minutes

Tip

Do not leave ciabatta rolls in the sandwich press for too long. The heated crust should be slightly crunchy on the outside and the filling should maintain its crispness.

- Preheat barbecue grill to medium
- Panini press, optional

2	zucchini, cut lengthwise into $\frac{1}{8}$-inch (3 mm) slices	2
2	red bell peppers, quartered lengthwise	2
5 oz	fresh goat cheese	150 g
	Juice of $\frac{1}{2}$ lemon	
	Freshly ground black pepper	
2 tbsp	chopped fresh oregano leaves	30 mL
4	small olive ciabatta rolls	4
4 tsp	olive oil	20 mL
4 tsp	toasted pine nuts	20 mL
1	package ($3\frac{1}{2}$ oz/100 g) fresh alfalfa sprouts	1

1. Place zucchini on preheated barbecue grill and grill, turning once, until golden and tender, about 5 minutes. Transfer to a plate.

2. Place bell peppers on grill with the skin side down and grill until skin is completely blackened and peppers are tender, about 8 minutes. Transfer to a plate and let cool until cool enough to handle. Peel off skins.

3. Preheat panini press, if using, or heat a heavy skillet over medium-low heat.

4. In a bowl, mash cheese, using a spatula, to make it easier to spread. Stir in lemon juice, pepper to taste, and oregano.

5. Cut ciabatta rolls in half and drizzle olive oil on both sides of each half. Spread cheese on bottom half, then add grilled vegetables, toasted pine nuts and alfalfa sprouts. Close sandwich with top half.

6. Place sandwiches in panini press or skillet and toast, flipping once if using skillet, until roll is toasted and filling is warmed through, about 5 minutes.

Croque Madame

Preparation time
15 minutes

Cooking time
35 minutes

- Preheat oven to 450°F (230°C)
- 13- by 9-inch (33 by 23 cm) glass baking dish, buttered

| 10 oz | Gruyère cheese (see Tip, page 218) | 300 g |

Béchamel Sauce

2 cups	milk	500 mL
2 tbsp	butter	30 mL
¼ cup	all-purpose flour	60 mL
	Salt	
	Cayenne pepper	
	Ground nutmeg	

8	slices bread	8
2	tomatoes, sliced	2
1 tbsp	butter	15 mL
4	eggs	4

1. Shred half of the Gruyère cheese and cut the remaining half into thin slices. Set both aside separately.

2. *Béchamel Sauce:* In a saucepan, bring milk almost to a boil over medium heat. In another saucepan, melt butter over medium heat. Sprinkle with flour and cook, stirring, for 1 minute to make a roux.

3. Gradually pour hot milk over roux, blending well with a whisk. Season with salt, cayenne pepper and nutmeg to taste. Bring to a boil. Reduce heat and boil gently, whisking, until thick, for 10 minutes. Remove from heat and stir in shredded Gruyère until melted and smooth. Set aside.

4. Lightly toast bread. Place on a work surface. Spread a little béchamel sauce on 4 of the slices of toast. Top with sliced Gruyère cheese and tomato slices, dividing equally. Spread with more béchamel sauce and top with remaining slices of toast.

5. Place sandwiches in prepared baking dish and spread tops and sides of sandwiches with a layer of béchamel sauce. Bake in preheated oven until golden brown, about 20 minutes.

6. Meanwhile, in a skillet, melt butter over medium-high heat. Fry eggs, sunny side up, until golden on the bottom and yolk is desired texture, 2 to 5 minutes. Place one egg on top of each croque madame.

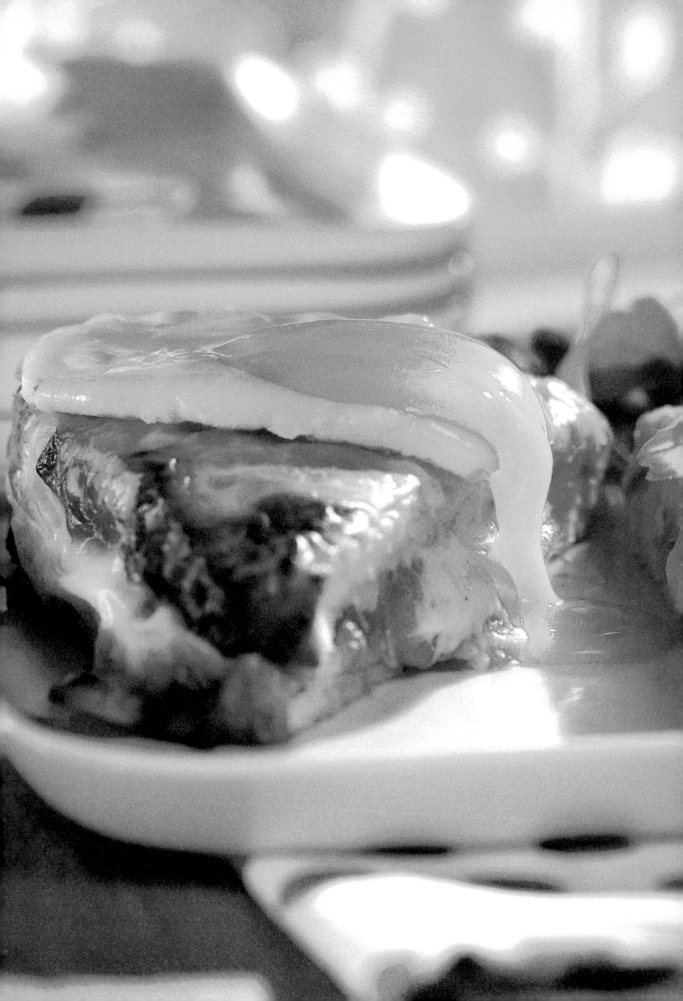

Crunchy Vegetable and Alfalfa Sprout Wraps

1 tbsp	olive oil	15 mL
1	small red onion, thinly sliced	1
1	red bell pepper, thinly sliced	1
1	large tomato, diced	1
	Salt and freshly ground black pepper	
12	spears asparagus	12
2	avocados	2
1/3 cup	sour cream or plain yogurt	75 mL
	Juice of 1/2 lemon	
4	large whole wheat or flax seed tortillas, warmed	4
1/2 cup	alfalfa sprouts	125 mL

1. In a skillet, heat oil over medium heat. Add red onion and cook, stirring, for 2 minutes. Reduce heat to medium-low and cook, stirring, until starting to caramelize, about 10 minutes. Stir in red bell pepper and tomato and cook, stirring, until onions are caramelized, about 15 minutes. Season with salt and pepper to taste.

2. Meanwhile, in a pot of boiling salted water, cook asparagus until tender-crisp, about 5 minutes. Drain and rinse under cold water to chill. Drain well and pat dry.

3. Cut avocados in half and remove pits. Scrape flesh from skins into a bowl. Using a fork, mash avocado with sour cream and lemon juice. Season with salt and pepper to taste.

4. Place warmed tortillas on a work surface. Divide avocado mixture among tortillas and spread thinly almost to the edge. Spoon onion mixture in a line along center of tortillas, dividing equally. Place 3 asparagus spears on top of each, then divide alfalfa sprouts equally on top. Fold up bottom of tortilla over filling, then fold in both sides and secure with a toothpick.

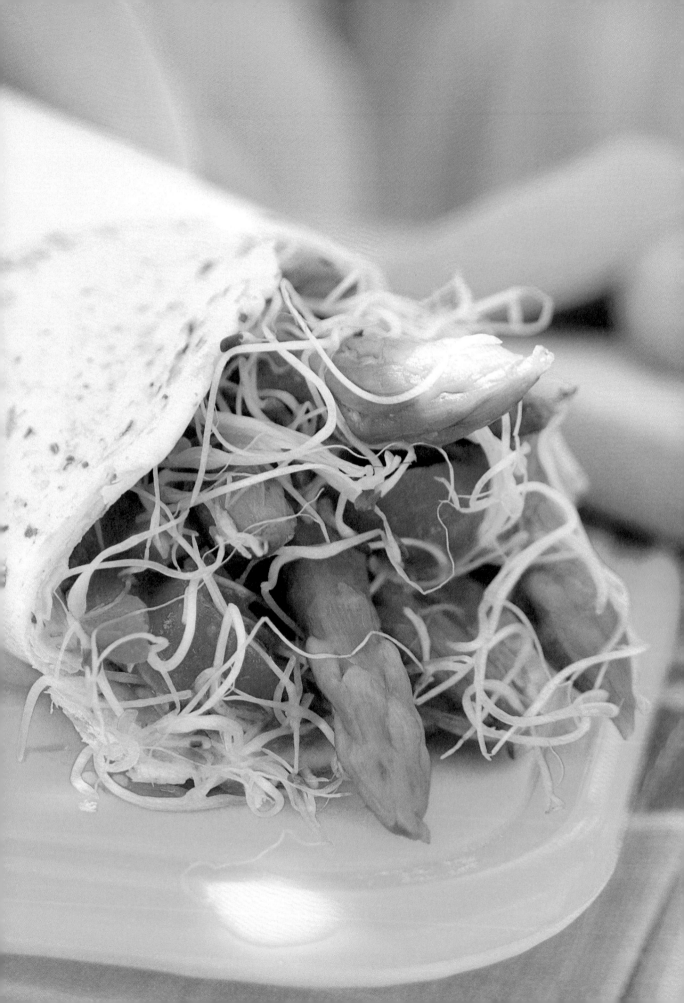

Sun-Dried Tomato, Brie and Arugula Panini

Serves 4

Preparation time
15 minutes

Cooking time
5 minutes

- Panini grill or large nonstick skillet
- Preheat panini grill to medium-high, if using, or preheat broiler

1	red bell pepper	1
2 tbsp	olive oil	30 mL
1	clove garlic, minced	1
1/3 cup	Sun-Dried Tomato Pesto (page 269) or store-bought	75 mL
4	panini rolls or ciabatta buns, split	4
5 oz	Brie cheese, thinly sliced	150 g
	Salt and freshly ground black pepper	
1 cup	arugula	250 mL

1. Cut bell pepper into wide strips. Place on preheated panini grill or on a baking sheet, and grill or broil, turning once, until browned and tender, about 8 minutes. Transfer to a bowl and let cool slightly. Peel off skin and discard.

2. Add oil and garlic to pepper and toss to coat. Let stand for 10 minutes to marinate.

3. Spread pesto on cut sides of rolls. Top with Brie and bell pepper, dividing equally and drizzling with any excess oil mixture. Season with salt and pepper to taste and top with arugula. Place tops on rolls to sandwich.

4. In batches as necessary, place on preheated panini grill or in a large skillet and heat, turning once if using skillet, until rolls are toasted and cheese is slightly melted. Serve hot.

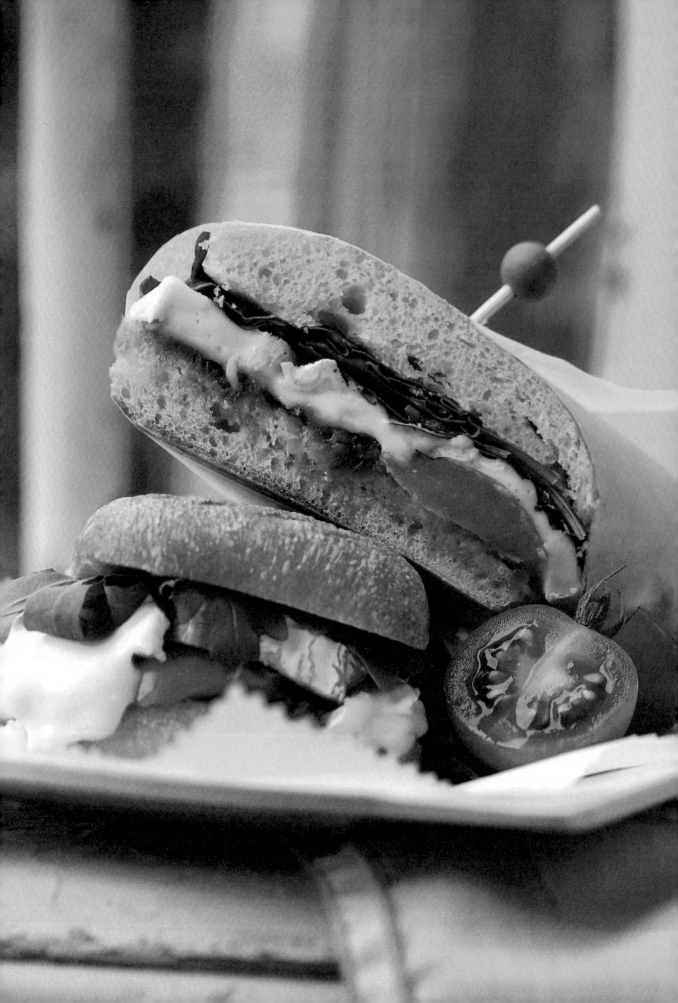

Quesadillas with Goat Cheese and Wild Mushrooms

Serves 4

Preparation time
15 minutes

Cooking time
10 minutes

● **Preheat oven to 400°F (200°C)**

2 tbsp	olive oil	30 mL
5 oz	wild or exotic mushrooms, such as chanterelles, sliced	150 g
¾ cup	thinly sliced onion	175 mL
1	red bell pepper, julienned	1
1 cup	cooked adzuki beans	250 mL
¼ cup	chopped fresh cilantro	60 mL
	Salt and freshly ground black pepper	
	Hot chile peppers, chopped	
4	large flour tortillas	4
3 oz	mozzarella cheese, shredded	90 g
4 oz	goat cheese, cut into pieces	125 g
	Sour cream	
	Guacamole	

1. In a large skillet, heat oil over medium-high heat. Add mushrooms and onion and cook, stirring, until onions are softened and mushrooms start to release their liquid, about 5 minutes. Add bell pepper and cook, stirring, until vegetables are just tender, about 3 minutes. Remove from heat.

2. Stir in adzuki beans and cilantro. Season with salt, pepper and hot peppers to taste.

3. Place two tortillas on a large baking sheet. Spread vegetable mixture evenly over tortillas. Sprinkle with mozzarella and goat cheese. Place remaining tortillas on top, pressing lightly.

4. Bake in preheated oven until filling is hot and cheese is melted, 10 to 15 minutes. Cut into wedges and serve with sour cream and guacamole.

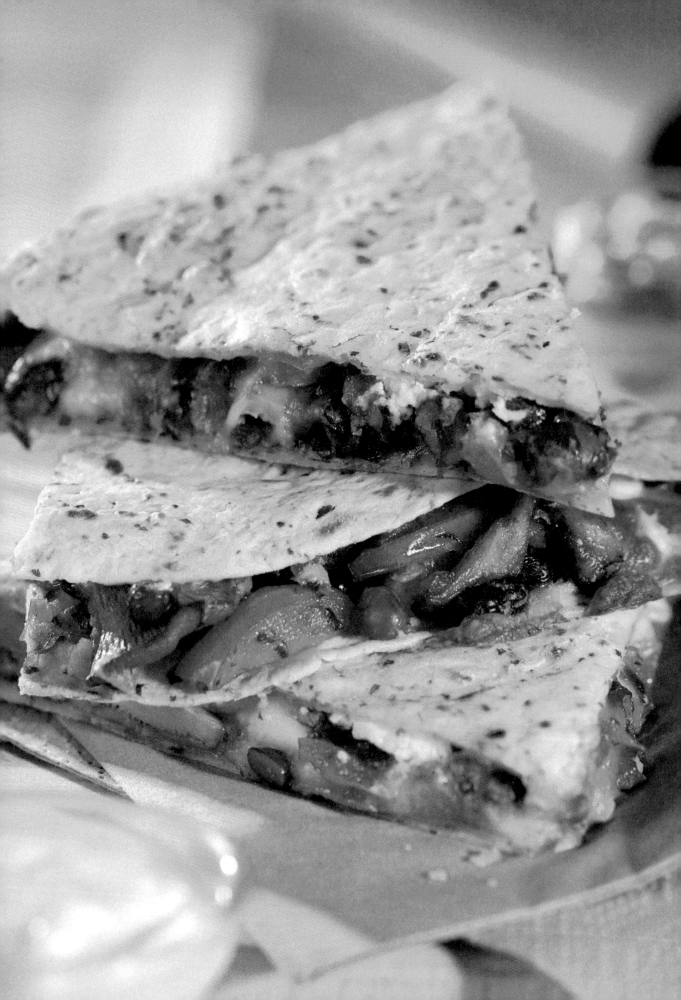

Buckwheat Crêpes with Pepper, Asparagus and Mushrooms

Serves 4

Preparation time
20 minutes

Chilling time
2 hours

Cooking time
15 minutes

Tips

For a more golden batter, add 1 or 2 eggs, 1 tsp (5 mL) honey or 1 cup (250 mL) milk in place of an equal volume of water.

For taste, one can add up to 1 cup (250 mL) all-purpose flour in place of an equal volume of buckwheat.

Adding 1 tsp (5 mL) oil will make the batter easier to handle.

2 cups	buckwheat flour	500 mL
1½ tsp	sea salt	7 mL
3 cups	water	750 mL

Filling

2 tbsp	butter or olive oil, divided	30 mL
1	bell pepper (any color), cut into strips	1
5 oz	mushrooms, sliced	150 g
1	small onion, thinly sliced	1
12	spears asparagus, trimmed, cut in half	12
5 oz	Gruyère cheese, shredded	150 g
	Salt and freshly ground black pepper	
4	eggs	4

1. In a large bowl, combine flour and salt. Gradually pour in 2½ cups (625 mL) water, mixing thoroughly with a wooden spoon, to obtain a thick batter.

2. Beat well, lifting the batter often to incorporate air. Cover and refrigerate for at least 2 hours or for up to 1 day. Just before using, thin batter as necessary with remaining water until mixture is the consistency of thick oil.

3. Heat a large skillet over medium-high heat. Ladle about ½ cup (125 mL) of batter per crêpe into skillet, swirling pan to thinly coat pan. Cook until bottom is golden and top looks dry, about 1 minute. Flip over and cook for 10 seconds. Transfer to a plate. Repeat, adjusting heat as necessary between crêpes.

4. In a large skillet, heat half of the butter over medium-high heat. Sauté bell pepper, mushrooms and onion until mushrooms start to brown, about 8 minutes. Add asparagus and sauté until tender-crisp, about 5 minutes. Transfer to a bowl, stir in cheese and season with salt and pepper to taste.

5. Add remaining butter to skillet and heat over medium-high heat. Fry eggs, sunny side up, until golden on the bottom and yolk is desired texture, 2 to 5 minutes. Season with salt and pepper to taste.

6. Place crêpes on serving plates and divide vegetable mixture among them. Top each with a fried egg. Fold edges over slightly to cover filling, leaving center exposed.

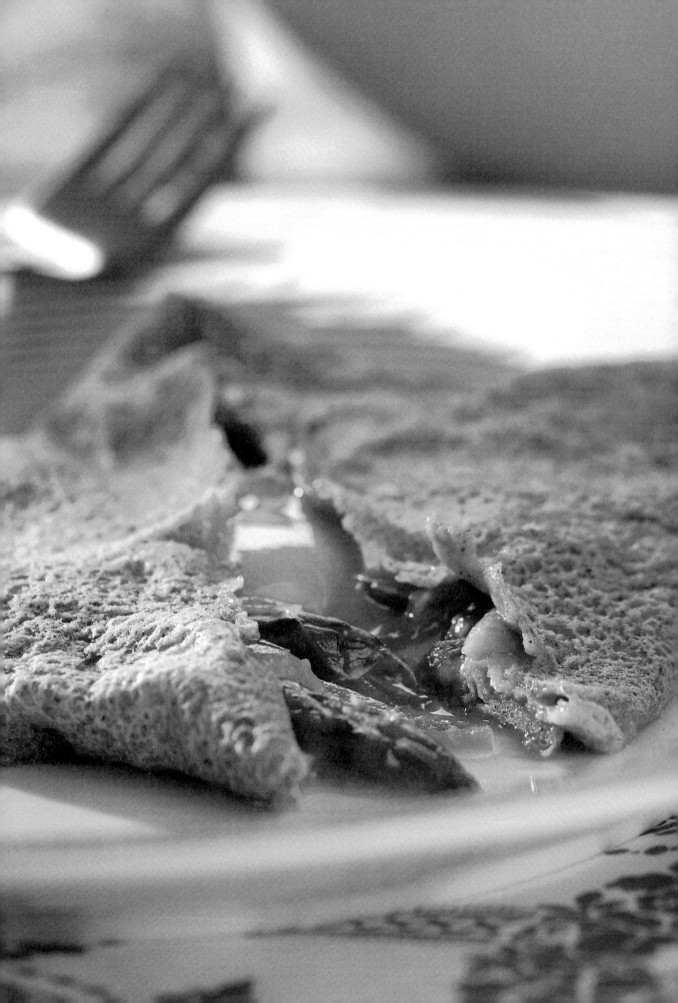

Cheese Fondue

Serves 4

Preparation time
40 minutes

Cooking time
25 minutes

Tip

Vacherin Fribourgeois is a Swiss cheese made from cow's milk with a washed rind. It is lightly pressed and aged for three to four months, giving it a semihard texture and a slightly pungent aroma and nutty flavor.

- Earthenware, ceramic or enameled cast-iron fondue pot with burner

1	head garlic	
3 cups	dry white wine	750 mL
1 tbsp	cornstarch (approx.)	15 mL
1½ lbs	Gruyère cheese, shredded	750 g
12 oz	Vacherin Fribourgeois cheese, another semi-firm washed-rind cheese or fontina cheese, shredded (see Tip, left)	375 g
⅓ cup	kirsch	75 mL
	Baguette, cut into bite-size pieces	

1. Cut 4 of the cloves of garlic in half and rub inside of fondue pot with cut sides of garlic.

2. Cut remaining garlic cloves into thin slices and place in fondue dish. Add white wine and bring to a boil over high heat. Reduce heat to keep wine at a simmer.

3. In a bowl, toss cornstarch with Gruyère cheese to evenly coat. Add by handfuls to simmering wine and stir constantly until cheese is melted (do not let boil).

4. Reduce heat to low and add Vacherin cheese. Simmer, stirring constantly, just until melted. Adjust thickness of mixture as needed, with a little cornstarch thinned with kirsch or with kirsch alone.

5. Place fondue dish over lit burner on table with baguette pieces for dipping.

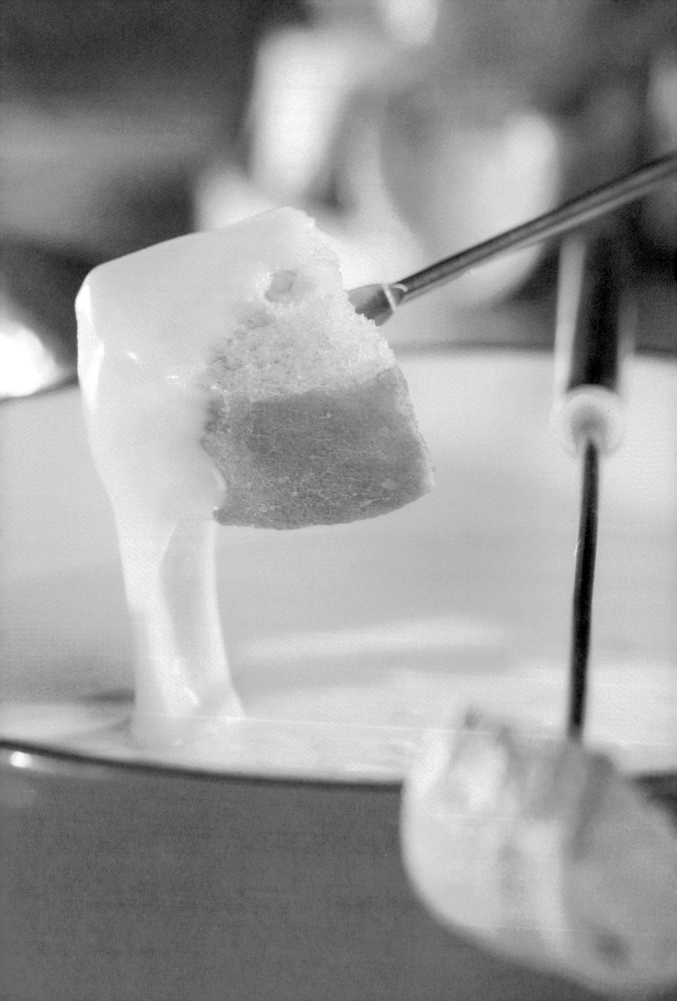

Frittata with Rapini and Chard

6	stalks rapini, cut into small sections	6
3	leaves Swiss chard (including stems)	3
8	eggs	8
	Salt and freshly ground black pepper	
2 tbsp	butter	30 mL

1. In a pot of boiling salted water, cook rapini until tender-crisp, about 8 minutes. Drain and let cool.

2. Separate leaves of Swiss chard from stems. Cut leaves into 1-inch (2.5 cm) squares. Dice stems into $\frac{1}{2}$-inch (1 cm) pieces. In another pot of boiling salted water, cook stems until tender-crisp, about 5 minutes. Using a mesh sieve, remove from boiling water and transfer to a colander to drain. Add leaves to boiling water and cook until wilted, about 3 minutes. Drain and let cool.

3. In a bowl, beat eggs until blended, then add salt and pepper to taste. Stir in rapini and Swiss chard, stems and leaves.

4. Heat a large skillet over medium heat. Add butter and swirl to coat. Pour in egg mixture. Cover and cook for 2 minutes. Slide frittata onto a large plate with the cooked side down. Invert skillet over plate, then flip over skillet and plate in one quick motion. Return skillet to heat and cook until eggs are set, about 2 minutes.

Stuffed Eggplants

- Preheat oven to 350°F (180°C)
- 13- by 9-inch (33 by 23 cm) glass baking dish

4	small eggplants	4
2 tsp	olive oil	10 mL
6 oz	soft goat cheese	175 g
1	egg	1
$\frac{1}{2}$ tsp	chopped fresh oregano	2 mL
	Salt and freshly ground black pepper	
	Bread crumbs	

1. Cut eggplants in half lengthwise. Pierce skin with the tip of a sharp knife. Drizzle cut sides with olive oil and place in baking dish. Bake in preheated oven until tender, for 20 to 30 minutes depending on size of eggplants. Leave oven on.

2. Using a spoon, scoop out eggplant flesh, leaving about $\frac{1}{4}$-inch (0.5 cm) thick walls and taking care not to break the skin. Cut flesh into large pieces. In a large bowl, combine eggplant flesh, cheese, egg and oregano. Season with salt and pepper to taste.

3. Stuff eggplant skins with eggplant mixture. Sprinkle with bread crumbs and return to baking dish. Bake until filling is hot and top is browned, about 15 minutes.

Eggplant Korma

Serves 4

Preparation time
10 minutes

Cooking time
20 minutes

1	eggplant	1
1/4 cup	vegetable oil	60 mL
2 tbsp	butter	30 mL
1/2	onion, thinly sliced	1/2
2	cloves garlic, chopped	2
1 tsp	minced fresh gingerroot	5 mL
1 tsp	ground turmeric	5 mL
1/2 tsp	ground cloves	2 mL
1/2 tsp	ground cinnamon	2 mL
Pinch	ground cumin	Pinch
Pinch	ground cardamom	Pinch
	Salt and freshly ground black pepper	
1/3 cup	plain yogurt	75 mL
6 tbsp	water	90 mL
1	large tomato, seeded and diced	1
4	sprigs cilantro, chopped	4
	Cooked basmati rice	

1. Remove stem of eggplant, then cut into sticks 2 inches (5 cm) long and 1/2 inch (1 cm) thick.

2. In a skillet, heat oil over high heat. Sauté eggplant, turning often to obtain a nice color, until tender (being sure to avoid burning it), about 10 minutes.

3. When eggplant is almost cooked, stir in butter, onion, garlic, ginger, turmeric, cloves, cinnamon, cumin and cardamom. Season with salt and pepper to taste. Cook, stirring, until spices are fragrant, about 2 minutes.

4. In a small bowl, combine yogurt and water. Add to eggplant mixture. Add tomato and cilantro and blend well. Serve with basmati rice.

Eggplant Parmigiana

Serves 4

Preparation time
30 minutes

Cooking time
30 minutes

- Preheat oven to 350°F (180°C)
- 8-inch (20 cm) square baking dish

1	large eggplant	1
	Salt	
4 cups	vegetable oil	1 L
	All-purpose flour	
2 cups	tomato sauce	500 mL
2 tbsp	chopped fresh basil	30 mL
1 tbsp	chopped fresh oregano or 1 tsp (5 mL) dried	15 mL
$\frac{1}{3}$ cup	shredded mozzarella cheese	75 mL
$\frac{1}{4}$ cup	grated vegetarian-friendly Parmesan cheese (see Tip, page 218) (approx.)	60 mL

1. Cut eggplant crosswise into slices about $\frac{1}{4}$ inch (0.5 cm) thick. Sprinkle slices lightly with salt and layer in a colander. Let drain for about 15 minutes. Pat dry with paper towels.

2. In a large saucepan, heat oil over medium heat. In batches, dip eggplant slices in flour to lightly coat both sides. Fry in oil, turning once, until golden, about 3 minutes. Using a slotted spoon, transfer to a baking sheet lined with paper towels and drain well. Repeat with remaining eggplant, adjusting heat as necessary between batches to prevent burning.

3. In a bowl, combine tomato sauce, basil and oregano. Spread a thin layer of tomato sauce in baking dish. Place a layer of eggplant on top and cover with more tomato sauce. Sprinkle with half of the mozzarella and Parmesan.

4. Repeat to make a second layer and, if there are enough ingredients remaining, a third. Top with a layer of Parmesan.

5. Bake in preheated oven until hot and bubbling, about 20 minutes. Let stand for 10 minutes before serving.

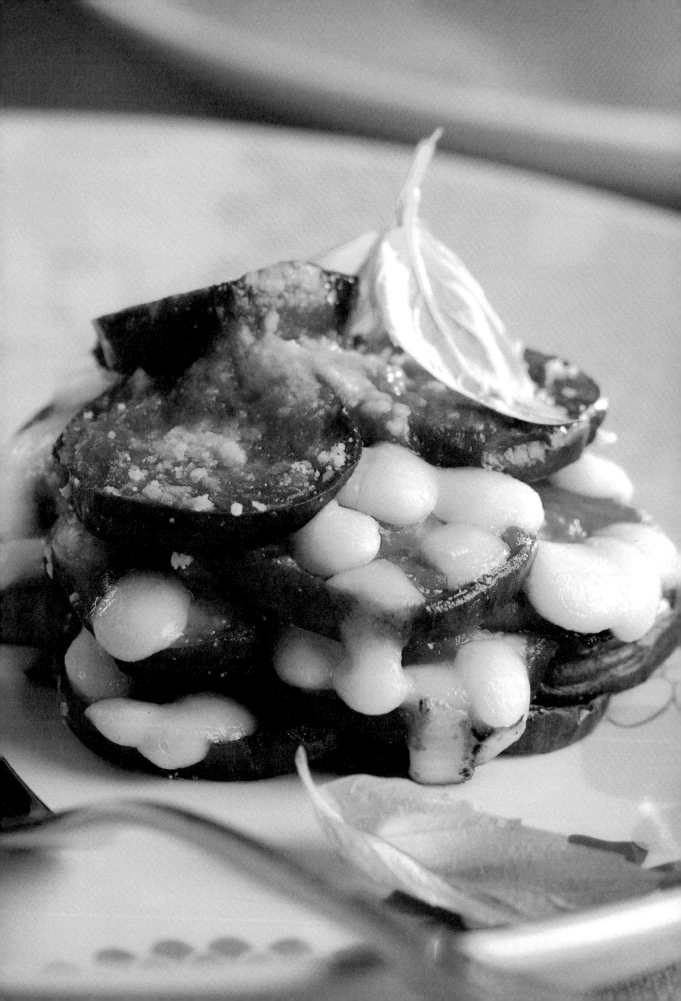

Stuffed Peppers

Serves 6

Preparation time
30 minutes

Cooking time
40 minutes

● **Preheat oven to 350°F (180°C)**

2 cups	milk	500 mL
¼ cup	butter	60 mL
⅓ cup	all-purpose flour	75 mL
	Salt and freshly ground black pepper	
6 tbsp	grated vegetarian-friendly Parmesan cheese (see Tip, page 218)	90 mL
1 cup	ricotta cheese	250 mL
6	egg yolks	6
8	egg whites	8
12	small red bell peppers	12

1. In a saucepan, bring milk almost to a boil over medium heat. In another saucepan, melt butter over medium heat. Sprinkle with flour and cook, stirring, for 1 minute to make a roux.

2. Gradually pour hot milk over roux, blending well with a whisk. Season with salt and pepper to taste. Bring to a boil. Reduce heat and boil gently, whisking, until thick, about 10 minutes. Remove from heat and stir in Parmesan and ricotta until melted and smooth. Transfer to a bowl and let cool to lukewarm. Whisk in egg yolks until blended and let cool completely.

3. In a large bowl, using an electric mixer, beat egg whites until frothy. Fold into cooled cheese mixture.

4. Cut about ½ inch (1 cm) from tops of peppers, retaining stems in tops. Scoop out cores and seeds from peppers. Fill with cheese mixture until three-quarters full and replace tops on peppers. Place on a baking sheet.

5. Bake in preheated oven until peppers are tender and filling is hot, about 30 minutes.

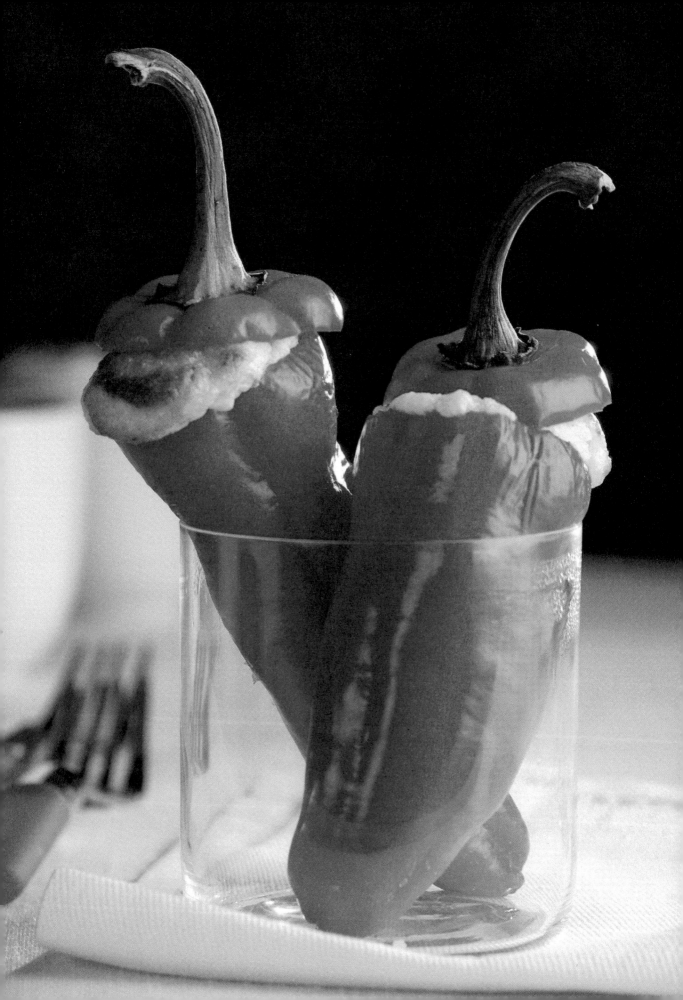

Gnocchi à la Romaine

Serves 4

Preparation time
50 minutes

Cooking time
25 minutes

Tip

These gnocchi are delicious with a tomato sauce.

- Large rimmed baking sheet, oiled
- 2-inch (5 cm) round cookie cutter
- Large shallow baking dish, buttered

2 cups	milk	500 mL
¼ cup	butter, divided	60 mL
	Salt and freshly ground black pepper	
	Ground nutmeg	
1 cup	semolina flour	250 mL
1 cup	grated vegetarian-friendly Parmesan cheese (see Tip, page 218)	250 mL
1	egg	1
2	egg yolks	2
	Vegetarian-friendly Parmesan cheese	

1. In a large saucepan, combine milk, 2 tbsp (30 mL) of the butter and salt, pepper and nutmeg to taste. Bring to a boil over medium-high heat. Remove from heat and gradually pour in semolina in a fine shower, stirring constantly.

2. Return to low heat and cook, stirring constantly with a wooden spoon, until thick, about 10 minutes. Remove from heat and stir in Parmesan cheese. Let cool slightly.

3. In a bowl, lightly beat egg and egg yolks. Stir into semolina mixture until well blended.

4. Pour onto prepared baking sheet and spread uniformly to a thickness of ¾ inches (2 cm). Cover with plastic wrap and let cool completely.

5. Meanwhile, preheat oven to 425°F (220°C).

6. Using a cookie cutter, cut out circles of dough and place in prepared baking dish. Sprinkle with Parmesan cheese and dot with small pieces of remaining butter.

7. Bake in preheated oven until cheese is melted, about 5 minutes.

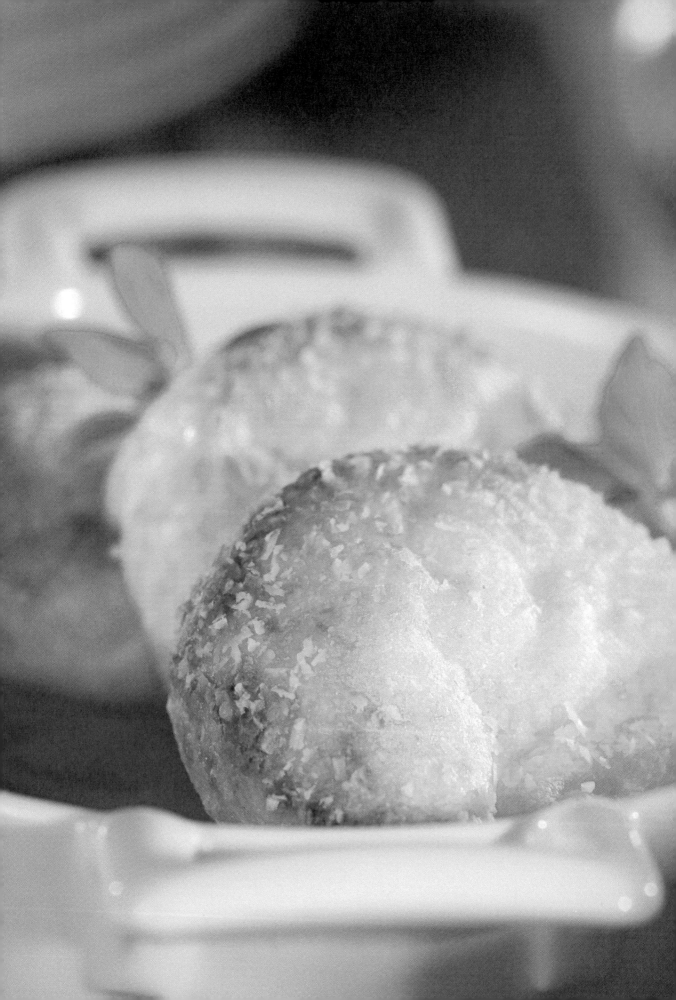

Pasta with Cherry Tomatoes and Ricotta

¼ cup	extra virgin olive oil, divided	60 mL
40	cherry tomatoes, cut in half	40
	Salt	
12 oz	gnocchetti sardi pasta or other short pasta	375 g
8 oz	ricotta cheese	250 g
2 oz	Pecorino Romano cheese, grated	60 g
2 tsp	cracked black peppercorns	10 mL

1. In a small saucepan, heat 2 tbsp (30 mL) of the oil over low heat. Add tomatoes and a pinch of salt and cook, stirring often, until softened and browned, about 10 minutes.

2. Meanwhile, in a large pot of boiling salted water, cook pasta according to package directions until al dente. Drain and transfer to a bowl.

3. Add tomatoes, ricotta and Pecorino Romano cheese to pasta and toss to combine. Drizzle with remaining olive oil and garnish with peppercorns.

Orecchiette Pasta with Rapini, Shiitake Mushrooms and Sun-Dried Tomatoes

12 oz	orecchiette pasta	375 g
½	bunch rapini, trimmed, cut into small pieces	½
6 tbsp	extra virgin olive oil, divided	90 mL
4	cloves garlic, minced	4
⅓ cup	thinly sliced shiitake mushroom caps	75 mL
⅓ cup	diced sun-dried tomatoes	75 mL
	Cracked black peppercorns	
⅓ cup	grated Pecorino Romano cheese	75 mL

1. In a large pot of boiling salted water, cook pasta according to package directions, adding rapini after 5 minutes, until pasta is al dente and rapini is tender. Drain well and transfer to a warmed bowl.

2. Meanwhile, in a skillet, heat ¼ cup (60 mL) of the oil over medium-high heat. Add garlic and cook, stirring, until softened but not browned, about 2 minutes. Add mushrooms and cook, stirring, until tender and starting to brown. Stir in sun-dried tomatoes and season with peppercorns to taste.

3. Spoon mushroom mixture on top of pasta mixture. Sprinkle with Pecorino Romano cheese and drizzle with remaining olive oil.

Linguine Canaletto

Serves 4

Preparation time
10 minutes

Cooking time
10 minutes

10 oz	linguine	300 g
3	carrots, thinly sliced	3
3	zucchini, thinly sliced	3
¾ cup	Vegetable Stock (page 128) or ready-to-use broth	175 mL
⅓ cup	butter, cut into pieces	75 mL
	Salt and freshly ground black pepper	
2 oz	vegetarian-friendly Parmesan cheese, grated (see Tip, page 218)	60 g
8	leaves fresh basil, finely chopped	8
2 tbsp	olive oil	30 mL

1. In a large pot of boiling salted water, cook pasta according to package directions until al dente. Add carrots and zucchini during the last minute of cooking time. Drain well.

2. Meanwhile, in a large skillet, bring vegetable stock, butter, and salt and pepper to taste to a boil over high heat, stirring until butter is melted. Add drained pasta and vegetables and heat, stirring gently to coat.

3. Divide pasta among serving bowls, sprinkle with Parmesan and basil and drizzle with olive oil.

Tagliatelle with Dried Mushrooms

Serves 4

Preparation time
10 minutes

Cooking time
10 minutes

3 oz	dried wild mushrooms, such as porcini	90 g
1 cup	hot Vegetable Stock (page 128) or ready-to-use broth	250 mL
12 oz	tagliatelle egg pasta	375 g
6 tbsp	butter	90 mL
	Freshly ground black pepper	
6 tbsp	grated Parmesan cheese, preferably Parmigiano-Reggiano	90 mL
	Chopped fresh Italian flat-leaf parsley	

1. In a heatproof bowl, soak mushrooms in hot vegetable stock until softened, about 20 minutes. Drain mushrooms, reserving stock. Chop mushrooms. Strain stock through a coffee filter or very fine mesh sieve to remove any grit. Set both aside separately.

2. Meanwhile, in a large pot of boiling salted water, cook pasta according to package directions until tender. Drain well.

3. In a large skillet, melt butter over medium-high heat. Add mushrooms and pepper to taste and cook, stirring, until starting to brown. Add reserved stock and bring to a boil. Add pasta and toss gently to coat. Stir in Parmesan and parsley until creamy.

Florentine-Style Cannelloni

Serves 4

Preparation time
50 minutes

Cooking time
30 minutes

- Preheat oven to 350°F (180°C)
- 8-inch (20 cm) square glass baking dish, buttered

8	fresh pasta sheets (each 4 to 5 inches/10 to 12.5 cm square)	8

Ricotta and Spinach Filling

1 lb	ricotta cheese	500 g
2	egg yolks	2
1 cup	fresh spinach, blanched, drained and chopped	250 mL
Pinch	ground nutmeg	Pinch
	Salt and freshly ground black pepper	
2 cups	Béchamel Sauce (page 259)	500 mL
½ cup	Tomato Basil Sauce (page 270) or store-bought	125 mL
3 tbsp	grated vegetarian-friendly Parmesan cheese (see Tip, page 218)	45 mL
3 tbsp	butter, cut into slivers	45 mL

1. In a large pot of boiling salted water, cook pasta sheets according to package directions until al dente. Drain well, then lay on a clean cloth spread on work surface.

2. *Ricotta and Spinach Filling:* In a large bowl, combine ricotta, egg yolks, spinach, nutmeg, and salt and pepper to taste.

3. Spoon one-eighth of the filling in a line along center of each pasta sheet and roll up into a cylinder.

4. Spread a thin layer of béchamel sauce on the bottom of prepared baking dish and place cannelloni on top, side by side with the seam sides down. Spread remaining béchamel sauce on top, then drizzle with tomato sauce. Sprinkle with Parmesan and top with slivers of butter.

5. Bake in preheated oven until filling is hot and sauce is bubbling, about 30 minutes. Let stand for 5 minutes before serving.

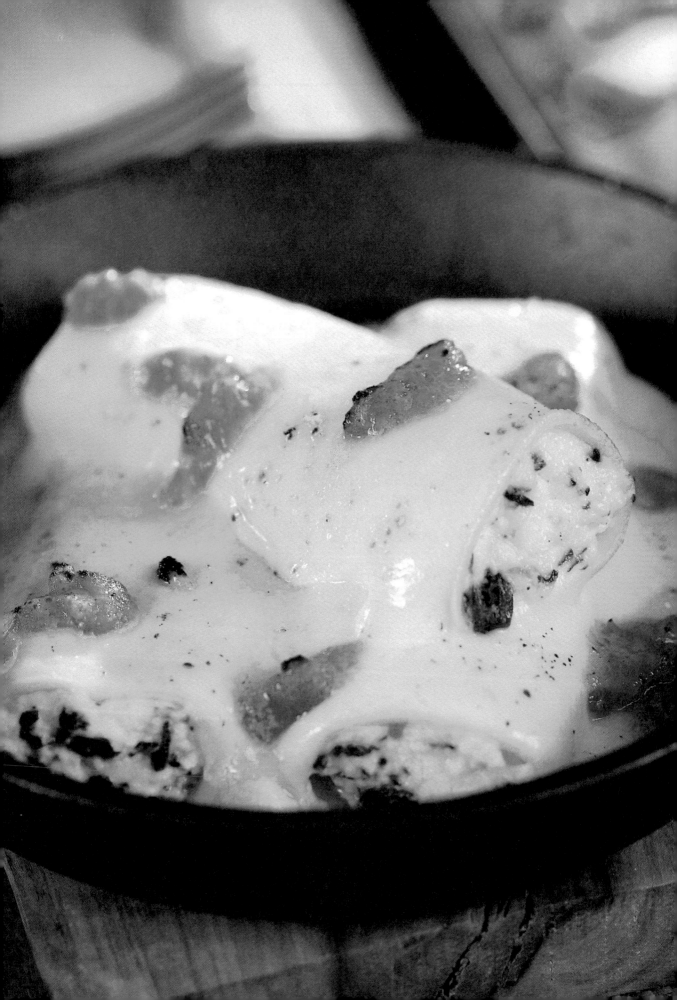

Lasagnette all'Ortolana

Preparation time
1 hour

Cooking time
40 minutes

- Preheat oven to 350°F (180°C)
- 11- by 7-inch (28 by 18 cm) glass baking dish, buttered

6 tbsp	extra virgin olive oil, divided	90 mL
2	zucchini, diced	2
½	eggplant, diced	½
1	red bell pepper, diced	1
1	yellow bell pepper, diced	1
1	stalk broccoli, cut into small florets, stem chopped	1
	Salt and freshly ground black pepper	
8	leaves fresh basil, chopped	8
12	egg pasta sheets, each 8 by 4 inches (20 by 10 cm)	12
4 cups	Béchamel Sauce (page 259)	1 L
5 oz	mozzarella cheese, shredded	150 g
4 oz	vegetarian-friendly Parmesan cheese, grated (see Tip, page 218)	125 g

1. In a skillet, heat 3 tbsp (45 mL) of the oil over high heat. Add zucchini and eggplant and cook, stirring, until tender and starting to brown, about 8 minutes. Transfer to a bowl.

2. Add remaining oil to skillet and heat over high heat. Add red pepper, yellow pepper and broccoli and cook, stirring, until tender and starting to brown, about 5 minutes. Add to zucchini mixture. Season with salt and pepper to taste and stir in basil. Set aside.

3. In a large pot of boiling water, in batches as necessary to avoid crowding, cook pasta sheets according to package directions until al dente. Rinse under cold water until chilled. Drain well.

4. Spread a thin layer of béchamel sauce in prepared baking dish. Place 2 of the pasta sheets on top, overlapping as necessary. Spread with a thin layer of béchamel, then top evenly with one-sixth of the vegetables, one-fifth of the mozzarella and one-sixth of the Parmesan cheese. Repeat layers four more times. Top with remaining noodles, then spread with remaining béchamel. Top with remaining vegetables and Parmesan.

5. Bake in preheated oven until hot, bubbling and golden brown on top, about 35 minutes. Let stand for 10 minutes before serving.

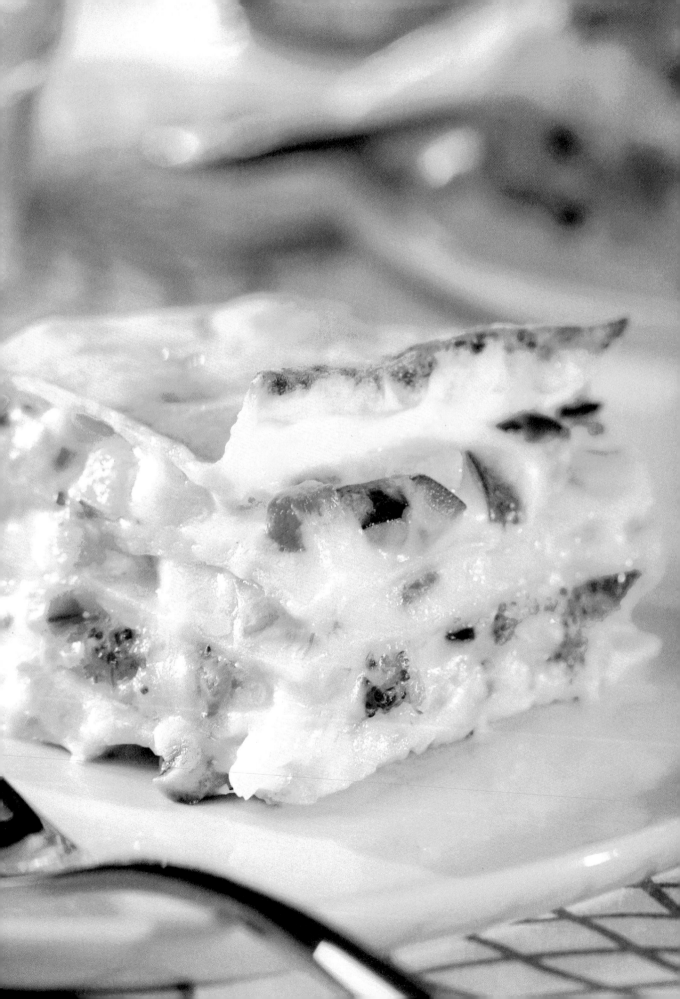

Chestnut Pappardelle with Pesto

- Pasta machine (see Tip, left)
- Crinkle cutter, optional

1 cup	bread flour	250 mL
⅔ cup	chestnut flour	150 mL
2	eggs	2
1	egg yolk	1
1 tsp	olive oil	5 mL
Pinch	salt	Pinch
	Pesto alla Genovese (page 268) or store-bought basil pesto	

1. In a bowl, combine bread and chestnut flours and make a well in the center. Add eggs, egg yolk, oil, 2 tsp (10 mL) water and a pinch of salt to the well. Stir together until a soft dough forms and holds together well, adding more water as necessary to moisten so dough comes together.

2. Transfer dough to a lightly floured work surface and knead until dough is smooth and very firm. If you have difficulty making it hold together, add a few drops of water.

3. Cover tightly with plastic wrap and refrigerate for 20 minutes.

4. Using pasta machine, roll out pasta according to manufacturer's directions to sheets approximately 12 inches (30 cm) in length. Using crinkle cutter or a sharp knife, cut lengthwise into ³⁄₄-inch (2 cm) wide strips.

5. In a large pot of boiling salted water, cook pasta until al dente, 3 to 4 minutes. Drain well and return to pot. Add pesto to taste and toss gently to coat.

Tagliolini with Dried Cranberries

Preparation time
10 minutes

Cooking time
10 minutes

Tip

Tagliolini are fresh egg pasta, the length of spaghetti but a square shape rather than round. You can make it using the Fresh Egg Pasta recipe on page 258 and using the thinnest setting in the cutting attachment of a pasta maker, or purchase it at Italian specialty shops or online. If you can't find it, use spaghettini or capellini. If using dried pasta, use 8 oz (250 g) and cook according to package directions.

6 tbsp	extra virgin olive oil, divided	90 mL
4	cloves garlic, chopped	4
¼ cup	dry white wine	60 mL
	Cayenne pepper or hot pepper flakes	
¾ cup	dried cranberries, chopped	175 mL
2 tbsp	chopped fresh Italian flat-leaf parsley leaves	30 mL
12 oz	fresh tagliolini pasta (see Tip, left)	375 g
	Salt	

1. In a large skillet, heat 2 tbsp (30 mL) of the oil over medium-low heat. Add garlic and cook, stirring, until softened. Add wine and bring to a boil, scraping up any brown bits stuck to pan.

2. Stir in cayenne to taste and cranberries. Reduce heat to low and cook, stirring, just until wine is evaporated. Stir in parsley and remove from heat.

3. In a large pot of boiling salted water, cook pasta until al dente, about 3 minutes. Drain, reserving 1 cup (250 mL) of the cooking water.

4. Return skillet to medium-high heat. Add pasta and cook, stirring and adding enough of the reserved cooking water just to moisten, until hot, about 2 minutes. Season with salt to taste.

5. Divide among warmed serving bowls and drizzle with remaining oil.

Pad Thai

Preparation time
30 minutes

Cooking time
15 minutes

7 oz	wide rice noodles	210 g
	Hot water	
1 tbsp	granulated sugar	15 mL
1 tsp	paprika	5 mL
¾ cup	water	175 mL
2 tbsp	tamari sauce	30 mL
3 tbsp	fish sauce	45 mL
	Juice of 1 lime	
4 tbsp	vegetable oil, divided	60 mL
4	eggs, beaten	4
10 oz	firm tofu, cut into strips	300 g
2	cloves garlic, minced	2
2	green onions, thinly sliced	2
1	bird's-eye chile pepper, chopped	1
2 cups	bean sprouts	500 mL
¼ cup	chopped fresh cilantro	60 mL
¼ cup	crushed peanuts	60 mL
1	lime, quartered	1

1. Place noodles in a large bowl and add hot water to cover by at least 2 inches (5 cm). Let soak until noodles are tender, about 15 minutes. Drain well.

2. In a bowl, combine sugar, paprika, water, tamari, fish sauce and lime juice. Set aside.

3. Heat a large wok or skillet over high heat. Add half of the oil and swirl to coat. Add eggs and cook, stirring, until just set, about 2 minutes. Transfer to a bowl.

4. Add remaining oil to wok and swirl to coat. Add tofu and stir-fry until well browned, about 5 minutes. Add garlic, green onions and chile pepper and stir-fry for 1 minute.

5. Add noodles and eggs to wok. Drizzle in sauce and stir-fry until noodles are well coated and hot, about 5 minutes. Stir in bean sprouts.

6. Arrange noodle mixture on serving dishes and garnish with cilantro and peanuts. Serve with lime wedges to squeeze overtop.

Barley Risotto with Cauliflower

Serves 4

Preparation time
20 minutes

Cooking time
50 minutes

5 cups	Vegetable Stock (page 128) or ready-to-use broth	1.25 L
¼ cup	butter, divided	60 mL
2 tbsp	finely chopped onion	30 mL
1 cup	pearl barley	250 mL
3 tbsp	dry white wine	45 mL
2 cups	finely chopped cauliflower	500 mL
	Salt	
2 tbsp	extra virgin olive oil	30 mL
2	plum (Roma) tomatoes, peeled and finely chopped	2
3 tbsp	grated vegetarian-friendly Parmesan cheese (see Tip, page 218)	45 mL

1. In a large saucepan, bring vegetables stock to a boil over high heat. Reduce heat to low, cover and keep stock hot.

2. In another large saucepan, melt half of the butter over medium-high heat. Add onion and cook, stirring, until browned, about 5 minutes. Stir in barley until well coated.

3. Add wine and cook, stirring, until evaporated. Stir in cauliflower and enough of the hot stock to cover barley. Season with salt to taste. Reduce heat and simmer, stirring often and adding more stock, ½ cup (125 mL) at a time, as previous addition is absorbed. Cook, adding stock, until barley is tender, about 40 minutes in total.

4. Meanwhile, in a small saucepan, heat oil over low heat. Add tomatoes and cook, stirring often, until very soft and thickened into a sauce.

5. Remove barley from heat and stir in remaining butter and Parmesan cheese. Divide among warmed serving bowls and garnish with tomato sauce.

Sweet Mama Squash Risotto

Preparation time
10 minutes

Cooking time
35 minutes

Tip

To roast squash: Cut a Sweet Mama or other winter squash in half and scrape out seeds. Place on a baking sheet, cut side down. Bake in 350°F (180°C) oven until tender, about 45 minutes. Let cool slightly. Scoop out squash pulp with a spoon, discarding skins, and mash with a potato masher or purée in a food processor.

6 cups	Vegetable Stock (page 128) or ready-to-use broth	1.5 L
¼ cup	butter, divided	60 mL
¼ cup	chopped onion	60 mL
1¼ cups	Vialone Nano, carnaroli or Arborio rice	300 mL
¼ cup	dry white wine	60 mL
1 cup	puréed roasted Sweet Mama squash (see Tip, left)	250 mL
	Salt and freshly ground black pepper	
1 oz	vegetarian-friendly Parmesan cheese, grated (see Tip, page 218)	30 g

1. In a saucepan, bring vegetable stock to a boil over high heat. Reduce heat to low, cover and keep stock hot.

2. In a large saucepan, melt half of the butter over medium heat. Add onion and cook, stirring, until golden brown, about 5 minutes. Add rice and cook, stirring, until rice is translucent, about 2 minutes.

3. Pour in wine and cook, stirring, until evaporated. Stir in squash. Season with salt and pepper to taste. Stir in enough of the hot stock to cover rice. Reduce heat and simmer, stirring often and adding more stock, ½ cup (125 mL) at a time, as previous addition is absorbed. Simmer, adding stock, until rice is al dente, about 30 minutes in total. Remove from heat and let stand for 1 minute.

4. Stir in remaining butter and Parmesan until melted. Add a little more stock, if necessary, to thin to a creamy, slightly loose consistency. Season with salt and pepper to taste.

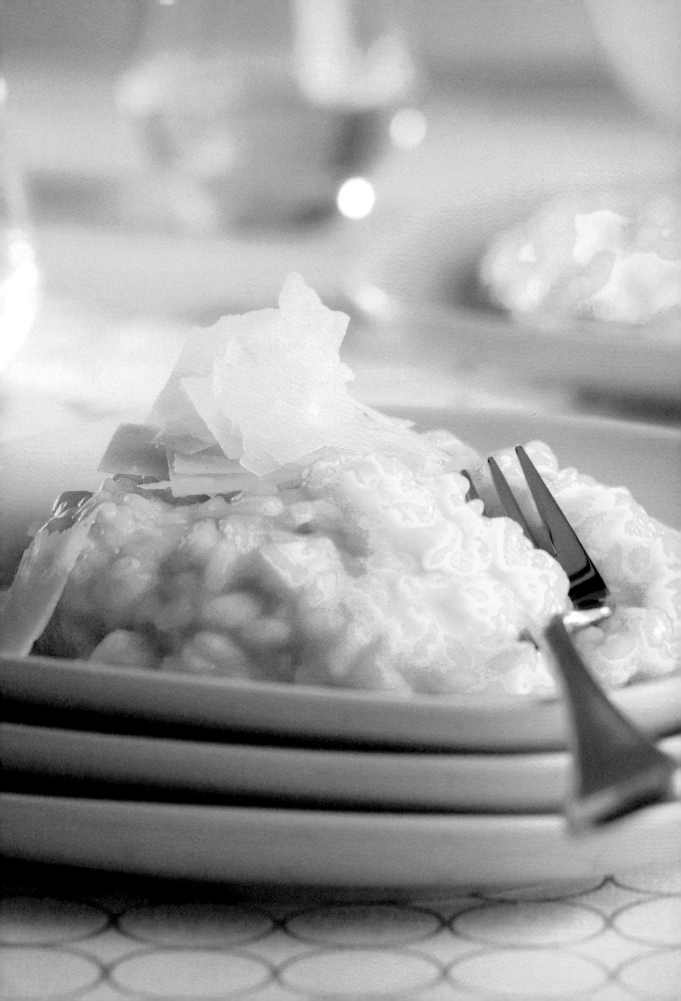

Quinoa Simmered with Fennel and Wild Mushrooms

Serves 4

Preparation time
30 minutes

Cooking time
45 minutes

Variation

The quinoa in this recipe can be replaced by millet.

2½ cups	Vegetable Stock (page 128) or reduced-sodium ready-to-use broth (approx.)	625 mL
½ tsp	anise seeds	2 mL
2 oz	dried porcini or other wild mushrooms	60 g
2 tbsp	olive oil, divided	30 mL
1	onion, finely chopped	1
2	cloves garlic, chopped	2
1	bulb fennel, trimmed and thinly sliced	1
1½ cups	quinoa, rinsed and drained	375 mL
	Salt and freshly ground black pepper	
1½ cups	chopped kale leaves	375 mL
1	small red bell pepper, julienned	1
2 tbsp	butter	30 mL
1 cup	frozen green peas, thawed	250 mL
2 tbsp	chopped Italian flat-leaf parsley	30 mL
2 tbsp	hazelnut oil	30 mL

1. In a saucepan, combine vegetable stock and anise seeds and bring to a boil over high heat. Reduce heat to low, cover and keep stock hot.

2. In a heatproof bowl, cover dried mushrooms with boiling water. Let stand until softened, about 20 minutes.

3. In another large saucepan, heat 1 tbsp (15 mL) of the oil over medium heat. Add onion and cook, stirring, until softened but not browned, about 5 minutes. Add garlic and fennel and cook, stirring, until softened, about 5 minutes.

4. Stir in quinoa until well coated. Season with salt and pepper to taste. Stir in enough of the hot stock to cover quinoa. Reduce heat and simmer, stirring often and adding more stock, ½ cup (125 mL) at a time, as previous addition is absorbed. Cook, adding stock, until quinoa is almost tender, about 20 minutes in total.

5. Meanwhile, in a pot of boiling salted water, boil kale until tender, about 5 minutes. Drain well.

6. In a skillet, heat remaining oil over medium-high heat. Add bell pepper and cook, stirring, until tender, about 5 minutes. Set aside.

7. Drain mushrooms and pat dry. In same skillet, melt butter over low heat. Add mushrooms and cook, stirring, until starting to brown (do not let them dry out).

8. Stir kale, bell pepper, mushrooms, peas, parsley and hazelnut oil into quinoa. Simmer, stirring, until vegetables are hot. Season with salt and pepper to taste.

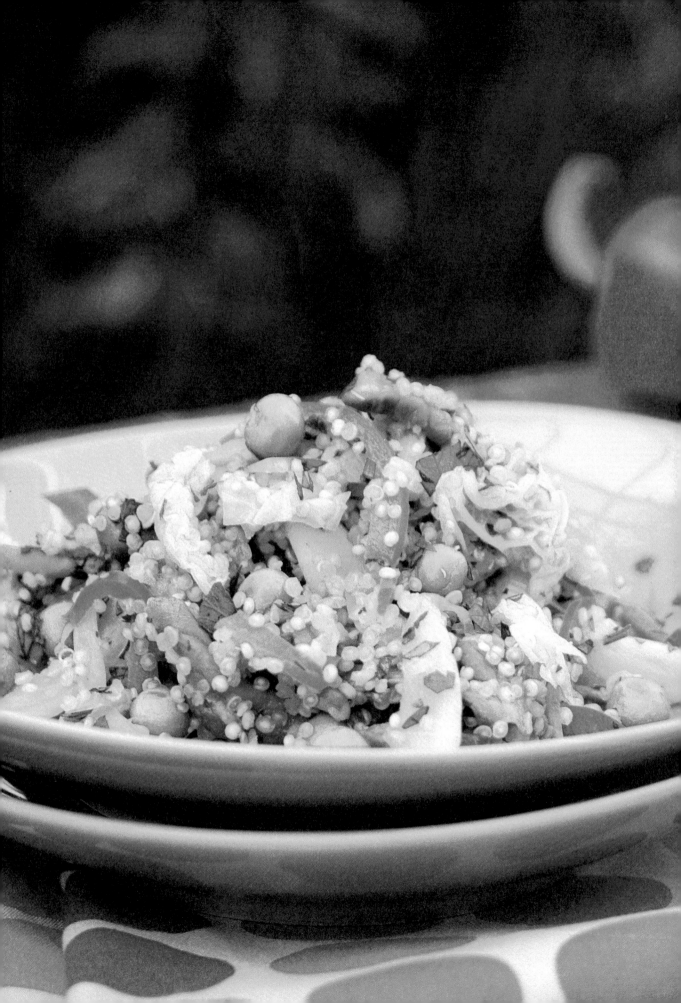

Spiced Vegetable and Chickpea Couscous

Serves 4

Preparation time
20 minutes

Cooking time
35 minutes

4 cups	Vegetable Stock (page 128) or reduced-sodium ready-to-use vegetable broth	1 L
1	clove garlic, crushed	1
2 tbsp	tomato paste	30 mL
1/4 tsp	ground nutmeg	1 mL
1/8 tsp	ground cumin	0.5 mL
1/8 tsp	ground cinnamon	0.5 mL
1	whole clove	1
	Salt and freshly ground black pepper	
	Cayenne pepper	
	Harissa	
	Ras el hanout	
4	large carrots, cut into 3/4-inch (2 cm) pieces	4
4	turnips, peeled and cut into 3/4-inch (2 cm) pieces	4
4	small zucchini, halved lengthwise and thinly sliced	4
2	green bell peppers, diced	2
1 cup	canned chickpeas, rinsed and drained	250 mL
1 cup	couscous	250 mL
2 tbsp	butter, cut into small pieces	30 mL

1. In a pot, combine vegetable stock, garlic, tomato paste, nutmeg, cumin, cinnamon, clove, and salt, black pepper, cayenne pepper, harissa and ras el hanout to taste. Bring to a boil over medium heat. Cover, reduce heat to low and simmer until flavors are blended, about 10 minutes. Remove garlic clove.

2. Transfer 1 1/4 cups (300 mL) of the broth to another saucepan. Set aside.

3. Add carrots and turnips to remaining broth in pot and bring to a boil over high heat. Cover, reduce heat to medium-low and simmer until vegetables are almost tender, about 20 minutes. Add zucchini, bell peppers and chickpeas. Cover and simmer until tender, about 5 minutes.

4. Meanwhile, bring saucepan of reserved broth to a boil over high heat. Gradually stir in couscous. Cover, remove from heat and let stand until softened and liquid is absorbed, about 5 minutes. Add butter and stir gently with a fork.

5. Mound couscous in 4 warmed serving bowls. Using a slotted spoon, remove vegetables from broth and spoon over couscous. Ladle just enough of the broth overtop to moisten. Serve remaining broth in separate warmed soup bowls and season with more harissa to taste.

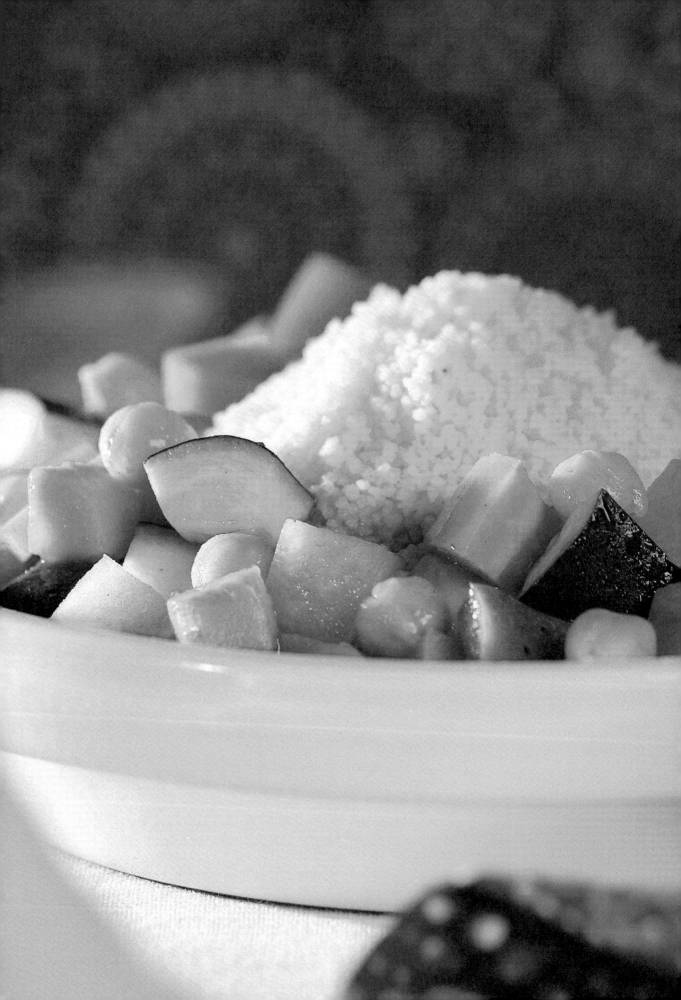

Papa Rellena

Preparation time
30 minutes

Cooking time
1 hour 10 minutes

Tips

Aji amarillo peppers are Peruvian hot chile peppers that are yellow to orange in color. They are available fresh, dried and in a paste form at Latin American grocery stores. If you can't find them fresh, substitute a tabasco pepper, 1 to 3 cayenne, serrano or Thai chile peppers or one-quarter of a Scotch bonnet or habanero pepper.

Cassava, also know as yuca, is a starchy root with thick, dark brown skin and white flesh. It must be cooked before consumption. It is used in many tropical and subtropical cuisines and can be found in some supermarkets and ethnic stores. The more familiar tapioca is made from cassava.

- Food mill or food processor

Salsa

1½ cups	thinly sliced red onion	375 mL
2	aji Amarillo chile peppers, julienned	2
6 tbsp	freshly squeezed lime juice	90 mL
3 tbsp	vegetable oil	45 mL
3 tbsp	white wine vinegar	45 mL
	Salt	
1 lb	yellow-fleshed potatoes, peeled (about 4)	500 g
1 lb	cassava, peeled and cut into chunks	500 g
1	egg, beaten	1
3 tbsp	vegetable oil	45 mL
	Salt and freshly ground black pepper	
1½ cups	Ratatouille (page 252) or store-bought	375 mL
½ cup	black olives, cut in half	125 mL
1 cup	all-purpose flour (approx.)	250 mL
2 cups	vegetable oil (approx.)	500 mL
1 tsp	chopped fresh parsley	15 mL

1. *Salsa:* In a bowl, combine onion, chiles, lime juice, oil, vinegar and salt to taste. Cover and let stand until onions are translucent, about 1 hour.

2. Meanwhile, place potatoes in a saucepan and add cold salted water to cover by 2 inches (5 cm). Bring to a boil over high heat. Reduce heat and boil gently until potatoes are tender, about 30 minutes. Drain well.

3. In another pot of boiling salted water, cook cassava until tender, about 30 minutes. Drain well.

4. Using a food mill or a food processor, purée potatoes and cassava until smooth. Transfer to a bowl, if necessary. Stir in egg and 3 tbsp (45 mL) oil. Season with salt and pepper to taste.

5. Using a sieve, drain excess liquid from ratatouille, discarding liquid. Place ratatouille in a bowl and stir in olives.

6. Divide mashed potato mixture into 16 equal portions. Working with one portion at a time, with floured hands, shape into an oval, 3 to 4 inches (7.5 to 10 cm) long. Place about 1 tbsp (15 mL) of the ratatouille mixture in the center and pinch potato mixture around filling to enclose into a croquette. Place on a floured baking sheet, turning to coat with flour. Repeat with remaining potato and filling.

7. In a skillet, heat oil over medium-high heat until very hot. Fry croquettes, in batches as necessary, turning once, until golden brown and filling is hot, about 5 minutes. Using a slotted spoon, remove from oil and place on a baking sheet lined with paper towels to drain. Add more oil to skillet and adjust heat as necessary between batches to prevent burning.

8. Just before serving, stir parsley into salsa. Serve croquettes hot with salsa on the side.

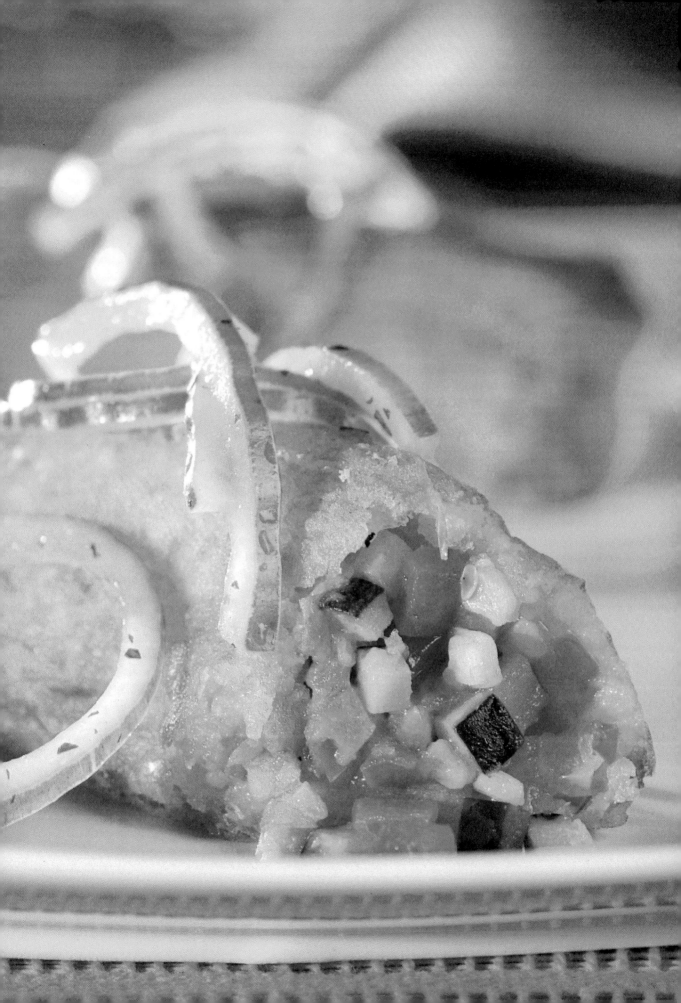

Vegetable Parmentier

Tip

A bouquet garni is a small bundle of aromatic herbs tied together with kitchen string. It is used to add flavor to a simmered or boiled mixture and is generally discarded before the dish is served. It often includes parsley, thyme and bay leaves but can also include any of your favorite herbs that complement the flavors of your dish.

- 8-cup (2 L) shallow baking dish, buttered

2 lbs	yellow-fleshed or oblong baking potatoes, peeled (about 8 small)	1 kg
2 tbsp	vegetable oil, divided	30 mL
1¼ cups	finely chopped onions	300 mL
1½ cups	finely diced carrots	375 mL
3	cloves garlic, chopped	3
1	red bell pepper, finely diced	1
1	bouquet garni (see Tip, left)	1
4 cups	cooked adzuki beans (2 cups/500 mL dried)	1 L
½ cup	water (approx.)	125 mL
10 oz	mushrooms, thinly sliced	300 g
	Salt and freshly ground black pepper	
2 tbsp	chopped fresh parsley	30 mL
¾ cup	butter, softened, divided	175 mL
½ cup	hot milk, optional	125 mL

1. Place potatoes in a saucepan and add cold salted water to cover by 2 inches (5 cm). Bring to a boil over high heat. Reduce heat and boil gently until potatoes are tender, about 30 minutes.

2. Meanwhile, in a saucepan, heat half of the oil over medium heat. Add onions and cook, stirring, until softened but not browned. Add carrots and cook, stirring, until starting to soften, about 5 minutes. Add garlic and bell pepper and cook, stirring, for 2 minutes. Stir in bouquet garni, beans and water. Reduce heat and simmer.

3. In a skillet, heat remaining oil over medium-high heat. Add mushrooms and cook, stirring, until tender and browned, about 8 minutes. Add to bean mixture and season with salt and pepper to taste. Simmer, stirring often and adding more water as necessary to prevent drying out, until carrots are tender and most of liquid is evaporated, about 10 minutes. Discard bouquet garni.

4. Meanwhile, preheat oven to 450°F (230°C).

5. Drain potatoes well and return to pot. Using a potato masher, mash potatoes, adding ½ cup (125 mL) of the butter and milk, if using, until potatoes are smooth. Season with salt and pepper to taste.

6. Spread half of the potatoes in prepared baking dish. Spread bean mixture over potatoes. Spread remaining potatoes on top. Cut remaining butter into small pieces and sprinkle over potatoes.

7. Bake in preheated oven for about 20 minutes or until hot and bubbling and topping is browned.

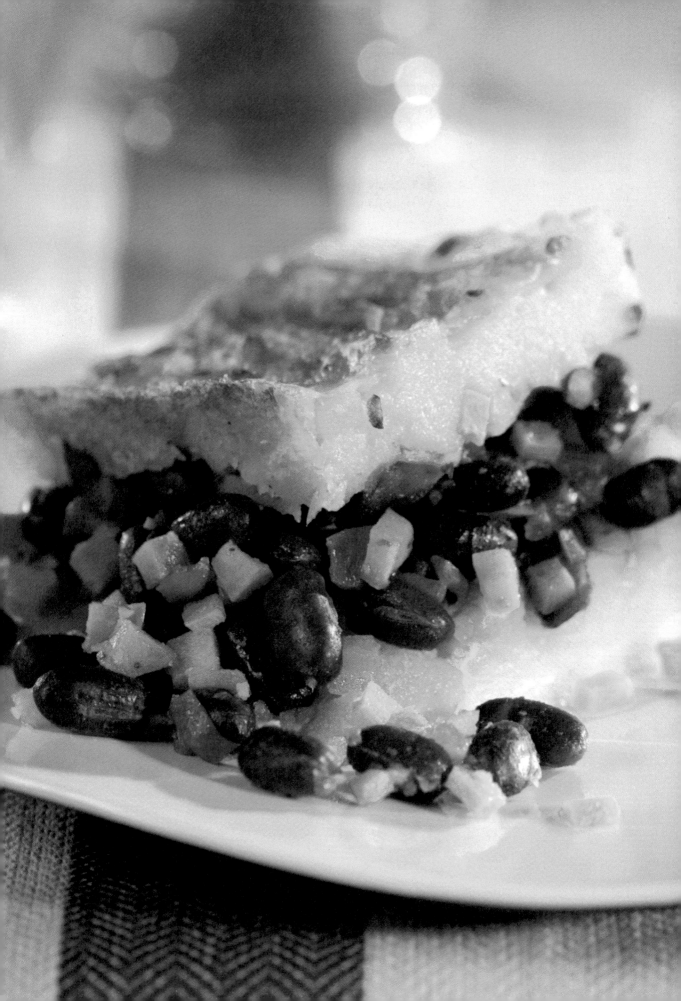

Asian-Style Sautéed Vegetables

Serves 4

Preparation time
45 minutes

Cooking time
15 minutes

2	carrots, cut into matchsticks	2
2	stalks celery, cut into matchsticks	2
1½ cups	broccoli florets	375 mL
2 cups	thinly sliced bok choy	500 mL
1½ cups	snow peas, trimmed	375 mL
2 tbsp	vegetable oil, divided	30 mL
7 oz	tofu, diced	210 g
1	large onion, thinly sliced	1
4	cloves garlic, minced	4
¼ cup	water	60 mL
5	green onions, sliced	5
1 cup	cooked or thawed frozen shelled edamame	250 mL
¼ cup	chopped fresh cilantro leaves	60 mL
¼ cup	oyster sauce	60 mL
3 tbsp	soy sauce	45 mL
2 tsp	black or white sesame seeds	10 mL
	Salt and freshly ground black pepper	

1. In a large pot of boiling salted water, blanch carrots, celery and broccoli for 1 minute. Using a sieve or slotted spoon, remove from water and drain well. In same pot, blanch bok choy and snow peas for 30 seconds. Drain well and set aside.

2. In a wok or large skillet, heat half of the oil over high heat. Add tofu and stir-fry until slightly browned and crispy, about 5 minutes. Transfer to a bowl.

3. Add remaining oil to wok and swirl to coat. Add onion and stir-fry for 1 minute. Add garlic, reserved carrots, celery, broccoli, bok choy and snow peas and water. Cook, stirring, until vegetables are starting to get tender, about 3 minutes.

4. Stir in green onions, edamame and cilantro. Pour in oyster sauce and soy sauce and toss to coat vegetables evenly. Stir-fry just until vegetables are tender-crisp. Stir in reserved tofu and sesame seeds. Season with salt and pepper to taste.

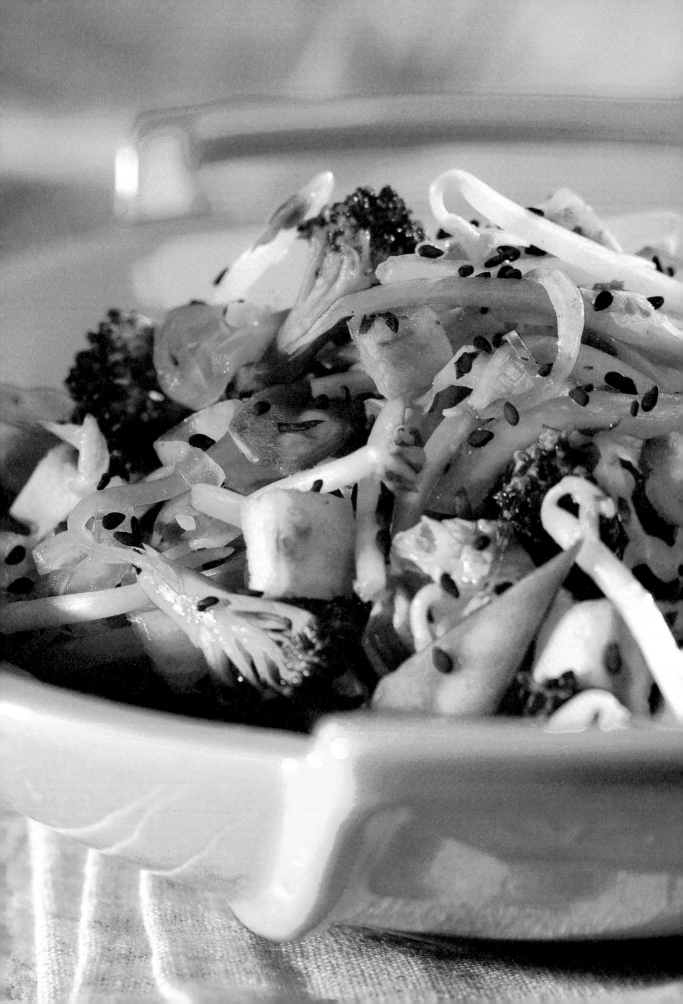

Polenta Pasticciata

Serves 4

Preparation time
30 minutes

Chilling time
1 hour

Cooking time
30 minutes

Tip

When buying cheese, read the label carefully and make sure to buy those that are not made from animal rennet.

- Preheat oven to 400°F (200°C)
- 13- by 9-inch (33 by 23 cm) metal baking pan or glass baking dish

Polenta

8 cups	water	2 L
1 tsp	salt	5 mL
2 tbsp	olive oil	30 mL
1¾ cups	cornmeal	425 mL
3 cups	tomato sauce	750 mL
8 oz	mozzarella cheese, shredded	250 g
4 oz	vegetarian-friendly Parmesan cheese, grated (see Tip, left)	125 g

1. In a large pot, bring water to a boil over high heat. Add salt and olive oil. Reduce heat to low and gradually pour cornmeal in a thin, steady stream into boiling water while whisking constantly. Simmer, stirring often with a wooden spoon, until polenta is soft and thick, about 20 minutes.

2. Spread one-third of the tomato sauce in baking dish. Cover with half of the hot polenta, using a large spoon to spread until fairly smooth. Spread half of the remaining tomato sauce on the polenta and sprinkle with half of the mozzarella cheese and half of the Parmesan. Spread remaining polenta on top, then spread with remaining tomato sauce and sprinkle with remaining cheeses. Cover and refrigerate for at least 1 hour, until set, or for up to 1 day.

3. Preheat oven to 400°F (200°C).

4. Uncover baking dish and bake in oven until hot in the center, cheese is melted and top starts to brown, 25 to 35 minutes. Let stand for 10 minutes before serving.

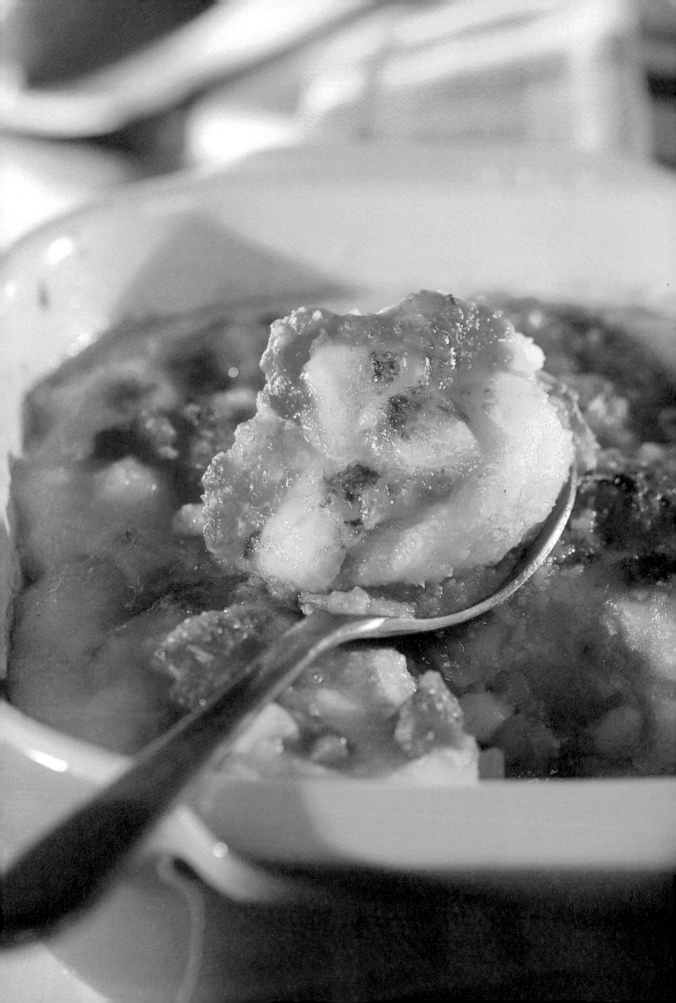

Pizza alla Marinara

Tip

When baking pizza in a domestic oven, it is best to use a preheated ceramic pizza stone, although a metal perforated pizza pan will do.

- Pizza stone, pizza pans or greased baking sheets (see Tip, left)

1 tsp	granulated sugar	5 mL
¾ cup + 2 tbsp	warm water (98°F/37°C)	205 mL
1½ tsp	active dry yeast	7 mL
2 cups	all-purpose flour (approx.)	500 mL
1½ tsp	salt	7 mL
3 tbsp	extra virgin olive oil, divided	45 mL
1 cup	tomato sauce	250 mL
4	leaves fresh basil, chopped	4
4	cloves garlic, chopped	4
Pinch	salt	Pinch
2 tbsp	chopped fresh parsley	30 mL
	Hot pepper flakes	

1. In a measuring cup or small bowl, combine sugar and water. Sprinkle yeast overtop and let stand until frothy, about 10 minutes.

2. In a bowl, combine flour and salt and make a well in the center. Pour yeast mixture and 1 tbsp (15 mL) of the oil into the well. Stir together until a soft dough forms.

3. Transfer dough to a lightly floured work surface and knead, adding more flour as necessary to prevent sticking, until dough is smooth and elastic, about 5 minutes. Place dough in an oiled bowl and turn to coat all over. Cover with a clean tea towel and let rise in a warm, draft-free place until doubled in bulk, about 40 minutes.

4. Cut dough into 4 equal pieces. Roll each piece into a ball. Cover and let rest for 10 minutes.

5. Preheat oven to 430°F (225°C). Preheat pizza stone, if using.

6. In a bowl, combine tomato sauce, basil, garlic, salt and remaining olive oil.

7. Shape each ball of dough into a circle ⅛ inch (3 mm) thick, letting it rest periodically while rolling if it feels too springy. Place on a baking sheet (to slide onto stone), pizza pans or prepared baking sheets. Divide tomato sauce equally among pizzas and spread over dough, leaving ¾ inch (2 cm) bare around the edges. Brush a little olive oil on the edges. Sprinkle parsley and hot pepper flakes on top.

8. Slide pizzas onto preheated pizza stones, if using. Bake, in batches as necessary, until crust is golden, 10 to 15 minutes per batch.

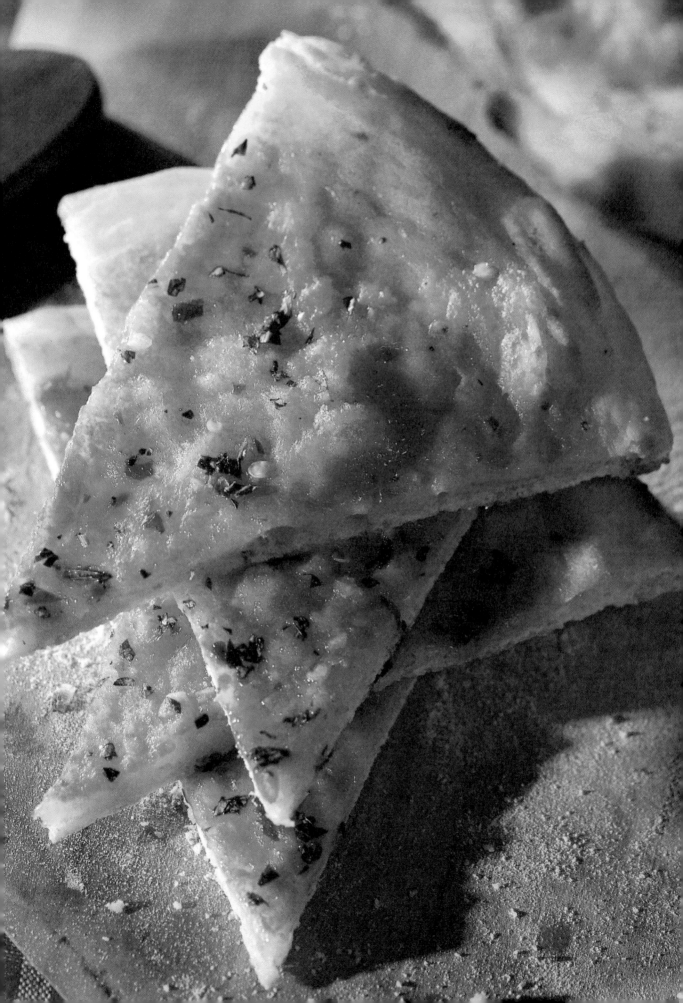

Neapolitan-Style Panzerotti

Serves 4

Preparation time
1 hour 45 minutes

Cooking time
20 minutes

- Candy/deep-fry thermometer

1 tsp	granulated sugar	5 mL
¾ cup + 2 tbsp	warm water (about 98°F/37°C)	205 mL
1½ tsp	active dry yeast	7 mL
2 cups	all-purpose flour (approx.)	500 mL
1½ tsp	salt	7 mL
3 tbsp	extra virgin olive oil, divided	45 mL
1 cup	chopped peeled tomatoes	250 mL
4	leaves fresh basil, chopped	4
	Salt	
4 oz	mozzarella cheese, diced	125 g
	Vegetable oil	

1. In a measuring cup or small bowl, combine sugar and water. Sprinkle yeast overtop and let stand until frothy, about 10 minutes.

2. In a bowl, combine flour and salt and make a well in the center. Pour yeast mixture and 1 tbsp (15 mL) of the oil into the well. Stir together until a soft dough forms.

3. Transfer dough to a lightly floured work surface and knead, adding more flour as necessary to prevent sticking, until dough is smooth and elastic, about 5 minutes. Place dough in an oiled bowl and turn to coat all over. Cover with a clean tea towel and let rise in a warm, draft-free place until doubled in bulk, about 40 minutes.

4. Meanwhile, in a bowl, combine tomatoes, basil, salt to taste and remaining oil. Set aside.

5. In a deep saucepan or deep-fryer, heat 3 inches (7.5 cm) of vegetable oil to 350°F (180°C).

6. Cut dough into 8 equal pieces and roll each into a ball. Working with one ball at a time, roll out to a very thin circle, about $\frac{1}{16}$ inch (2 mm) thick. Spoon about 2 tbsp (30 mL) of the tomato mixture in the center and top with one-eighth of the mozzarella. Fold one side over the filling to make a half-moon shape, pinching edges to seal. Repeat with remaining dough and filling.

7. In batches as necessary, fry panzerotti in hot oil, turning once, until dough is golden brown and filling is hot, about 5 minutes per side. Using a slotted spoon, remove panzerotti from oil and place on a baking sheet lined with paper towels to drain. Serve hot.

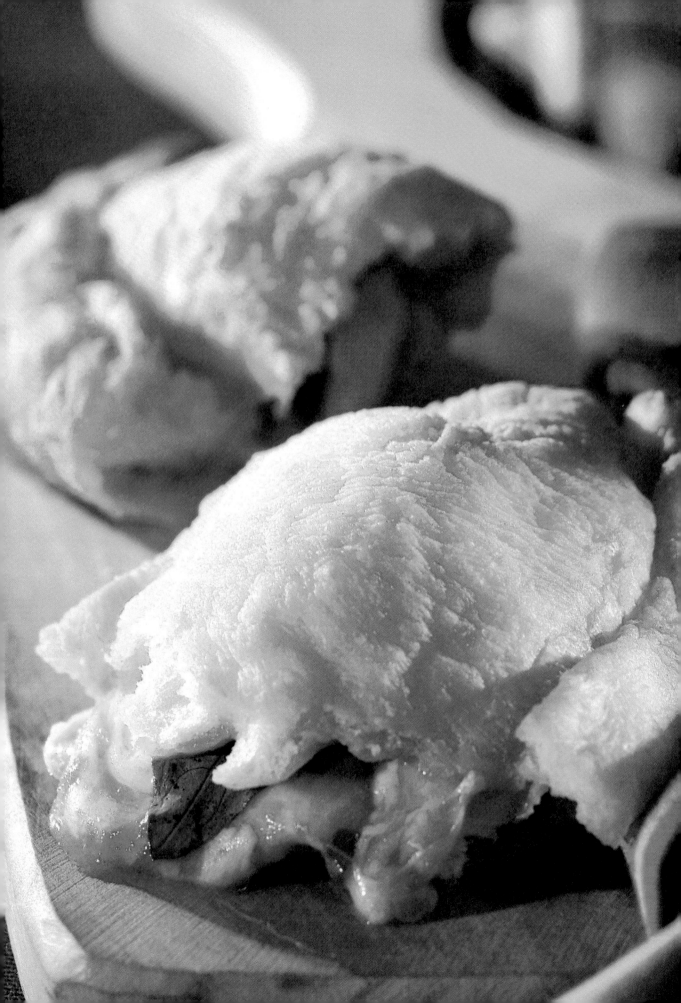

Sautéed Vegetables and Bean Sprouts (page 254)

Sides

Fried Rice

Serves 4

Preparation time
45 minutes

Cooking time
35 minutes

Tip
You can use leftover
rice cooked the
day before to make
this recipe.

- Preheat oven to 350°F (180°C)
- Ovenproof saucepan

2 tbsp	vegetable oil, divided	30 mL
1 cup	finely chopped onions	250 mL
2 cups	basmati rice	500 mL
2¾ cups	water	675 mL
	Salt and freshly ground black pepper	
2	eggs	2
1 cup	diced carrots	250 mL
1 cup	diced red bell peppers	250 mL
1 cup	diced zucchini	250 mL
2 tsp	chopped garlic	10 mL
¼ cup	thinly sliced green onions	60 mL
1 tbsp	grated fresh gingerroot	15 mL
1½ tsp	soy sauce	7 mL
	Sesame oil	
1 cup	cooked or frozen green peas, thawed if frozen	250 mL
¾ cup	cooked or frozen shelled edamame, thawed if frozen	175 mL

1. In an ovenproof saucepan, heat half of the oil over medium-low heat. Add onions and cook, stirring, until softened but not browned, about 5 minutes. Stir in rice until well coated in oil and translucent. Add water and salt and pepper to taste. Bring to a boil over high heat.

2. Cover saucepan and transfer to oven. Bake until rice is tender and most of liquid is absorbed, about 18 minutes.

3. Meanwhile, in a bowl, whisk eggs until blended. In a large skillet, heat half of the remaining oil over medium heat. Pour in eggs and cook, without stirring, until set. Transfer to a cutting board and cut into thin strips. Set aside.

4. Return skillet to low heat and add remaining oil. Add carrots and cook, stirring, until softened but not browned, about 5 minutes. Increase heat to high and add bell peppers and zucchini and cook, stirring, until tender, about 3 minutes. Add garlic and green onions and cook, stirring, for 1 minute.

5. Stir in rice, ginger, soy sauce, and sesame oil to taste. Add egg strips, peas and edamame and stir gently until heated through. Season with salt and pepper to taste.

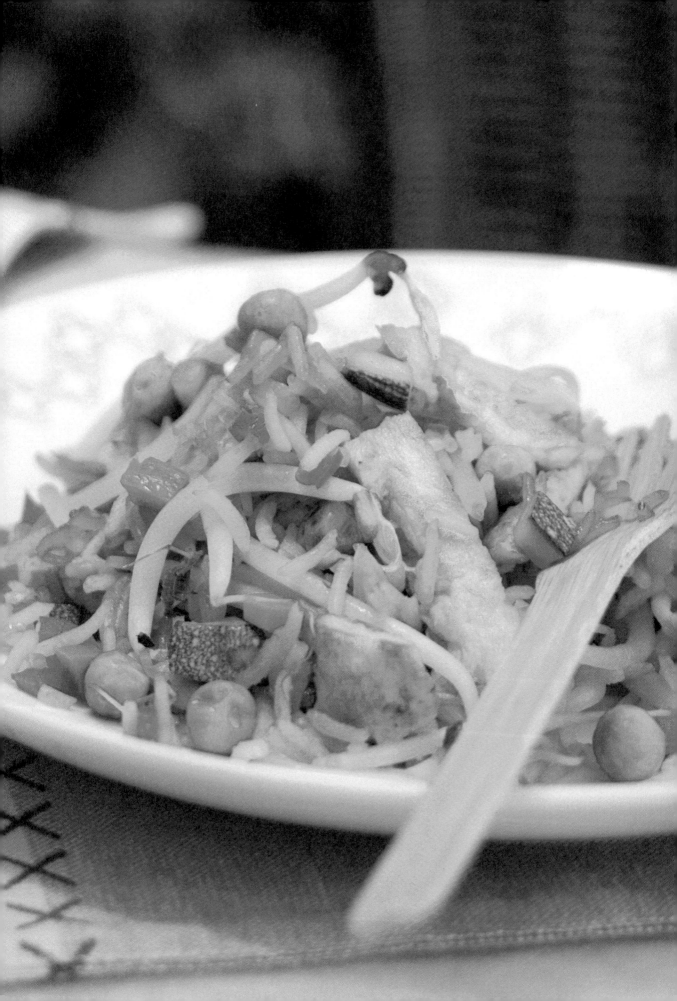

Sweet Moroccan-Style Couscous

Serves 4

Preparation time
10 minutes

Cooking time
20 minutes

Tip

This recipe makes an excellent dessert minus the garlic.

2 cups	Vegetable Stock (page 128) or reduced-sodium ready-to-use vegetable broth	500 mL
1	small clove garlic, crushed	1
2 tbsp	packed brown sugar	30 mL
$\frac{1}{8}$ tsp	ground nutmeg	0.5 mL
Pinch	ground cumin	Pinch
Pinch	ground cinnamon	Pinch
1	whole clove	1
	Salt and freshly ground black pepper	
	Cayenne pepper	
1 cup	pitted prunes	250 mL
1 cup	dried apricots	250 mL
1 cup	pitted dates	250 mL
$\frac{1}{2}$ cup	raisins	125 mL
8	dried figs	8
1 cup	couscous	250 mL
2 tbsp	butter, cut into pieces	30 mL
$\frac{1}{2}$ cup	toasted slivered almonds	125 mL
1 tbsp	confectioner's (icing) sugar	15 mL

1. In a pot, combine vegetable stock, garlic, brown sugar, nutmeg, cumin, cinnamon, clove, and salt, black pepper and cayenne pepper to taste. Bring to a boil over medium heat. Cover, reduce heat to low and simmer until flavors are blended, about 10 minutes. Remove from heat and remove garlic clove.

2. Transfer $1\frac{1}{4}$ cups (300 mL) of the broth to another saucepan. Set aside.

3. Add prunes, apricots, dates, raisins and figs to remaining broth in pot. Cover and let stand until fruit is soft and plump, about 10 minutes.

4. Meanwhile, bring saucepan of reserved broth to a boil over high heat. Gradually stir in couscous. Cover, remove from heat and let stand until couscous is softened and liquid is absorbed, about 5 minutes. Add butter and stir gently with a fork.

5. Mound couscous in 4 warmed serving bowls. Using a slotted spoon, remove fruit from broth and spoon over couscous. Ladle just enough of the broth overtop to moisten. Sprinkle with almonds and confectioner's sugar.

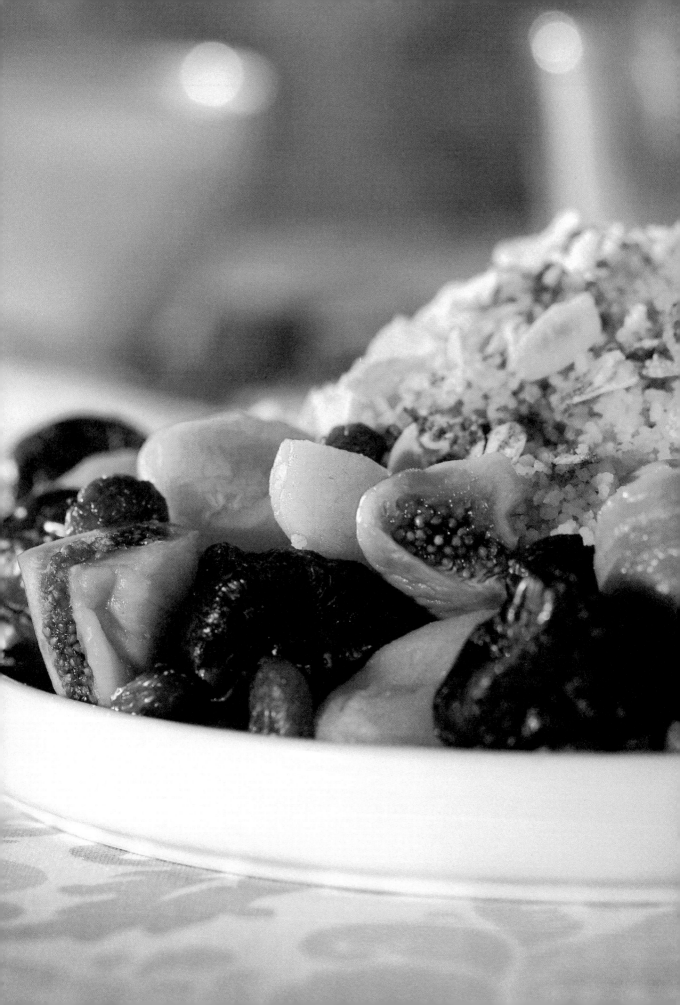

Greek-Style Vegetables

Tip

To "turn" a vegetable means to pare pieces into a regular, rounded football-like shape to improve its presentation and facilitate cooking. You can cut the vegetables into chunks for a more casual presentation.

4	artichokes	4
	Juice of 1 lemon, divided	
1 tbsp	olive oil	15 mL
1	onion, chopped	1
1	clove garlic, minced	1
1 lb	cauliflower florets	500 g
1	bouquet garni (see Tip, page 214)	1
1 tsp	coriander seeds	5 mL
	Salt	
	Whole black peppercorns	
2 tsp	white wine	10 mL
2	zucchini, each about 8 oz (250 g), cut into chunks (see Tip, left)	2
1 lb	mushrooms, such as button, quartered	500 g

1. Remove all the leaves from each artichoke and scoop out the fuzzy purple choke. Cut off stem and trim until only tender bottom remains. As you work, place trimmed artichokes in a bowl with 1 tbsp (15 mL) of the lemon juice and water to cover. Set aside.

2. In a large sauté pan or skillet with a lid, heat oil over medium heat. Add onion and garlic and cook, stirring, until softened but not browned, about 5 minutes.

3. Drain artichokes and add to pan with cauliflower, bouquet garni, coriander seeds, and salt and peppercorns to taste. Stir in wine and $\frac{1}{2}$ cup (125 mL) water and bring to a boil. Cover, reduce heat to low and simmer until cauliflower starts to soften, about 10 minutes.

4. Stir in zucchini, cover and simmer for 3 minutes. Stir in mushrooms, cover and simmer until vegetables are tender-crisp, about 5 minutes longer. Using a slotted spoon, transfer vegetables to a bowl, leaving liquid and bouquet garni in pan.

5. Increase heat and bring liquid left in pan to a boil. Boil gently until reduced and flavorful. Season with remaining lemon juice to taste. Discard bouquet garni and pour dressing over vegetables. Cover and refrigerate until chilled, about 2 hours. Serve cold.

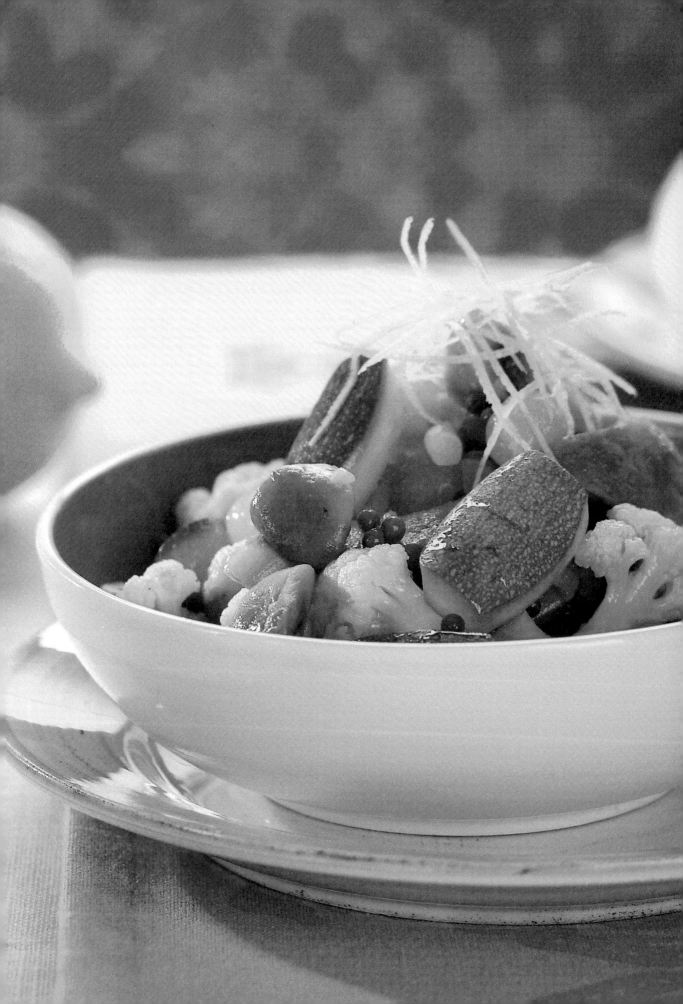

Bassano del Grappa White Asparagus

See photo, opposite

Serves 4

Preparation time
20 minutes

Cooking time
17 minutes

Tip

This simple traditional way of preparing asparagus is typical of Bassano del Grappa, Igor Brotto's native city in the province of Venice, renowned for the white asparagus cultivated there. This recipe highlights the delicate natural bitterness of the vegetable.

24	spears white asparagus	24
4	eggs	4
	Salt and freshly ground pepper	
1 tbsp	red wine vinegar	15 mL
¼ cup	extra virgin olive oil	60 mL

1. Using a vegetable peeler, peel asparagus, except for the tips, taking care not to break them. Cut about 1 inch (2.5 cm) off the bottom to remove the tough and fibrous stem.

2. In a pot of boiling salted water over medium heat, boil asparagus gently until tips are tender without breaking and stems are firm, about 15 minutes. Drain well.

3. Meanwhile, place eggs in a saucepan and add cold water to cover. Bring to a boil over high heat. Remove from heat, cover and let stand for 17 minutes to hard-cook. Run under cold water just until cool enough to handle. Drain and peel while still hot.

4. In a bowl, using a fork, immediately mash eggs. Add salt and pepper to taste. Stir in vinegar and olive oil until a creamy sauce is obtained.

5. Arrange asparagus in individual dishes and serve immediately with the warm sauce on the side. (You can also pour the sauce over the asparagus.)

Red Cabbage with Apples

Serves 4

Preparation time
20 minutes

Cooking time
45 minutes

3 tbsp	butter	45 mL
¾ cup	finely chopped onion	175 mL
8 oz	red cabbage, trimmed and cut into thin strips	250 g
	Salt and freshly ground black pepper	
1 tbsp	red wine vinegar	15 mL
4	Golden Delicious or other sweet, firm apples	4
1 tbsp	packed brown sugar	15 mL

1. In a saucepan, melt butter over medium heat. Add onion and cook, stirring, until softened but not browned, about 3 minutes. Stir in cabbage and season with salt and pepper to taste. Stir in vinegar and 1 to 2 tbsp (15 to 30 mL) water, if necessary, to prevent burning. Reduce heat to low, cover and cook until cabbage is soft, about 45 minutes, adding more water if mixture gets too dry.

2. Meanwhile, peel apples and cut into ½-inch (1 cm) pieces.

3. Stir apples and brown sugar into cabbage mixture. Cover and cook until apples are tender, 15 to 20 minutes.

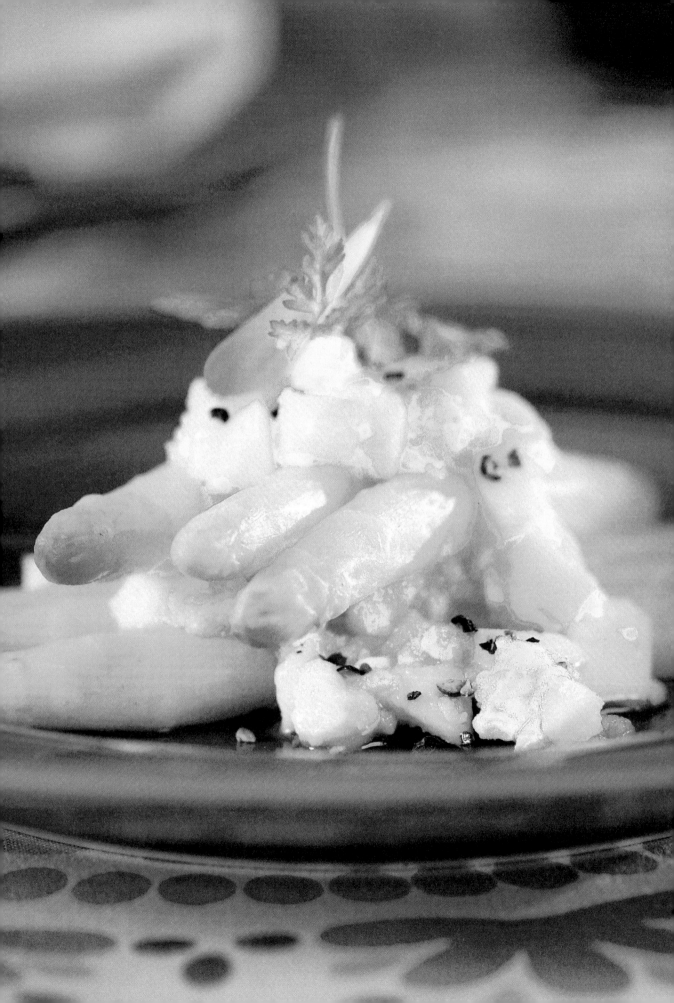

Endives au Gratin

Serves 4

Preparation time
55 minutes

Cooking time
35 minutes

Tip

When buying cheese, read the label carefully and make sure to buy those that are not made from animal rennet.

Variation

You can substitute grated vegetarian-friendly Parmesan cheese for some of the Gruyère cheese.

- Preheat oven to 475°F (250°C)
- Baking dish, buttered

2 lbs	Belgian endives (about 4 large)	1 kg
1 tbsp	butter	15 mL
	Juice of ½ lemon	
¼ cup	water	60 mL
	Salt	

Mornay Sauce

2 cups	milk	500 mL
3 tbsp	butter	45 mL
3 tbsp	all-purpose flour	45 mL
	Salt	
	Cayenne pepper	
	Nutmeg	
7 oz	Gruyère cheese, shredded, divided (see Tip, left)	210 g

1. Remove thick outer leaves from endives. In a saucepan, combine endives, butter, lemon juice, water, and salt to taste. Bring to a boil over medium-high heat. Reduce heat to low, cover and simmer for 20 to 30 minutes or until fork-tender. Drain well and set aside.

2. *Mornay Sauce:* In a saucepan, bring milk almost to a boil over medium heat. In another saucepan, melt butter over medium heat. Sprinkle with flour and cook, stirring, for 1 minute to make a roux.

3. Gradually pour hot milk over roux, blending well with a whisk. Season with salt, cayenne pepper and nutmeg to taste. Bring to a boil. Reduce heat and boil gently, whisking, until thick, about 10 minutes. Remove from heat and stir in shredded Gruyère until melted and smooth.

4. Squeeze endives to remove as much water as possible. Arrange in prepared baking dish so endives are side by side. Top with Mornay sauce. Sprinkle with remaining Gruyère cheese.

5. Bake in preheated oven until cheese is melted and top is browned, about 5 minutes.

Braised Endives in Maple Syrup

2 tbsp	butter, divided	30 mL
6	small Belgian endives, cut in half lengthwise	6
	Salt	
1 tbsp	pure maple syrup	15 mL
1 tsp	freshly squeezed lemon juice	5 mL

1. In a skillet, melt half the butter over medium heat. Add endives, cut sides facing down. Sprinkle with salt to taste and drizzle with maple syrup and lemon juice.

2. Pour in enough water to come halfway up sides of endives. Cut remaining butter into small pieces and scatter overtop. Cover and boil until endives are almost tender, about 10 minutes.

3. Uncover and boil until sauce is slightly reduced and endives are tender, 5 to 10 minutes. Serve endives with sauce spooned overtop.

Jerusalem Artichokes en Papillote

Tip

"En papillote" means enclosed in a wrapping, sometimes in parchment paper but in this case foil. The food steams and bakes within the wrapping.

● **Preheat oven to 300°F (150°C)**

2 lbs	Jerusalem artichokes	1 kg
2 tbsp	olive oil	30 mL
4	whole cloves garlic	4
1	sprig thyme	1
	Salt and freshly ground black pepper	
¼ cup	butter	60 mL
1 tbsp	finely chopped fresh chives	15 mL

1. Scrub Jerusalem artichokes thoroughly under running water. In a pot of boiling salted water, boil artichokes for 10 minutes. Drain well.

2. Place artichokes in foil (see Tip, left). Sprinkle with olive oil, garlic cloves, thyme, and salt and pepper to taste.

3. Seal papillote well and place on a baking sheet or in a baking dish. Bake in preheated oven for 1 hour to 1 hour 30 minutes.

4. When Jerusalem artichokes are completely cooked, remove from oven and open papillote. Let cool for a few minutes before peeling them, but they should still be hot. Cut into large pieces.

5. In a skillet, melt butter over medium heat. Add artichoke pieces and sauté until soft but not browned. Adjust seasoning and add chives.

Frico

1 tbsp	butter	15 mL
½	onion, finely chopped	½
2 tbsp	olive oil	30 mL
2	medium-size potatoes, diced	2
	Salt and freshly ground black pepper	
10 oz	Montasio cheese, shredded (see Tip, left)	300 g

1. In a nonstick skillet, melt butter over low heat. Add onion and cook, stirring, until softened but not browned, about 8 minutes. Transfer to a bowl and set aside.

2. In same skillet, heat olive oil over medium heat. Add potatoes and cook, stirring, until tender and golden brown, about 10 minutes. Season with salt and pepper to taste.

3. Stir reserved onions and cheese into potatoes and spread out in an even layer. Reduce heat to low and cook until cheese is melted and a golden brown crust forms on the bottom. Invert a plate on top of the skillet and flip frico onto plate. Slide back into skillet and cook until second side is golden brown and crisp. Slide onto a cutting board and cut into wedges or break into chips.

Garlic Scape Tomato Fondue

Serves 4

Preparation time
10 minutes

Cooking time
20 minutes

Tip

Garlic scapes are the seed stalks of growing garlic that shoot up from the bulb in the spring. Look for them at farmers' markets and specialty produce shops.

¼ cup	extra virgin olive oil	60 mL
1	large tomato, peeled, seeded and diced	1
	Salt and freshly ground black pepper	
8 oz	garlic scapes (see Tip, left)	250 g
2	large leaves fresh basil	2

1. In a saucepan, heat olive oil over low heat. Add tomato and cook, stirring, until a saucy texture, about 15 minutes. Season with salt and pepper to taste.

2. Meanwhile, in a pot of boiling salted water, boil garlic scapes until tender-crisp, about 5 minutes. Drain well.

3. Add garlic scapes to tomato sauce and simmer until tender, about 5 minutes. Serve garnished with basil leaves.

Gratin Dauphinois

Serves 4

Preparation time
15 minutes

Cooking time
40 minutes

Tip

Yellow-fleshed potatoes or oblong baking potatoes, such as russets, are best for this recipe, so the cream is absorbed while they bake. Waxy, round or new potatoes don't absorb the cream as well.

- Preheat oven to 400°F (200°C)
- 6-cup (1.5 L) baking dish

2 tsp	butter, softened	10 mL
1	clove garlic, minced	1
1½ lbs	yellow-fleshed or oblong baking potatoes (see Tip, left)	750 g
	Salt and freshly ground black pepper	
	Grated nutmeg	
1½ cups	heavy or whipping (35%) cream	375 mL

1. In a small bowl, combine butter and garlic and brush evenly in baking dish.

2. Peel potatoes, if desired, and cut into thin slices, about ⅛ inch (3 mm) thick. Layer in prepared baking dish, overlapping as necessary and seasoning each layer with salt, pepper and nutmeg. Pour cream evenly over potatoes and use a spatula to press potatoes down.

3. Bake in preheated oven until potatoes are tender and top is lightly browned, about 40 minutes. Let stand for 10 minutes before serving.

Cauliflower with Cheese Sauce

- Preheat oven to 400°F (200°C)
- 6-cup (1.5 L) baking dish, buttered

10 oz	cauliflower, cut into florets	300 g

Mornay Sauce

4 tbsp	butter, divided	60 mL
3 tbsp	all-purpose flour	45 mL
2 cups	milk	500 mL
	Salt	
	Cayenne pepper	
	Grated nutmeg	
5 oz	Gruyère cheese, shredded, divided	150 g

1. In a pot of boiling salted water, boil cauliflower until starting to soften, about 3 minutes. Drain well and spread on a baking sheet lined with paper towels to drain.

2. *Mornay Sauce:* In a saucepan, bring milk almost to a boil over medium heat. In another saucepan, melt 3 tbsp (45 mL) of the butter over medium heat. Sprinkle with flour and cook, stirring, for 1 minute to make a roux.

3. Gradually pour hot milk over roux, blending well with a whisk. Season with salt, cayenne pepper and nutmeg to taste. Bring to a boil. Reduce heat and boil gently, whisking, until thick, about 10 minutes. Remove from heat and stir in half of the shredded Gruyère, until melted and smooth.

4. Transfer cauliflower to prepared baking dish and pour Mornay sauce evenly overtop. Sprinkle with remaining cheese. Cut remaining butter into small pieces and sprinkle overtop.

5. Bake in preheated oven until cauliflower is tender and top is slightly browned, about 20 minutes.

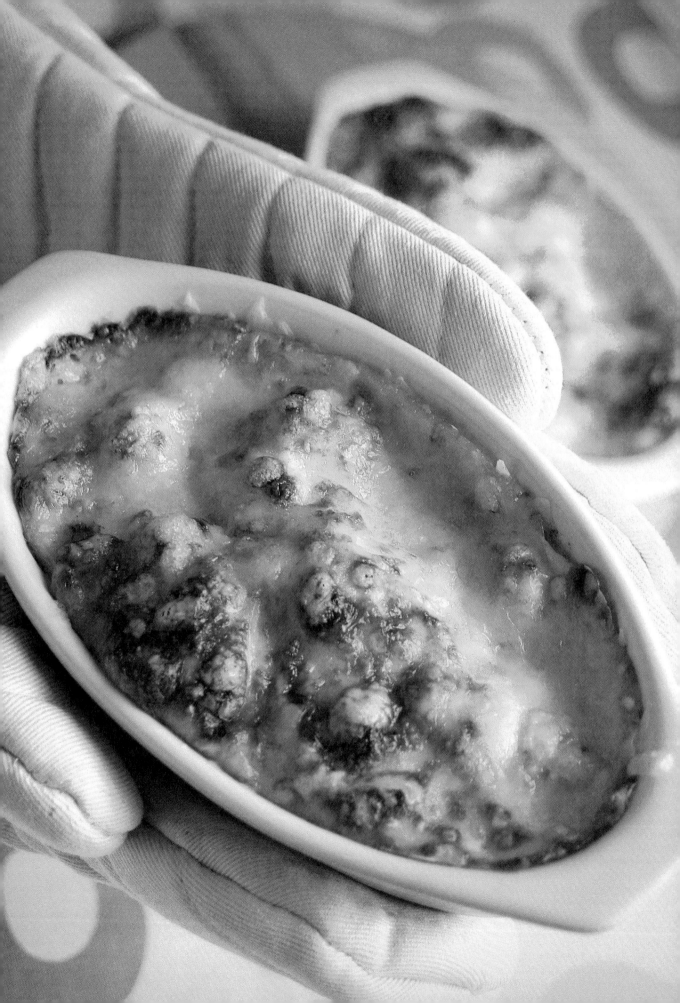

Mixed Baby Vegetable Fricassee

Serves 4

Preparation time
30 minutes

Cooking time
about 1 hour

1	bunch small white turnips	1
1	bunch baby carrots with tops	1
½ cup	sweet green peas	125 mL
8	baby new potatoes	8
2 tbsp	olive oil	30 mL
2 tbsp	butter	30 mL
1	sprig thyme	1
8	cippolini onions	8
½ cup	chopped parsley root	125 mL
	Salt and freshly ground black pepper	

1. Trim off all but ½ inch (1 cm) of the green tops of turnips and carrots. Scrub well if skins are thin and tender or peel, if desired.

2. Place turnips in a saucepan and add enough cold salted water to cover by 2 inches (5 cm). Bring to a boil over high heat. Reduce heat and boil gently for 10 minutes. Add carrots and boil gently until turnips and carrots are tender, about 10 minutes. Add peas and boil until peas are tender, 2 to 3 minutes. Drain well.

3. Place potatoes in another pot and add cold salted water to cover by 1 inch (2.5 cm). Bring to a boil over high heat. Reduce heat and boil gently until slightly tender, 5 to 10 minutes. Drain well.

4. In a large skillet, heat oil and butter over medium-high heat. Add potatoes and thyme and fry, stirring often, until starting to brown and are tender, about 10 minutes. Using tongs, transfer potatoes to a plate, leaving butter and oil in pan.

5. Add onions to pan and reduce heat to low. Cook, stirring often, until onions are tender and browned, about 10 minutes. Increase heat to medium-high and add parsley root. Cook, stirring, until tender, about 5 minutes. Add turnips, carrots, peas and potatoes to pan and season with salt and pepper to taste. Cook, stirring, until heated through. Discard thyme sprig.

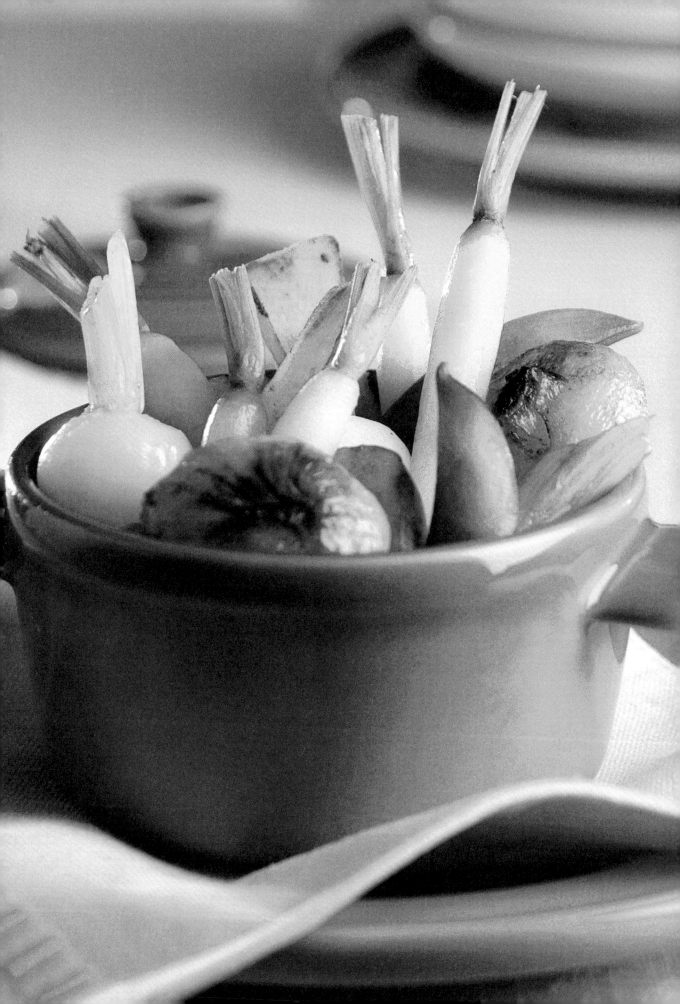

Grilled Vegetables

Serves 4

Preparation time
40 minutes

Cooking time
1 hour

Marinating time
1 hour

Tip

For the professional restaurant look on your grilled vegetables, place vegetables (this works best for the zucchini, eggplant and sweet potatoes) on grill grates on a slight angle. Once grill marks form, rotate the vegetable 90 degrees so the grill marks form a crosshatch pattern. Flip over and repeat on the second side.

4	green onions, trimmed	4
2 tbsp	olive oil	30 mL
1 tbsp	balsamic vinegar	15 mL
2 tsp	chopped fresh oregano	10 mL
1 tsp	chopped fresh thyme	5 mL
1 tsp	chopped fresh rosemary	5 mL
	Salt and freshly ground black pepper	
1	small zucchini, sliced lengthwise	1
1	small red bell pepper, cut lengthwise into triangles	1
$\frac{1}{2}$	small eggplant, sliced lengthwise	$\frac{1}{2}$
2 oz	oyster mushrooms	60 g
1	small sweet potato, unpeeled	1
2 tbsp	all-purpose flour (approx.)	30 mL

1. In a pot of boiling salted water, blanch green onions until bright green, about 2 minutes. Drain well and rinse under cold water to cool. Pat dry.

2. In a large shallow dish, combine oil, vinegar, oregano, thyme and rosemary. Season with salt and pepper to taste. Add green onions, zucchini, bell pepper, eggplant and mushrooms and turn to coat with marinade. Cover and marinate at room temperature for 30 minutes.

3. Preheat barbecue grill to medium-high heat.

4. Remove vegetables from marinade, shaking off and reserving excess marinade. Grill green onions, zucchini, bell pepper, eggplant and mushrooms, turning once, until tender and grill-marked, 5 to 10 minutes. Return to dish with remaining marinade and turn gently to coat. Let marinate at room temperature for 1 hour.

5. Meanwhile, preheat oven to 350°F (180°C).

6. Pierce sweet potato all over with a fork. Bake in preheated oven until just tender, about 40 minutes. Cut crosswise into $\frac{1}{2}$-inch (1 cm) thick slices.

7. Reheat grill to medium-high heat and grease grill.

8. Spread flour on a plate and dip sweet potato slices into flour, lightly coating both sides. Shake off excess. Place sweet potato on greased grill. Grill, turning once, until golden on both sides, about 5 minutes.

9. Arrange grilled vegetables on a large platter in a decorative fashion.

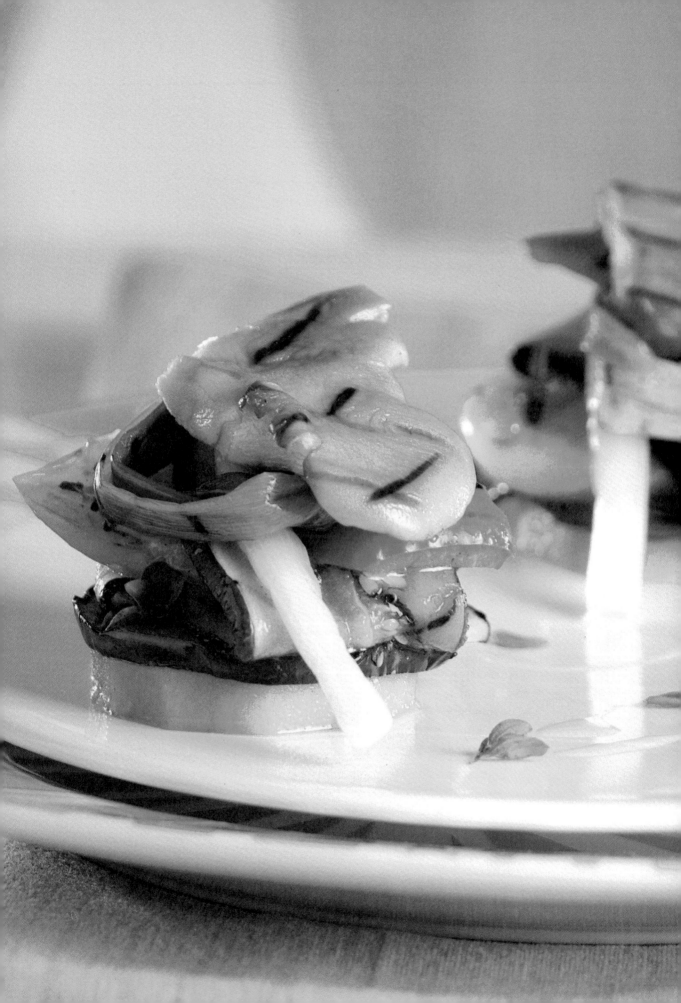

Sautéed Pattypan Squash

Serves 4			
	3 tbsp	extra virgin olive oil	45 mL
	16	small pattypan squash, quartered	16
Preparation time 10 minutes		Salt and freshly crushed black peppercorns	
	1	clove garlic, chopped	1
Cooking time 10 minutes	4	leaves fresh basil, chopped	4
	1 tbsp	chopped fresh marjoram	15 mL

1. In a skillet, heat olive oil over medium-high heat. Add squash and season with salt and pepper to taste. Cook, stirring, until squash is tender and golden brown, about 8 minutes.

2. Stir in garlic, basil and marjoram and cook, stirring, until garlic is fragrant, about 1 minute.

Seasoned Green Peas

Serves 4			
	2 tbsp	olive oil	30 mL
	½ cup	finely chopped French shallots	125 mL
Preparation time 45 minutes	1	clove garlic, chopped	1
	1	large tomato, peeled, seeded and diced	1
Cooking time 35 minutes	¼ cup	butter	60 mL
	1	onion, finely chopped	1
	4	leaves lettuce, shredded	4
	1	bulb fennel, trimmed and thinly sliced	1
	1	bouquet garni (see Tip, page 214)	1
	2 cups	fresh or frozen green peas (thawed if frozen)	500 mL
	2 tbsp	water	30 mL
		Salt and freshly ground black pepper	
		Granulated sugar	

1. In a saucepan, heat olive oil over medium heat. Add shallots and cook, stirring, until softened but not browned, about 3 minutes. Add garlic and tomato and cook, stirring, until tomatoes are very soft but not reduced to a purée, about 10 minutes. Set aside.

2. Meanwhile, in a large skillet, melt butter over medium heat. Add onion and cook, stirring, until softened but not browned, about 3 minutes.

3. Stir in lettuce, fennel, bouquet garni and fresh peas (if using thawed frozen peas, add for last 5 minutes of cooking). Season with salt, pepper and sugar to taste. Reduce heat and simmer, stirring occasionally, until fennel and peas are tender, about 10 minutes.

4. Stir in tomato mixture and simmer, stirring, until hot and bubbly.

Roasted New Potatoes with Oregano and Parmesan Cheese

- Preheat oven to 300°F (150°C)
- 8-cup (2 L) shallow baking dish, greased

2 lbs	new (grelot) potatoes	1 kg
1	red onion, thinly sliced	1
2 tbsp	chopped fresh oregano	30 mL
3 oz	vegetarian-friendly Parmesan cheese, grated (see Tip, page 234)	90 g
½ cup	bread crumbs	125 mL
¼ cup	olive oil	60 mL
	Salt and freshly ground black pepper	

1. Scrub potatoes under running water. If potatoes are large, cut in half.

2. In a bowl, combine potatoes, red onion, oregano, cheese, bread crumbs, olive oil, and salt and pepper to taste. Spread in prepared baking dish.

3. Bake in preheated oven, stirring often, until potatoes are tender and browned, about 1 hour and 15 minutes.

Mashed Sweet Potatoes with Beurre Noisette

Tip

For the best flavor, we recommend freshly grating whole nutmeg rather than using pre-ground nutmeg. You can buy whole nutmeg at spice shops, online and at well-stocked supermarkets.

- Preheat oven to 350°F (180°C)
- Baking sheet, lined with foil

2½ lbs	sweet potatoes (about 3 large)	1.25 kg
3 tbsp	olive oil	45 mL
	Salt and freshly ground black pepper	
1	sprig thyme	1
3	cloves garlic	3
6 tbsp	butter	90 mL
	Freshly grated nutmeg (see Tip, left)	

1. Place sweet potatoes in center of prepared baking sheet, drizzle with olive oil and season with salt and pepper to taste. Place thyme and garlic between potatoes. Fold up foil to enclose potatoes and seal edges.

2. Bake in preheated oven until potatoes are tender, about 2 hours.

3. Meanwhile, to make beurre noisette, in a small saucepan, cook butter over medium heat until a hazelnut-brown color, reducing heat as necessary to prevent burning. Remove from heat and keep warm.

4. Peel skins from potatoes and place flesh in a large bowl. Using a potato masher, mash potatoes, gradually adding beurre noisette. Season with nutmeg, salt and pepper to taste.

Stuffed Potatoes

See photo, opposite

Serves 4

Preparation time
45 minutes

Cooking time
30 minutes

- Preheat oven to 350°F (180°C)
- Rimmed baking sheet, parchment paper

4	medium yellow-fleshed potatoes (about 1½ lbs/750 g)	4
4	yellow tomatoes, peeled and cut in half lengthwise	4
4 tbsp	extra virgin olive oil, divided	60 mL
	Salt and freshly ground black pepper	
4	stems fresh chives, finely chopped	4

1. Scrub potatoes under cold running water and pierce all over with a fork. Bake in preheated oven until tender, about 45 minutes.

2. Meanwhile, place tomatoes cut side down on prepared baking sheet. Drizzle with half of the olive oil and season with salt and pepper. Bake until very soft, about 20 minutes. Transfer to a bowl and mash lightly.

3. Cut potatoes in half and scoop flesh into a bowl, leaving ¼-inch (0.5 cm) thick walls.

4. Mash potato flesh in bowl until smooth. Stir in half of the crushed tomatoes and remaining olive oil. Season with salt and pepper to taste. Spoon into potato shells, heaping as necessary. Drizzle remaining crushed tomatoes on top and sprinkle with chives.

Potato and Mango Purée with Tarragon

Serves 4

Preparation time
15 minutes

Cooking time
20 minutes

2 lbs	yellow-fleshed potatoes, peeled and cut into chunks	1 kg
1¼ cups	butter, cut into pieces and softened	300 mL
1 cup	puréed mango (see Tip, left)	250 mL
1 tsp	chopped fresh tarragon	5 mL
	Heavy or whipping (35%) cream, optional	
	Salt	

Tip

For the mango purée, peel and purée 2 very ripe mangos in a food processor or with an immersion blender, then measure 1 cup (250 mL) purée. Alternatively, you can use drained canned mango or thawed frozen mango.

1. Place potatoes in a large pot and add cold salted water to cover. Bring to a boil over high heat. Reduce heat and boil gently until potatoes are tender, about 20 minutes.

2. Drain potatoes well and return to pot over low heat. Using a potato masher, mash potatoes, incorporating butter. Stir in mango purée and tarragon, adding a little cream, if desired, for a softer consistency. Season with salt to taste.

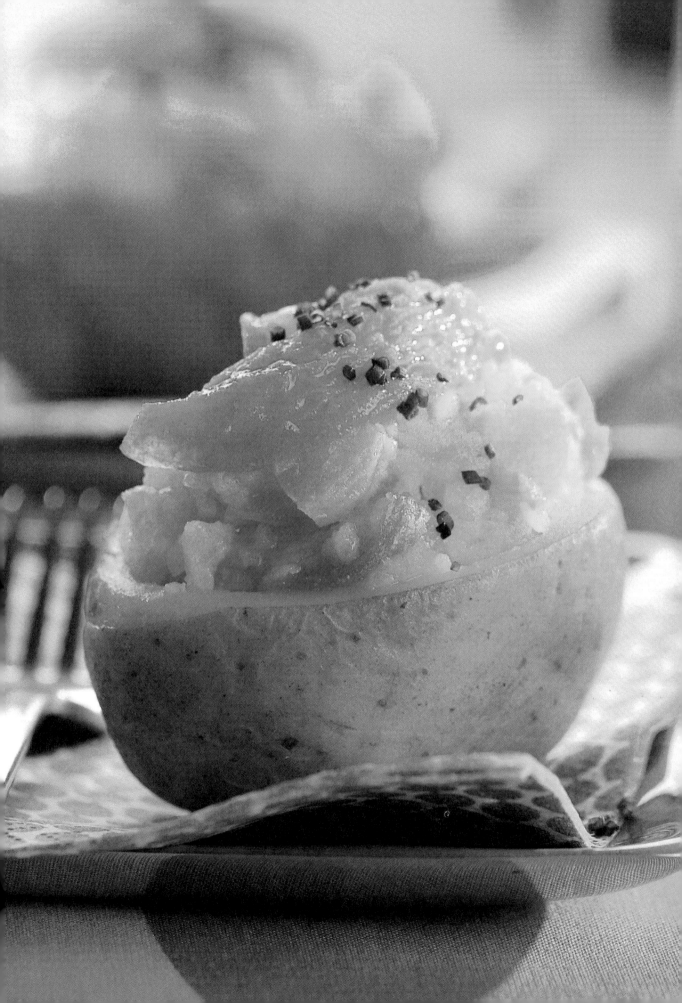

Mashed Potatoes with Goat Cheese, Sun-Dried Tomatoes and Basil

Serves 4

Preparation time
20 minutes

Cooking time
20 minutes

Tips

It's important not to cut potatoes into small pieces before boiling them, as they risk turning soggy. Cut them into large chunks, keeping the size as uniform as possible.

It's important to avoid boiling the potatoes too vigorously, to prevent them from breaking apart, which will make them lose some of their starch.

2 lbs	yellow-fleshed potatoes, peeled and cut into chunks (see Tips, left)	1 kg
7 oz	soft goat cheese	210 g
	Heavy or whipping (35%) cream	
¾ cup	butter, cut into pieces and softened (approx.)	175 mL
⅓ cup	diced sun-dried tomatoes	75 mL
¼ cup	finely chopped fresh basil	60 mL
	Salt	

1. Place potatoes in a large pot and add cold salted water to cover. Bring to a boil over high heat. Reduce heat and boil gently until potatoes are tender, about 20 minutes.

2. Meanwhile, in a bowl, mash goat cheese, adding just enough cream to make a slightly soft, creamy consistency.

3. Drain potatoes and return to pot over low heat. Using a potato masher, mash potatoes, adding cheese mixture and enough of the butter to make a soft, creamy consistency. Stir in tomatoes and basil and season with salt to taste.

Funghi Trifolati

Serves 4

Preparation time
10 minutes

Cooking time
8 minutes

6 tbsp	extra virgin olive oil	90 mL
4 oz	button mushrooms, thinly sliced	125 g
4 oz	oyster mushrooms, thinly sliced	125 g
4 oz	shiitake mushrooms, stems removed, caps thinly sliced	125 g
	Salt and freshly crushed black peppercorns	
2	large cloves garlic, chopped	2
¼ cup	chopped fresh Italian flat-leaf parsley	60 mL

1. In a large skillet, heat olive oil over medium-high heat. Add mushrooms and cook, stirring, until tender and starting to brown, about 7 minutes. Season with salt and peppercorns to taste.

2. Stir in garlic and parsley and cook, stirring, until garlic is fragrant, about 1 minute.

Beurre Noisette Chestnut Purée

1	can (30 oz/860 g) water-packed peeled whole chestnuts, drained	1
1 cup	heavy or whipping (35%) cream	250 mL
1	sprig savory	1
¼ cup	butter	60 mL
	Salt and freshly ground black pepper	

1. In a saucepan, combine chestnuts, cream and savory. Bring to a simmer over medium heat, stirring often. Simmer until chestnuts are hot and softened, about 10 minutes.

2. Drain chestnuts and place in a bowl, reserving cream and discarding savory sprig. Return cream to saucepan and bring to a boil over medium-high heat. Reduce heat and boil, stirring often, until cream is reduced by about half.

3. Meanwhile, to make beurre noisette, in a small saucepan, cook butter over medium heat until a hazelnut-brown color, reducing heat as necessary to prevent burning. Remove from heat and keep warm.

4. Using an electric mixer, beat chestnuts until smooth. Beat in beurre noisette and enough of the reduced cream to make a creamy consistency. Season with salt and pepper to taste.

Caramelized Herbed Salsify

Tip

Salsify is a root vegetable that looks similar to parsnip with white flesh and gray or golden skin, or the less common black-skinned version. It is also known as oyster plant for its slight similarity in flavor to fresh oysters.

4 cups	water	1 L
	Juice of 1 lemon	
2 lbs	salsify (see Tip, left)	1 kg
2 tbsp	olive oil	30 mL
¼ cup	butter, divided	60 mL
1	sprig rosemary	1
1	sprig savory	1
	Salt and freshly ground black pepper	

1. In a bowl, combine water and lemon juice. Peel salsify, adding to lemon water as you work to prevent browning. Cut into pieces about 4 inches (10 cm) long, returning to lemon water as they're cut. Drain well and pat dry.

2. In a large skillet, heat olive oil and half of the butter over medium-high heat. Add salsify, rosemary and savory, stirring to coat. Reduce heat to low and cook, stirring often, until salsify is tender and caramelized, about 30 minutes. Stir in remaining butter and a little water, if necessary, to moisten. Season with salt and pepper to taste.

Vegetable and Mushroom Ragoût

Serves 4

Preparation time
35 minutes

Cooking time
45 minutes

Tip

We like to use a mixture of wild mushrooms such as pieds bleus, pieds-de-mouton and black trumpets for this recipe. However, you can use any mixture you prefer.

Variation

We like to add about 1½ oz (45 g) salicorne (also called salicornia, samphire or glasswort), a succulent plant that grows in salt marshes, on beaches and in mangroves. It has a fresh green, salty flavor similar to young asparagus. Boil it in unsalted water until bright green and tender, then drain well. Add with the vegetables in Step 5.

4	small yellow beets	4
4	small red beets	4
4	baby fennel bulbs	4
¼ cup	butter, divided	60 mL
8	pearl onions, peeled (about 4 oz/125 g)	8
	Salt	
	Granulated sugar	
9 oz	wild or exotic mushrooms, sliced if necessary (see Tip, left)	270 g
4	baby zucchini, sliced	4
4	baby pattypan squash	4
	Freshly ground pepper	
	Chopped fresh Italian flat-leaf parsley	

1. Place yellow beets and red beets in two separate saucepans and add cold salted water to cover. Bring to a boil over high heat. Reduce heat and boil gently until the skin is easy to remove and beets are tender, 30 to 45 minutes. (Cooking time will vary according to the size of the beets.) Drain and let cool. Trim off remaining stems and tap roots. Peel off skins and cut beets into quarters.

2. Meanwhile, trim root end and any stalks off fennel bulbs. In a pot of boiling water, blanch fennel bulbs until starting to get tender, about 5 minutes. Drain well.

3. In a large skillet, melt 1 tbsp (15 mL) of the butter over medium heat. Add onions and cook, stirring, until outsides start to soften, about 5 minutes. Add ¼ cup (60 mL) water and season with salt and sugar to taste. Reduce heat to medium-low and simmer, stirring often, until liquid is evaporated and onions are soft and golden, about 20 minutes. Transfer to a bowl.

4. In same skillet, melt 2 tbsp (30 mL) of the remaining butter over high heat. Add mushrooms and cook, stirring, until tender and golden brown, about 8 minutes.

5. Add fennel, onions, zucchini and pattypan squash and enough water to make a thin layer in the skillet. Reduce heat and simmer, stirring often and adding more water as necessary to keep pan moist, until vegetables are tender, about 15 minutes.

6. Stir in beets and season with salt and pepper to taste. Simmer, stirring, until beets are heated through. Stir in remaining butter until melted and sprinkle with parsley.

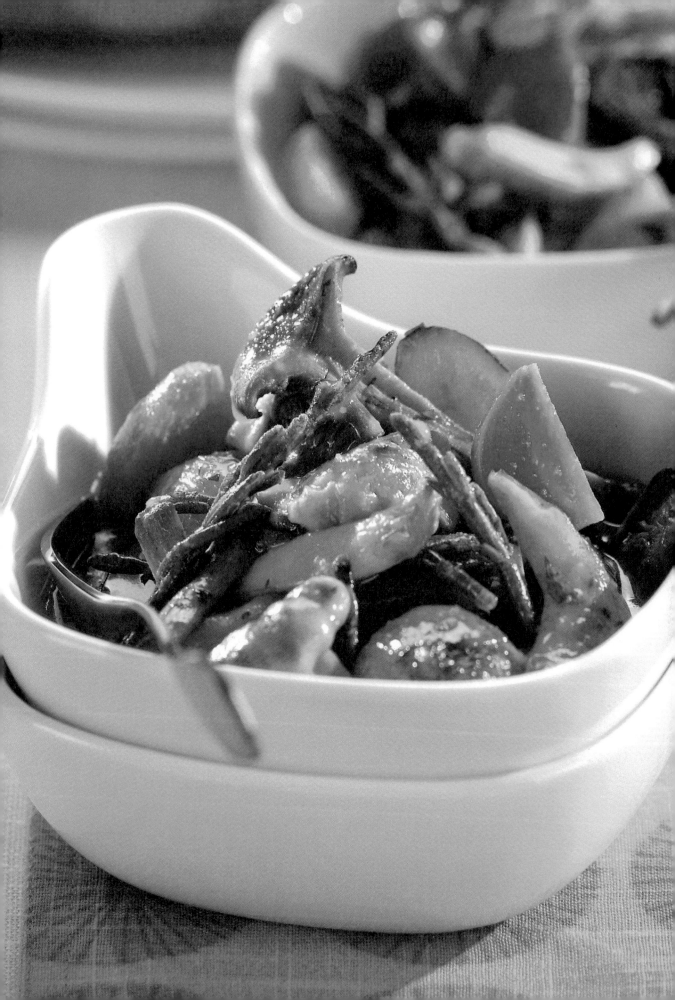

Ratatouille

See photo, opposite

Serves 4

Preparation time
40 minutes

Cooking time
20 minutes

Tip

Ratatouille has many uses in recipes and as a sauce. It can be served hot or cold.

2 tbsp	olive oil	30 mL
1	onion, diced	1
½	small eggplant, diced	½
1	small red bell pepper, diced	1
1	small green bell pepper, diced	1
1	tomato, diced	1
2	cloves garlic, chopped	2
1	bouquet garni (see Tip, page 214)	1
	Salt and freshly ground black pepper	

1. In a saucepan, heat oil over medium heat. Add onion and cook, stirring, until softened, about 5 minutes. Add eggplant and cook, stirring, until liquid is released and eggplant starts to brown, about 5 minutes.

2. Stir in red and green bell peppers and cook, stirring, until peppers start to soften, about 3 minutes. Stir in tomato, garlic and bouquet garni and season with salt and pepper to taste.

3. Reduce heat and simmer, stirring often, until vegetables are soft and ratatouille is thickened, about 15 minutes or until desired consistency. Discard bouquet garni.

Grilled Treviso Radicchio

Serves 4

Preparation time
5 minutes

Cooking time
20 minutes

Tip

Treviso is a highly prized variety of radicchio grown in the province of Treviso, in the Veneto region. It is a seasonal product available there from November to March. Its white stems are very straight and surrounded by a very thin red leaf that is not fully developed. In Italy it is given the name *spadone*, which means "broadsword."

- Preheat barbecue grill or grill pan to medium-high
- Preheat oven to 350°F (180°C)
- Shallow baking dish

2	heads Treviso radicchio (see Tip, left)	2
¼ cup	olive oil, divided	60 mL
	Salt and freshly ground black pepper	

1. Trim off root end and any damaged outer leaves of radicchio heads and rinse well. Cut lengthwise into quarters and place in a bowl. Add half of the olive oil and season with salt to taste. Toss to coat.

2. Place radicchio wedges, cut side down, on preheated grill. Grill just until grill marks appear, about 3 minutes. Turn to mark remaining cut side (do not let burn). Transfer to baking dish.

3. Bake in preheated oven until radicchio is tender, about 15 minutes. Drizzle with remaining olive oil and season with pepper to taste.

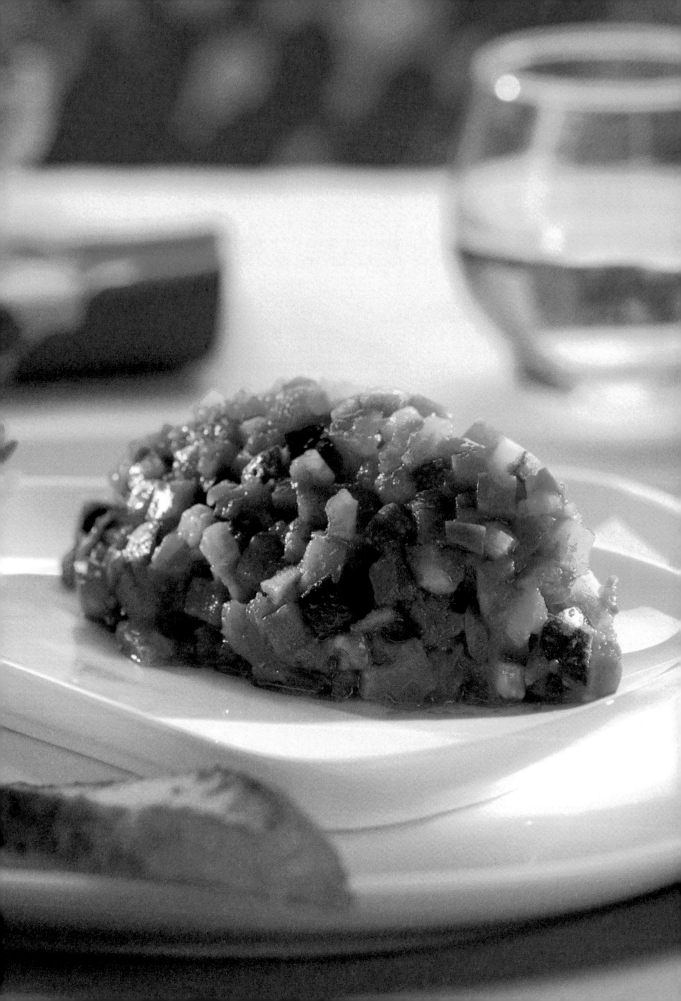

Sautéed Vegetables and Bean Sprouts

Serves 4		

Preparation time
15 minutes

Cooking time
5 minutes

¼ cup	vegetable oil	60 mL
1	carrot, cut into strips	1
1	stalk celery, thinly sliced	1
2½ oz	shiitake mushroom caps	75 g
1	head broccoli, cut into florets	1
½	red bell pepper, thinly sliced	½
2	baby bok choy, trimmed	2
½	can (14 to 15 oz/400 to 425 mL) baby corn, drained	½
1	can (8 oz/227 mL) sliced water chestnuts, drained	1
	Salt and freshly ground black pepper	
¼ cup	mirin	60 mL
2 cups	bean sprouts	500 mL

1. In a wok or large skillet, heat oil over high heat. Add carrot and celery and stir-fry for 1 minute. Add mushrooms and broccoli and stir-fry for 1 minute.

2. Add bell pepper, bok choy, baby corn and water chestnuts and stir-fry just until vegetables are tender-crisp, about 2 minutes. Season with salt and pepper to taste and stir in mirin. Add bean sprouts and stir-fry just until wilted, about 30 seconds.

Rice Pilaf with Cardamom

Serves 4 to 8		

Preparation time
5 minutes

Cooking time
20 minutes

- Preheat oven to 400°F (200°C)
- Ovenproof saucepan with lid

½ cup	butter, divided	125 mL
1 cup	finely chopped onions	250 mL
2 cups	basmati rice	500 mL
2¾ cups	water, Vegetable Stock (page 128) or ready-to-use-broth	675 mL
1	bouquet garni (see Tip, page 214)	1
	Salt and freshly ground black pepper	
	Ground cardamom	

1. In ovenproof saucepan, melt half of the butter over medium heat. Add onions and cook, stirring, until softened but not browned, about 5 minutes. Add rice and cook, stirring, until well coated with butter, about 2 minutes.

2. Stir in water and bouquet garni and season with salt, pepper and cardamom to taste. Bring to a boil.

3. Cover pan and transfer to preheated oven. Bake until rice is tender, about 18 minutes. Let stand, covered, for 5 minutes. Fluff with a fork and gently stir in remaining butter until melted. Discard bouquet garni.

Risi e Bisi

Tip
This dish is halfway between a risotto and a soup. It is eaten with a spoon.

4 cups	Vegetable Stock (page 128) or ready-to-use broth	1 L
1/4 cup	butter	60 mL
3 tbsp	finely chopped onion	45 mL
1 1/4 cups	Vialone Nano, carnaroli or Arborio rice	300 mL
1/4 cup	dry white wine	60 mL
1 1/2 cups	green peas	375 mL
Pinch	fennel seeds	Pinch
	Salt and freshly ground black pepper	
2 oz	Grana Padano cheese, grated	60 g

1. In a saucepan, bring vegetable stock to a boil over high heat. Reduce heat to low, cover and keep stock hot.

2. In a large saucepan, melt butter over medium heat. Add onion and cook, stirring, until softened but not browned, about 3 minutes. Add rice and cook, stirring, until rice is translucent, about 2 minutes.

3. Pour in wine and cook, stirring, until evaporated. Stir in green peas and fennel seeds. Season with salt and pepper to taste. Stir in enough of the hot stock to cover rice. Reduce heat and simmer, stirring often and adding more stock, 1/2 cup (125 mL) at a time, as previous addition is absorbed. Simmer, adding stock, until rice is al dente, about 30 minutes total.

4. Remove from heat and stir in cheese. Add a little more stock, if necessary, to thin to a creamy, slightly loose consistency, as this dish must be more liquid than an ordinary risotto. Season with salt and pepper to taste.

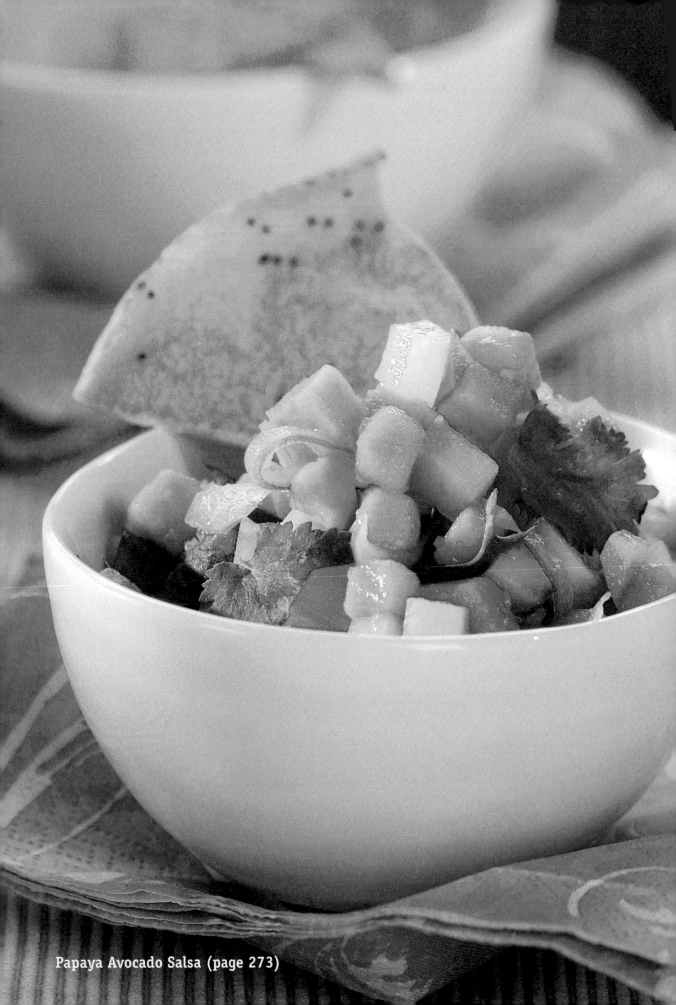

Papaya Avocado Salsa (page 273)

Basics and Condiments

Fresh Egg Pasta

Tip
You can use this egg dough in recipes calling for fresh pasta.

1 cup	all-purpose flour	250 mL
1 cup	durum wheat semolina	250 mL
2	eggs	2
1	egg yolk	1
1 tbsp	olive oil	15 mL
Pinch	salt	Pinch

1. In a bowl, combine all-purpose flour and semolina and make a well in the center. Add eggs, egg yolk, oil, 1 tbsp (15 mL) water and pinch of salt to well. Stir together until a soft dough forms, adding more water as necessary to moisten so dough comes together.

2. Transfer dough to a lightly floured work surface and knead until smooth and very firm. If you have difficulty making it hold together, add a few drops of water.

3. Cover tightly with plastic wrap and refrigerate for 30 minutes.

4. Roll out and cook according to recipe directions calling for fresh pasta.

Roasted Pepper and Tomato Sauté

Variation
Chakchuka: This recipe is easily adapted to the Tunisian dish chakchuka (also spelled shakshouka). Chakchuka, which means "a mixture," is most often served with eggs that are cooked beside the tomato and pepper sauce. It is perfect for breakfast or a light lunch.

● **Preheat barbecue to medium-high or preheat broiler**

4	bell peppers of various colors	4
1/3 cup	extra virgin olive oil	75 mL
1/2	onion, thinly sliced	1/2
4	cloves garlic, thinly sliced	4
2	tomatoes, peeled, seeded and chopped	2
	Fresh hot chile pepper, minced	
	Salt	

1. Place bell peppers on preheated grill (or place on a baking sheet and place under the broiler) and grill or broil, turning often, until skin is blackened all over and pepper is tender, about 20 minutes. Transfer to a bowl, cover and let cool. Remove skins, cores and seeds and cut peppers into large strips.

2. In a skillet, heat oil over medium heat. Add onion and cook, stirring, until translucent, about 5 minutes. Add garlic and cook, stirring, until onion starts to brown. Add tomatoes and cook, stirring often, until softened, about 5 minutes.

3. Stir in bell peppers. Add chile pepper and salt to taste. Reduce heat to low and cook, stirring, until peppers are warmed through and flavors are blended.

Pipérade

Serves 4

Preparation time
30 minutes

Cooking time
15 minutes

2 tbsp	olive oil	30 mL
2	large onions, thinly sliced	2
2	green bell peppers, cut into large strips	2
3	cloves garlic, chopped	3
1	bouquet garni (see Tip, page 214)	1
1 lb 6 oz	tomatoes, peeled, seeded and cut in large pieces (about 4)	675 g
Pinch	piment d'Espelette or cayenne pepper	Pinch
	Salt and freshly ground black pepper	
	Sugar, optional	

1. In a large skillet, heat olive oil over medium heat. Add onions and bell peppers and cook, stirring, until starting to soften, about 5 minutes. Add garlic and bouquet garni and cook, stirring, until onions are soft and starting to brown, about 5 minutes.

2. Stir in tomatoes and season with Espelette pepper and salt and black pepper to taste. Increase heat to high and cook, stirring, until liquid evaporates and sauce is thick, about 10 minutes. Stir in sugar as needed, depending on acidity of tomatoes. Discard bouquet garni.

Béchamel Sauce

**Makes about
1½ cups
(375 mL)**

Preparation time
5 minutes

Cooking time
20 minutes

2 cups	milk	500 mL
3 tbsp	butter	45 mL
3 tbsp	all-purpose flour	45 mL
Pinch	freshly grated nutmeg	Pinch
	Salt and freshly ground black pepper	

1. In a saucepan, bring milk almost to a boil over medium heat.

2. In another saucepan, melt butter over medium heat. Sprinkle with flour and cook, stirring, for 1 minute to make a roux.

3. Gradually pour hot milk over roux, blending well with a whisk. Season with nutmeg and salt and pepper to taste. Bring to a boil. Reduce heat and boil gently, whisking, until thick, about 10 minutes.

Spiced Squash Compote

**Makes 4 cups
(1 L)**

Preparation time
15 minutes

Cooking time
1 hour

Tips

To sterilize canning jars, immerse in a pot of simmering, not boiling, water for 10 minutes or wash, using the sterilizing cycle, in dishwasher. Keep hot until filling.

This compote is an excellent accompaniment to cheeses, especially aged firm cheeses.

- Two pint (500 mL) canning jars

2¼ lbs	winter squash, such as turban or Sweet Mama squash (1 medium), peeled and cut into cubes	1.125 kg
2⅓ cups	granulated sugar	575 mL
2 tsp	salt	10 mL
1 cup	water	250 mL
½ cup	freshly squeezed lemon juice	125 mL
1 tsp	black peppercorns	5 mL
6	whole cloves	6
2	star anise	2
1 tsp	ground cinnamon	5 mL

1. In a pot, combine squash, sugar, salt, water and lemon juice and bring to a boil over medium heat, stirring often. Reduce heat and simmer, stirring often, until squash is softened.

2. Meanwhile, in a mortar using a pestle or in a spice grinder, grind peppercorns, cloves and star anise until powdered.

3. Stir spice mixture and cinnamon into squash and cook over low heat, stirring often, until mixture is thick and jam-like, about 30 minutes.

4. Meanwhile, sterilize canning jars (see Tips, left). Empty water from jar and fill with compote. Seal jar with tight-fitting lid and refrigerate for at least 3 days. Store in the refrigerator for up to 3 weeks.

Red Pepper Coulis

**Makes about
½ cup
(125 mL)**

Preparation time
10 minutes

Cooking time
30 minutes

- Blender or food processor

2 tbsp	butter	30 mL
¼ cup	finely chopped French shallots	60 mL
1	red bell pepper, chopped	1
¼ cup	water	60 mL
	Salt	

1. In a small saucepan, melt butter over medium heat. Add shallots and cook, stirring, until softened but not browned, about 3 minutes.

2. Add bell pepper and cook, stirring, until softened but not browned, about 5 minutes. Add water, reduce heat and simmer, stirring often, until pepper is very soft, about 15 minutes.

3. Transfer to a blender or food processor and purée until smooth. Strain through a sieve into a bowl and season with salt to taste. Use immediately or cover and refrigerate for up to 3 days.

Preserved Lemons

**Makes about
1 quart (1 L)**

Preparation time
20 minutes

Tip
To use, scrape flesh from the peel and discard. Rinse peel, then cut into thin strips or as directed in your recipe.

- One quart (1 L) canning jar with lid, sterilized (see Tips, page 260)

2 lbs	lemons (about 6)	1 kg
¾ cup	coarse salt	175 mL
	Warm water	
¼ tsp	coriander seeds	1 mL
¼ tsp	black peppercorns	1 mL
	Freshly squeezed lemon juice	

1. Scrub lemons under running water. Cut off both ends of each lemon. Starting at one end, cut a deep incision almost but not all the way through to opposite end of each lemon. At opposite end, cut another incision perpendicular to the first one.

2. Holding one lemon over the canning jar, spoon salt into each incision, then place lemon in the jar. Repeat with remaining lemons, packing into jar. Add enough warm water to the jar to cover lemons, pressing to immerse. Add coriander seeds and peppercorns.

3. Seal jar with tight-fitting lid and store in a cool, dark place for 7 days, checking to make sure lemons are immersed in liquid. If necessary, add lemon juice to cover lemons.

4. Store for 3 weeks longer, until lemons are translucent. The lemons are now ready to use. For longer storage, store in refrigerator for up to 1 year. As you use the lemons, add more lemon juice to jar to keep remaining lemons immersed.

Ground Cherry and Cranberry Chutney

Serves 4

Preparation time
20 minutes

Cooking time
1 hour

See photo, page 263

1¼ lbs	ground cherries (cape gooseberries), husks removed	625 g
10 oz	cranberries	300 g
1 cup	packed brown sugar	250 mL
1 cup	white vinegar	250 mL
2 tbsp	grated fresh gingerroot	30 mL

1. In a saucepan, combine ground cherries, cranberries, brown sugar, vinegar and ginger. Bring to a boil over medium heat, stirring often. Reduce heat and simmer, stirring often, until thick and jam-like, about 1 hour. Serve hot or transfer to an airtight container and refrigerate for up to 2 weeks.

Spaghetti Squash Chutney with Currants and Lime

See photo, opposite

Tip

If available, use wild lime (also known as Makrut and kaffir), a small green citrus fruit, smaller and more acidic than a lemon. Use only the green part for the zest.

2 lbs	spaghetti squash	1 kg
2 cups	granulated sugar	500 mL
½ cup	currants	125 mL
2 tsp	salt	10 mL
2 cups	white wine vinegar	500 mL
2 cups	water	500 mL
	Zest of 1 lime (see Tip, left)	

1. Peel squash and cut in half lengthwise. Scoop out seeds. Cut squash into sections ½ inch (1 cm) thick and 2 inches (5 cm) long.

2. In a saucepan, combine squash, sugar, currants, salt, vinegar and water. Bring to a boil over medium heat, stirring often. Reduce heat and simmer, stirring often, until squash is very soft and breaking apart, about 1½ hours.

3. Stir in lime zest and simmer for 5 minutes. Serve hot or transfer to an airtight container and refrigerate for up to 2 weeks.

Mango Chutney

See photo, opposite

Tip

Special vegetable peelers are available that are designed to remove just the very thin layer of skin from bell peppers. Look for them at specialty kitchenware stores. If you don't have one, you can leave the peel on, or roast the pepper (see page 258, bottom, Step 1) then peel off the skin.

2	mangos (about 1 lb/500 g), cut into ½-inch (1 cm) cubes	2
1	red bell pepper, peeled and julienned (see Tip, left)	1
½ cup	packed brown sugar	125 mL
⅔ cup	white vinegar	150 mL
1 tsp	mustard seeds, slightly crushed	5 mL

1. In a saucepan, combine mangos, bell pepper, brown sugar, vinegar and mustard seeds. Bring to a boil over medium heat, stirring often. Reduce heat and simmer, stirring often, until thick and jam-like, about 1 hour. Serve hot or transfer to an airtight container and refrigerate for up to 2 weeks.

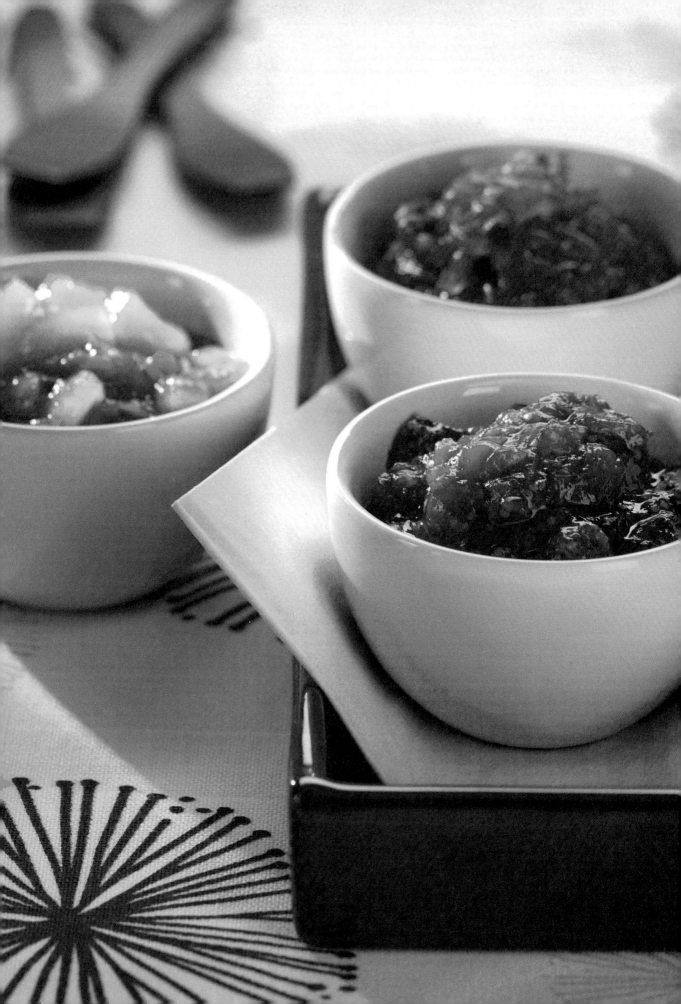

Squash Chips

Tip

For frying, it is best to use peanut oil, as it can tolerate higher temperatures than other vegetable oils before it starts to smoke and deteriorate.

• Candy/deep-fry thermometer

4 cups	vegetable oil, preferably peanut oil (see Tip, left)	1 L
1	buttercup or Sweet Mama squash	1
	Salt	

1. In a deep skillet, Dutch oven or deep-fryer, heat oil over medium heat until about 340°F (170°C).

2. Cut stem from squash. Cut squash in half lengthwise and scoop out seeds. Place cut side down and cut crosswise into very thin slices.

3. Add squash slices, in batches, to hot oil and fry until golden and crisp. Using a slotted spoon, remove from oil and place on a baking sheet lined with paper towels to drain. Season with salt to taste.

Pineapple Chips

Tip

The drying time in the oven can vary considerably. A convection oven, for example, will be much faster and more efficient.

• Preheat oven to 210°F (100°C)
• Baking sheets, lined with parchment paper

1	pineapple	1
3½ cups	granulated sugar	875 mL
4 cups	water	1 L

1. Cut leaves and root end from pineapple. Using a serrated knife, cut off peel. Use a paring knife to remove all spikes and eyes. Cut crosswise into very thin slices and trim out core.

2. In a large saucepan, combine sugar and water and bring to a boil over medium heat, stirring to dissolve sugar. Add half of the pineapple slices to syrup. Reduce heat and boil gently for 3 minutes. Using a slotted spoon, remove pineapple from syrup, draining well. Place on prepared baking sheets, without touching. Repeat with remaining pineapple slices.

3. Dry pineapple slices in preheated oven until firm and dried through, about 3 hours. Slide parchment paper onto wire racks and let pineapple cool completely. Store in a cookie tin at room temperature for up to 3 days.

Peanut Satay Sauce

Serves 4

Preparation time
15 minutes

Cooking time
5 minutes

Tip

A smoother mixture can be obtained by chopping the peanuts in the mini chopper or food processor.

• **Mortar and pestle, mini chopper or food processor**

1 cup	unsalted roasted peanuts	125 mL
¼ cup	sesame seeds	60 mL
3 tbsp	packed brown sugar	45 mL
2 tbsp	soy sauce	30 mL
¾ cup	water	175 mL
	Sambal oelek or hot pepper flakes	

1. In mortar, using pestle, crush peanuts until finely ground (or pulse in a mini chopper or food processor).

2. In a small saucepan, combine peanuts, sesame seeds, brown sugar, soy sauce, water, and sambal oelek to taste. Bring to a simmer over medium heat, stirring often. Reduce heat and simmer, stirring, until thickened, about 5 minutes. Serve warm.

Tapenade

Serves 4

Preparation time
15 minutes

Tip

It is important to use olives of the highest quality possible.

• **Food mill, mortar and pestle or food processor**

10 oz	pitted black olives (see Tip, left)	300 g
3	cloves garlic	3
⅓ cup	drained capers	75 mL
¾ cup	olive oil (approx.)	175 mL
	Juice of 1 lemon	
	Salt and freshly ground black pepper	

1. Using food mill, in mortar using a pestle or in food processor, purée olives, garlic and capers. Transfer to a bowl, if necessary. Gradually stir in olive oil until incorporated. Season with lemon juice and salt and pepper to taste. Stir well. Serve immediately or cover and refrigerate for up to 1 week.

Sweet-and-Sour Pearl Onions

**Makes
about 3 cups
(750 mL)**

Preparation time
30 minutes

Cooking time
5 minutes

See photo, opposite

- Three 8-oz (250 mL) canning jars with lids, sterilized (see Tips, page 260)

½ cup	salt	125 mL
½ cup	granulated sugar	125 mL
4 cups	white wine vinegar	1 L
¼ cup	corn oil	60 mL
2 lbs	pearl onions, peeled	1 kg

1. In a pot, combine salt, sugar, vinegar and oil. Bring just to a boil over medium heat, stirring to dissolve sugar and salt. Add onions and return to a boil.

2. Using a slotted spoon, pack onions into canning jars. Pour in pickling liquid to cover. Insert a narrow spatula between onions to remove any air bubbles and add more liquid as necessary. Seal jars with lids and refrigerate for at least 3 days to blend flavors. Store in refrigerator for up to 1 month.

Marinated Sun-Dried Tomatoes

**Makes
40 sun-dried
tomatoes**

Preparation time
1 hour

Tip

The tomatoes must always remain covered by oil to prevent mold from developing. Garlic in oil should never be stored for more than 1 week. To keep these tomatoes longer (for up to 1 month), omit the garlic from the layers and just add fresh minced garlic to taste as you use them.

- One quart (1 L) glass jar with lid, sterilized

40	sun-dried tomato halves	40
4	cloves garlic, sliced	4
2 tbsp	drained capers	30 mL
⅔ cup	olive oil (approx.)	150 mL

1. In glass jar, layer tomatoes, garlic and capers, then sprinkle with olive oil, alternating ingredients as you fill jar (you must add oil to each layer). Use a fork to press down on tomatoes to remove air between layers, and add more oil as necessary to cover tomatoes.

2. Seal jar and refrigerate for at least 2 days before using or for up to 1 week (see Tip, left).

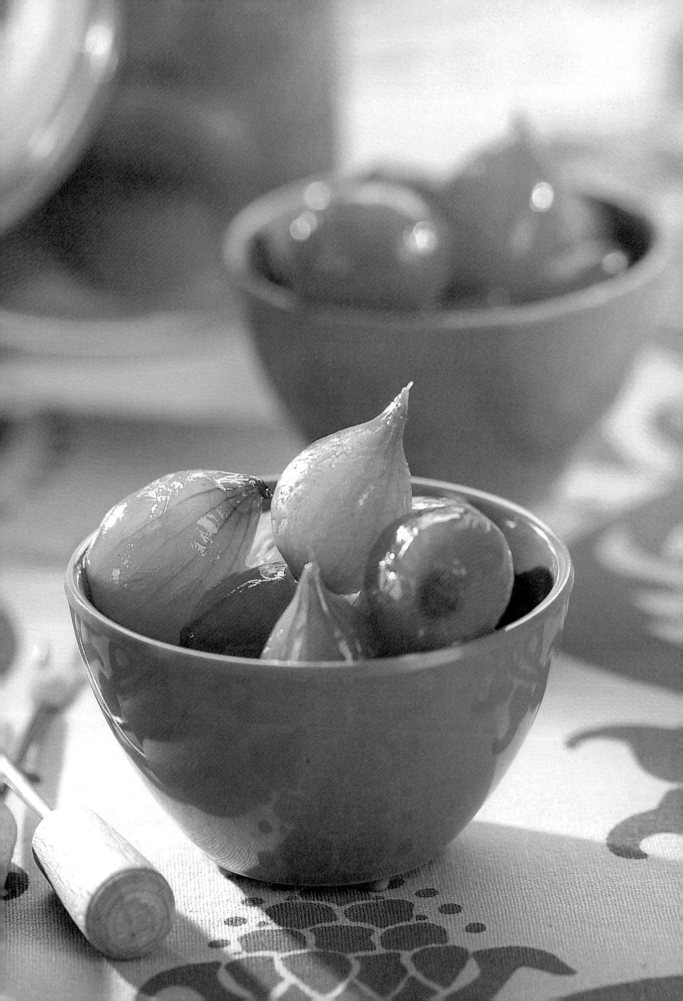

Arugula Pesto

Serves 4

Preparation time
15 minutes

Tip
When buying cheese, read the label carefully and make sure to buy those that are not made from animal rennet.

- **Food processor**

2	bunches arugula	2
¼ cup	pine nuts	60 mL
2	cloves garlic	2
2 oz	vegetarian-friendly Parmesan cheese, grated (see Tip, left)	60 g
1 tsp	salt	5 mL
¾ cup	extra virgin olive oil	175 mL

1. Remove and discard any arugula stems that are too tough.

2. In food processor, combine arugula, pine nuts, garlic, Parmesan and salt. Pulse until finely chopped, stopping occasionally to scrape down sides of bowl.

3. With motor running, gradually add olive oil through hole in feed tube and process until blended. Use immediately or transfer to an airtight container and refrigerate for up to 2 days.

Pesto alla Genovese

Serves 4

Preparation time
15 minutes

- **Food processor**

3 cups	fresh basil leaves	750 mL
2 tbsp	toasted pine nuts	30 mL
2 tbsp	grated vegetarian-friendly Parmesan cheese (see Tip, above)	30 mL
2 tbsp	grated Pecorino Romano cheese	30 mL
1 tsp	coarse salt	5 mL
2	cloves garlic	2
2	small ice cubes	2
¼ cup	extra virgin olive oil	60 mL

1. In food processor, combine basil, pine nuts, Parmesan, Romano, salt, garlic and ice cubes. Pulse until finely chopped, stopping occasionally to scrape down sides of bowl.

2. With motor running, gradually add olive oil through hole in feed tube and process until blended. Use immediately or transfer to an airtight container and refrigerate for up to 2 days.

Sun-Dried Tomato Pesto

● **Food processor**

8 oz	sun-dried tomatoes	250 g
	Warm water	
½ cup	extra virgin olive oil, divided	125 mL
2	cloves garlic, chopped	2
1	slice stale bread without crusts, crumbled	1
2 tbsp	drained capers	30 mL

1. Place tomatoes in a bowl and add warm water to cover. Let stand until tomatoes are soft and plump, about 20 minutes. Drain.

2. Meanwhile, in a skillet, heat 2 tbsp (30 mL) of the oil over medium-low heat. Add garlic and cook, stirring, until garlic is translucent, about 2 minutes. Add bread and cook, stirring, until golden, about 2 minutes. Remove from heat.

3. In food processor, combine tomatoes, garlic mixture and capers and pulse until finely chopped, stopping occasionally to scrape down bowl.

4. With motor running, gradually add remaining olive oil through hole in feed tube and process until blended. Use immediately or transfer to an airtight container and refrigerate for up to 2 days.

Nut Paste

● **Preheat oven to 375°F (190°C)**
● **Mortar and pestle**

¾ cup	walnuts	175 mL
½ cup	hazelnuts	125 mL
½ cup	shelled pistachios	125 mL
½ cup	pine nuts	125 mL
6 tbsp	liquid honey	90 mL

1. Spread walnuts and hazelnuts on a baking sheet and toast in preheated oven for 5 minutes. Add pistachios and pine nuts and toast until nuts are golden brown and fragrant, about 4 minutes. Transfer to mortar and crush with pestle.

2. Transfer to a bowl and stir in honey to make a semi-firm paste. Use immediately or transfer to an airtight container and store at room temperature for up to 1 week.

Fresh Garden Tomato Sauce

Serves 4

Preparation time
20 minutes

See photo, opposite

Tip

This sauce is a wonderful way to highlight the freshness and quality of the products you grow in your vegetable garden. Serve it with egg tagliatelle covered generously in Parmesan — an ideal meal that you will surely enjoy eating in your garden.

4	tomatoes, diced	4
¼ cup	chopped fresh basil	60 mL
¼ cup	chopped fresh parsley	60 mL
1	clove garlic, minced	1
1 tsp	black peppercorns, crushed	5 mL
	Salt	
½ cup	extra virgin olive oil	125 mL

1. In a bowl, combine tomatoes, basil, parsley, garlic, pepper, and salt to taste. Add oil and toss to combine. Let stand for 10 minutes before serving.

Tomato Basil Sauce

Serves 4

Preparation time
10 minutes

Cooking time
35 minutes

- **Food mill or food processor**

4	tomatoes, peeled	4
3 tbsp	olive oil	45 mL
2	cloves garlic, minced	2
2 tbsp	chopped onion	30 mL
2 tbsp	chopped celery	30 mL
2 tbsp	chopped carrot	30 mL
	Salt and freshly ground black pepper	
4	leaves fresh basil, chopped	4

1. Using food mill or in a food processor, purée tomatoes. Set aside.

2. In a saucepan, heat oil over medium heat. Add garlic, onion, celery and carrot and cook, stirring, until softened, about 5 minutes.

3. Stir in tomatoes and season with salt and pepper to taste. Bring to a boil, stirring often. Reduce heat and simmer, stirring often, until thickened, about 30 minutes. Stir in basil.

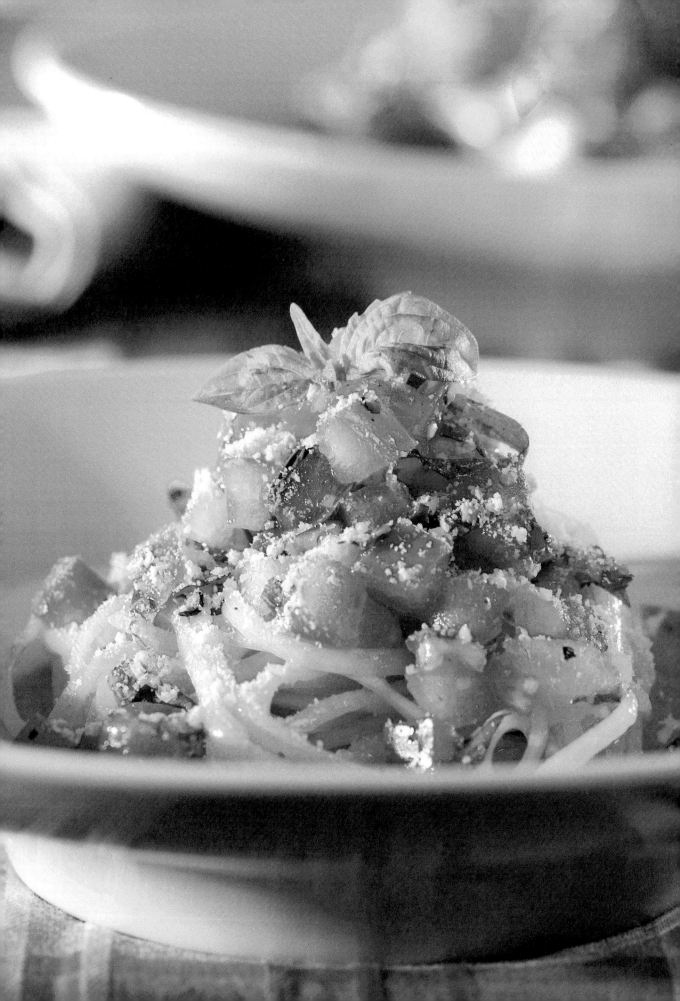

Mango Cilantro Salsa

1	mango, julienned	1
½ cup	diced red bell pepper	125 mL
1 tbsp	finely chopped French shallot	15 mL
¼ tsp	finely chopped fresh chive	1 mL
¼ tsp	chopped fresh cilantro	1 mL
½ tsp	freshly squeezed lime juice	2 mL
½ tsp	olive oil	2 mL
	Salt and freshly ground black pepper	

1. In a bowl, combine mango, bell pepper, shallot, chive and cilantro. Add lime juice and olive oil, then salt and pepper to taste, and toss to coat.

2. Cover and marinate at room temperature for at least 2 hours before serving or refrigerate for up to 8 hours.

Tomato Salsa

1	large tomato, seeded and diced	1
2 tbsp	finely chopped French shallot	30 mL
2	cloves garlic, minced	2
¼ tsp	finely chopped fresh chive	1 mL
10	leaves fresh basil, chopped	10
	Fresh Italian flat-leaf parsley, chopped	
1 tbsp	drained chopped capers	15 mL
½ tsp	sherry vinegar	2 mL
	Olive oil	
	Salt and freshly ground black pepper	

1. In a bowl, combine tomato, shallot, garlic, chive, basil, parsley to taste, and capers. Add vinegar and oil to taste. Season with salt and pepper to taste and toss to coat. Cover and refrigerate for 30 minutes before serving.

Papaya Avocado Salsa

Serves 4

Preparation time
15 minutes

Marinating time
30 minutes

1	medium papaya, diced	1
1	avocado, diced	1
1	tomato, diced	1
½	yellow bell pepper	½
½ cup	finely chopped red onion	125 mL
¼ cup	chopped fresh cilantro	60 mL
	Salt	
	Juice of 1 lime	
	Fresh hot chile pepper, chopped	
3 tbsp	extra virgin olive oil	45 mL

1. In a bowl, combine papaya, avocado, tomato, bell pepper, red onion and cilantro. Add salt, lime juice and chile pepper to taste. Add oil and toss to coat. Cover and refrigerate for 30 minutes before serving.

Green Apple Confit

Serves 4

Preparation time
40 minutes

Cooking time
2 minutes

Chilling time
2 hours

Tip

This apple confit is a great accompaniment to a cheese platter.

1½ cups	granulated sugar	375 mL
2 cups	water	500 mL
4	Granny Smith or other green apples, diced	4
1 tsp	powdered wasabi	5 mL
Pinch	salt	Pinch

1. In a saucepan, combine sugar and water and bring to a boil over medium-high heat, stirring to dissolve sugar. Add apples and boil for 1 minute.

2. Drain apples and spread on a rimmed baking sheet to cool.

3. Transfer apples to a bowl and season with wasabi and salt. Cover and refrigerate for at least 2 hours for flavors to meld or for up to 2 days.

Fried Sage

See photo, opposite

Serves 4		
Preparation time 10 minutes		
Cooking time 10 minutes		

Tip

It is important to rinse the sage leaves well, then pat completely dry so the batter will stick to them.

• Candy/deep-fry thermometer

½ cup	all-purpose flour	125 mL
2 tbsp	grated vegetarian-friendly Parmesan cheese (see Tip, page 268)	30 mL
¾ cup	milk	175 mL
¼ cup	beer	60 mL
2	eggs, separated	2
1	bunch fresh sage, stems removed	1
2 cups	olive oil	500 mL
	Salt	

1. In a bowl, whisk together flour, Parmesan, milk, beer and egg yolks. Let stand for 10 minutes.

2. In another bowl, using an electric mixer or whisk, beat egg whites until stiff peaks form. Fold into batter until blended. Cover and refrigerate for up to 1 hour.

3. In deep skillet, heat oil to 350°F (180°C). Dip each sage leaf into batter, then fry in hot oil, in batches to avoid crowding pan, until golden and crisp. Using a slotted spoon, transfer to a plate lined with paper towels to drain. Repeat with remaining sage.

4. Season with salt and serve hot.

Raspberry Vinegar

Serves 4		
Preparation time 10 minutes		
Infusing time 2 weeks		
Cooking time 10 minutes		

• One quart (1 L) canning jar, sterilized (see Tips, page 260)

1 lb	raspberries	500 g
2 cups	white wine vinegar, divided	500 mL
½ cup	granulated sugar	125 mL

1. In a bowl, using a potato masher, crush raspberries with half of the vinegar. Pour into sterilized jar and add remaining vinegar. Cover with lid and store in a cool, dark place for 2 weeks for flavor to infuse.

2. Strain vinegar through a fine-mesh sieve into a saucepan, discarding solids. Stir in sugar and bring to a boil over medium heat, stirring until sugar is dissolved.

3. Sterilize jar. Return vinegar to jar and seal with lid. Use immediately or store in a cool, dark place for up to 6 months.

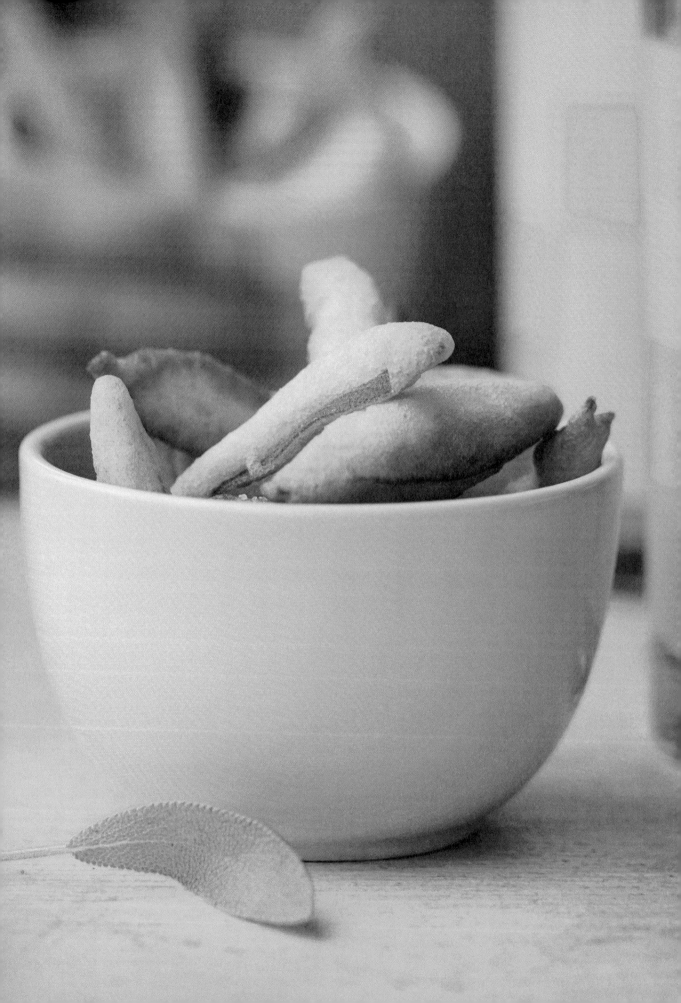

Apricot and Lavender Tart (page 310)

Desserts

Custard Fritters

Serves 4

Preparation time
1 hour

Chilling time
4 hours

Cooking time
10 minutes

• Candy/deep-fry thermometer

2 cups	milk	500 mL
1/2 cup	granulated sugar, divided	125 mL
4	egg yolks	4
Pinch	salt	Pinch
1/2 cup	all-purpose flour	125 mL
	Finely grated zest of 1 lemon	
	Vegetable oil	

Coating

1/3 cup	all-purpose flour	75 mL
2	eggs, beaten	2
1 1/2 cups	fine bread crumbs, toasted	375 mL
1/4 cup	granulated sugar	60 mL

1. In a saucepan, combine milk and 3 tbsp (45 mL) of the sugar. Heat over medium heat, stirring often, until almost boiling.

2. Meanwhile, in a bowl, whisk together remaining sugar, egg yolks and salt until pale and creamy. Whisk in flour and lemon zest.

3. Gradually whisk yolk mixture into hot milk. Reduce heat to low and cook, stirring, until thick, about 5 minutes (if cream starts to stick to bottom of pan, remove from heat and avoid scraping bottom). Pour into a small baking dish so that it is about 3/4 inch (2 cm) deep. Let cool for 20 minutes.

4. Place plastic wrap directly on the surface and refrigerate until chilled and firm, about 4 hours.

5. In a deep skillet, Dutch oven or deep-fryer, heat 3 inches (7.5 cm) oil over medium heat until about 350°F (180°C).

6. Cut custard into diamond shapes.

7. *Coating:* Place flour in one shallow dish, beaten eggs in another and bread crumbs in a third dish. Dip custard pieces first into flour, then egg, then coat in crumbs, shaking off excess.

8. Drop fritters, in batches, into hot oil and fry, turning once, until golden and hot inside, about 5 minutes. Using a slotted spoon, remove from oil and place on a baking sheet lined with paper towels to drain. Adjust heat as necessary between batches to prevent burning. Serve fritters hot, sprinkled with sugar.

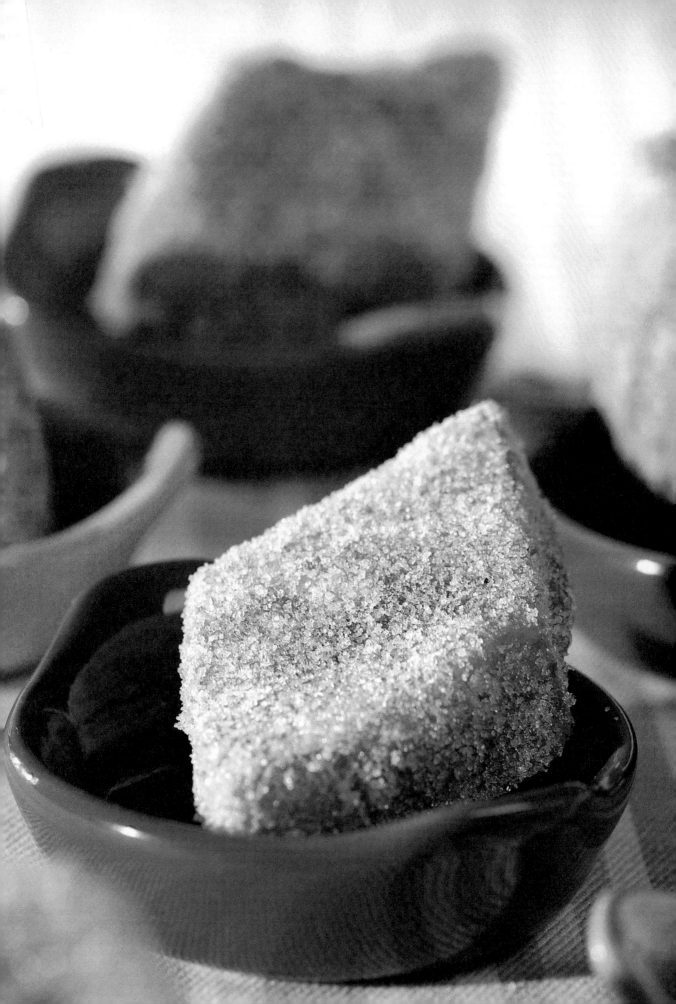

Apple Fritters

Tip

These fritters can be served with ice cream and/or chocolate sauce.

Variation

Banana Fritters: Use the same recipe, but replace apples with bananas, the calvados with rum and leave out the cinnamon and lemon.

- Candy/deep-fry thermometer

Batter

¾ cup	all-purpose flour	175 mL
Pinch	salt	Pinch
1	egg yolk	1
6 tbsp	beer	90 mL
2	egg whites	2
1½ lbs	Golden Delicious or other sweet, firm apples	750 g
	Juice of 1 lemon	
2 tbsp	granulated sugar	30 mL
	Ground cinnamon	
1 tbsp	Calvados	15 mL
1 tbsp	confectioner's (icing) sugar	15 mL
	Vegetable oil	

1. In a bowl, combine flour and salt. Make a well in the center and add egg yolk and beer. Stir until blended and smooth. Cover and refrigerate batter for 1 hour.

2. Meanwhile, peel and core apples. Cut crosswise into ¼-inch (0.5 cm) thick slices and place in a bowl with lemon juice as you cut. Sprinkle with granulated sugar and cinnamon to taste. Stir in Calvados. Cover and refrigerate for 1 hour, gently stirring often.

3. In a deep skillet, Dutch oven or deep-fryer, heat oil over medium-high heat to about 425°F (220°C).

4. In another bowl, using an electric mixer or whisk, beat egg whites to form stiff peaks. Fold into batter.

5. Drain apple slices and pat dry. Working in batches to avoid overcrowding, dip apple slices into batter and fry in hot oil, turning once, until cooked inside and deep golden, about 2 minutes per side. Using a slotted spoon, remove from oil and place on a plate lined with paper towels to drain. Adjust heat as necessary between batches to prevent burning. Serve fritters hot, sprinkled with confectioner's sugar.

Baklava

- Preheat oven to 350°F (180°C)
- 13- by 9-inch (33 by 23 cm) metal baking pan, buttered

1 cup	chopped almonds	250 mL
1 cup	chopped walnuts	250 mL
½ cup	granulated sugar	125 mL
1 tsp	ground cinnamon	5 mL
1 lb	phyllo pastry dough (about 22 sheets)	500 g
1½ cups	butter, melted	375 mL

Syrup

3 cups	granulated sugar	750 mL
1 tsp	ground cinnamon	5 mL
2	whole cloves	2
2 cups	water	500 mL
1 cup	honey	250 mL

1. In a bowl, combine almonds, walnuts, sugar and cinnamon.

2. Place 1 sheet of phyllo in prepared baking pan, trimming to fit as necessary. Brush with butter. Repeat with 2 more sheets. Sprinkle with about one-fifth of the nut mixture.

3. Top with 3 more sheets of phyllo, buttering each as you layer. Sprinkle with one-quarter of the remaining nut mixture. Repeat layering 3 more times, using 9 more phyllo sheets and remaining nut mixture.

4. Layer remaining phyllo sheets on top, buttering each as you layer. Using the tip of a sharp knife, score the top layers of phyllo lengthwise to make 6 rows. Score on a diagonal to make 4 rows, creating about 24 diamonds.

5. Bake in preheated oven until pastry is golden and crisp, 50 to 60 minutes.

6. *Syrup:* Meanwhile, in a saucepan, combine sugar, cinnamon, cloves, water and honey. Bring to a boil over medium heat, stirring to dissolve sugar. Reduce heat and boil gently until slightly reduced and syrupy, about 10 minutes. Discard cloves.

7. Pour boiling syrup evenly over hot baklava. Let cool completely in pan on a wire rack. Cover and let stand at room temperature for 24 hours. Cut along score marks into diamonds.

Nut Cookies with Caramelized Fruit and Nuts

Tips

The nut cookie can be cooled, wrapped and stored at room temperature for up to 2 days. The caramelized fruit and nut mixture can be covered and stored at room temperature for up to 8 hours.

This is also nice served with a scoop of ice cream on the side — fig ice cream is a particular favorite.

- Preheat oven to 325°F (160°C)
- 8- by 4-inch (20 by 10 cm) metal loaf pan, lined with parchment paper, leaving 2-inch (5 cm) overhang at each end

Nut Cookies

3 tbsp	ground almonds (almond flour or meal)	45 mL
2 tbsp	all-purpose flour	30 mL
½ cup	chopped nuts	125 mL
3	egg whites	3
½ cup	granulated sugar	125 mL

Caramelized Fruit and Nuts

1 tbsp	honey	15 mL
	Juice of ½ lemon	
1	pear, diced	1
2 tbsp	raisins	30 mL
4	dried figs, chopped	4
¼ cup	packed dried apricots, chopped	60 mL
¼ cup	chopped nuts	60 mL

1. *Nut Cookies:* In a bowl, whisk together ground almonds and all-purpose flour. Stir in nuts.

2. In another bowl, using an electric mixer or a whisk, beat egg whites until foamy. Gradually beat in sugar and continue beating until stiff peaks form. Fold into nut mixture. Spread in prepared pan.

3. Bake in preheated oven until golden and firm, about 40 minutes. Remove from pan, using parchment overhang as handles. Transfer to a wire rack and let cool completely.

4. *Caramelized Fruit and Nuts:* In a small skillet, bring honey to a boil over medium heat. Boil, swirling pan often, until honey starts to caramelize. Carefully pour in lemon juice (it will splatter). Reduce heat to medium-low. Add pears and raisins and cook, stirring frequently, until pears are tender and caramelized, about 10 minutes. Transfer to a bowl. Stir in figs, apricots and nuts and let cool.

5. To serve, cut nut cookie into 4 equal pieces and place each on an individual serving plate. Spoon caramelized fruit and nut mixture with a little of the accumulated juice on top.

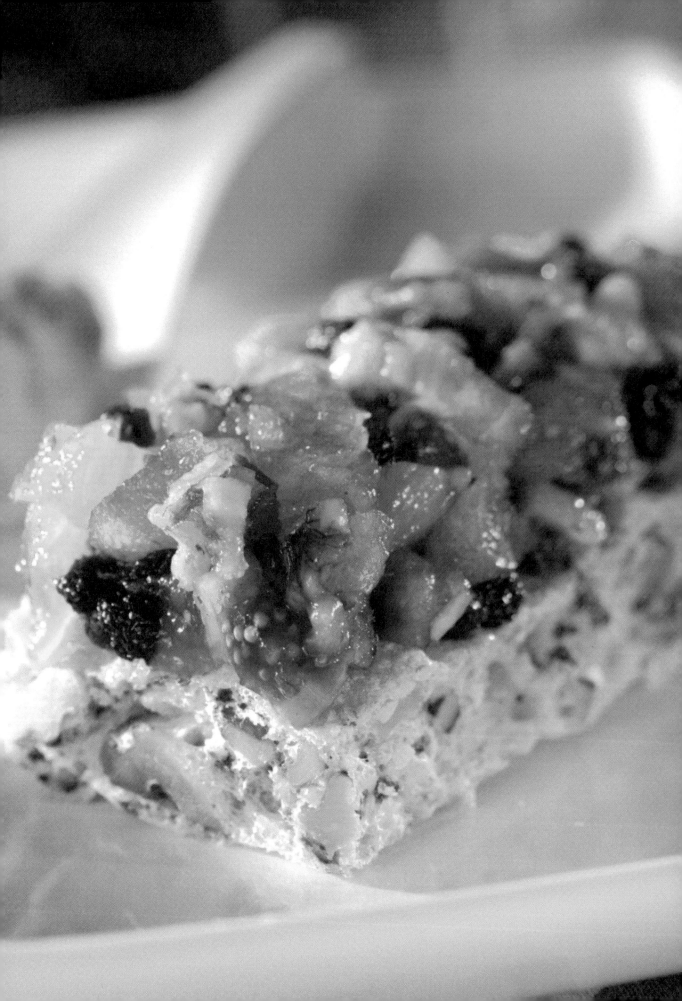

Almond Biscotti

Makes about 34 biscotti

Preparation time
45 minutes

Chilling time
45 minutes

Freezing time
30 minutes

Cooking time
1 hour 10 minutes

Tips

To toast chopped almonds: Spread almonds on a baking sheet and bake in 375°F (180°C) oven until golden and fragrant, 5 to 8 minutes.

You can buy whole almonds blanched (peeled) or blanch them yourself. *To blanch almonds:* Place almonds in a heatproof bowl and pour in boiling water to cover. Let stand until water is just lukewarm. Drain almonds and squeeze out of their skins. Place on a baking sheet lined with paper towels and pat dry. Once dry, toast as for chopped almonds, increasing the time to 8 to 12 minutes.

● Baking sheets, lined with parchment paper

2½ cups	all-purpose flour	625 mL
2 tsp	baking powder	10 mL
Pinch	salt	Pinch
½ cup	butter, softened	125 mL
1 cup	granulated sugar	250 mL
4	eggs	4
½ cup	chopped almonds, toasted (see Tips, left)	125 mL
	Zest of ½ orange	
	Zest of ½ lemon	
2 tsp	vanilla extract	10 mL
1 cup	blanched whole almonds, toasted (see Tips, left)	250 mL

1. In a bowl, sift together flour, baking powder and salt.

2. In a large bowl, using an electric mixer, beat butter and sugar until light and fluffy. Beat in eggs, one at a time, between each addition. On low speed, gradually beat in flour mixture just until blended.

3. Beat in chopped almonds, orange zest, lemon zest and vanilla. Using a wooden spoon, stir in whole almonds. Cover and refrigerate dough until firm, about 45 minutes.

4. On a lightly floured work surface, divide dough in half. With floured hands, shape each piece into a baguette-shaped log about 2 inches (5 cm) wide. Wrap with plastic wrap and place on a baking sheet. Freeze until slightly firm, about 30 minutes.

5. Preheat oven to 375°F (190°C).

6. Unwrap dough and place on prepared baking sheet at least 3 inches (7.5 cm) apart. Bake in preheated oven until firm and golden, about 25 minutes. Let cool on baking sheet on a wire rack for 10 minutes. Reduce oven temperature to 325°F (160°C).

7. Transfer cooled logs to cutting board and cut on a slight diagonal into ½-inch (1 cm) thick slices. Place, cut side down, on baking sheets.

8. Bake until dry and crisp, turning halfway though, about 30 minutes. Let cool on wire rack.

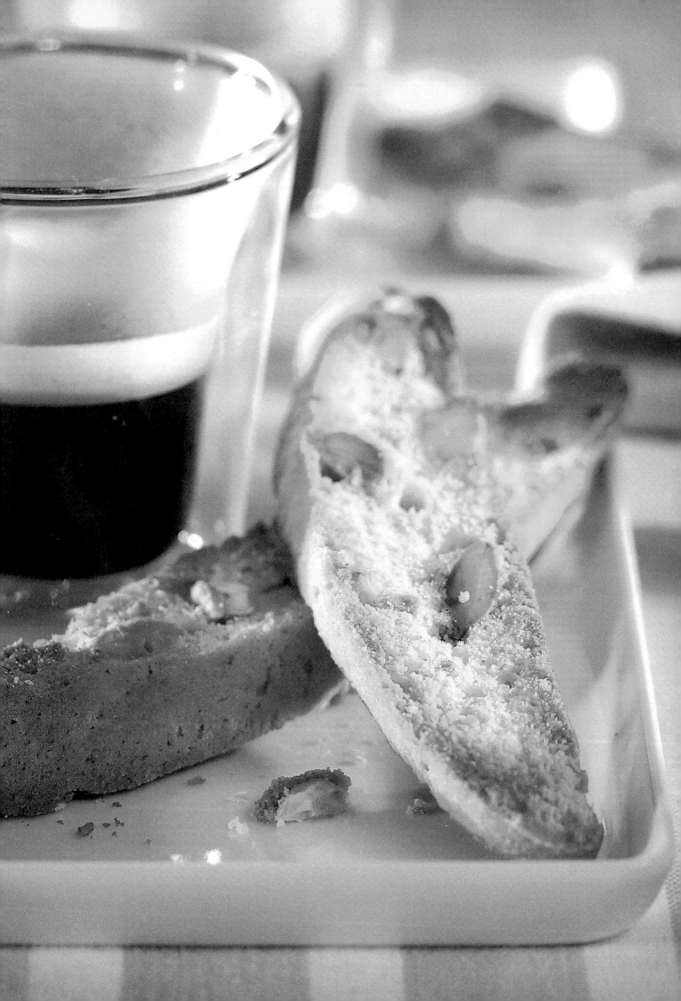

Orange-Scented Amaretti

- Preheat oven to 300°F (150°C)
- Food processor
- Baking sheets, lined with parchment paper

1 lb	almonds (3¼ cups/800 mL)	500 g
	Boiling water	
2 cups	granulated sugar	500 mL
3	egg whites, at room temperature	3
	Zest of 1 orange	

1. Place almonds in a heatproof bowl and pour in boiling water to cover. Let stand until water is just lukewarm. Drain almonds and squeeze out of skins. Place on a baking sheet lined with paper towels and pat dry.

2. In food processor, combine almonds and sugar and process until almonds are very finely chopped but not powdery. Transfer to a bowl.

3. In another bowl, using electric mixer or a whisk, beat egg whites until foamy and soft peaks form. Add to almond mixture with orange zest and fold until well blended.

4. Scoop by heaping tablespoonfuls (15 mL) and roll tightly into 1¼-inch (3.5 cm) balls. Place on prepared baking sheets at least 2 inches (5 cm) apart.

5. Bake in preheated oven, switching position of baking sheets on racks partway through, until cookies are light brown, firm on top and fairly dry around the edges, about 30 minutes. Let cool on baking sheets on wire racks.

Cranberry Muffins

**Makes
12 muffins**

Preparation time
20 minutes

Cooking time
25 to 30 minutes

- Preheat oven to 350°F (180°C)
- 12-cup muffin pan, lined with paper liners

¾ cup	dried cranberries	175 mL
	Boiling water	
2 cups	all-purpose flour	500 mL
1 tbsp	baking powder	15 mL
¼ tsp	salt	1 mL
2	eggs	2
⅔ cup	packed brown sugar	150 mL
1 cup	milk	250 mL
½ cup	butter, melted	125 mL
1 tsp	vanilla extract	5 mL

1. In a heatproof bowl, cover cranberries with boiling water and let soak until plump, about 10 minutes. Drain well and pat dry.

2. In a large bowl, combine flour, baking powder and salt.

3. In another bowl, whisk together eggs and brown sugar. Whisk in milk, butter and vanilla until blended. Pour over flour mixture and sprinkle with cranberries. Stir just until moistened.

4. Scoop into prepared muffin pan, dividing equally.

5. Bake in preheated oven until tops spring back when lightly touched, 25 to 30 minutes. Let cool in pan on a wire rack for 5 minutes. Transfer to rack to cool completely.

Caramelized Nectarines Scented with Vanilla

Serves 4

Preparation time
15 minutes

Cooking time
10 minutes

3 tbsp	butter	45 mL
6	nectarines, cut into eighths	6
1	vanilla bean, slit lengthwise	1
¼ cup	packed brown sugar	60 mL
2 tbsp	brandy, optional	30 mL

1. In a skillet, melt butter over high heat. Add nectarines and cook, stirring, until starting to soften, about 2 minutes. Scrape seeds from vanilla bean into skillet. Add pod to skillet and stir in brown sugar. Reduce heat to prevent sugar from burning and cook, stirring, until nectarines are tender. Discard vanilla pod.

2. If using, sprinkle with brandy and ignite. Spoon nectarines and syrup into heatproof serving dishes.

Roasted Pineapple with Vanilla

See photo, opposite

Serves 4

Preparation time
15 minutes

Cooking time
25 minutes

Chilling time
48 hours

Tips

The syrup drained from the pineapple can be mixed with sparkling water or fruit juice for a refreshing drink.

The vanilla bean sticks can be dried, then added to a container of granulated sugar to make vanilla sugar.

● **Large glass baking dish**

1	pineapple	1
2	vanilla beans (see Tips, left)	2
1 cup	granulated sugar	250 mL
1 cup	honey	250 mL
	Vanilla ice cream, frozen yogurt or pineapple sorbet	

1. Peel pineapple and cut crosswise into slices about $1/2$ inch (1 cm) thick. Remove core.

2. Cut vanilla beans in half lengthwise, then cut into sticks about $1/2$ inch (1 cm) long.

3. Insert about 6 sticks vanilla into each pineapple slice at regular intervals. Place pineapple slices in baking dish and sprinkle evenly with sugar. Cover and refrigerate for 48 hours, turning pineapple slices every 12 hours.

4. Drain liquid from pineapple and remove vanilla beans (discard beans and liquid or reserve for another use).

5. In a large skillet, heat honey over medium heat until warmed and very fluid. Add pineapple slices and spoon honey over top. Reduce heat and simmer, spooning honey over pineapple often, until pineapple is heated and tender, about 10 minutes.

6. Serve pineapple hot, topped with ice cream.

Clementines with Basil and Cocoa Sorbet

Serves 4

Preparation time
20 minutes

Chilling time
4 to 6 hours

● **Shallow baking dish**

10	clementines	10
$2/3$ cup	granulated sugar	150 mL
$3/4$ cup	water	175 mL
10	fresh basil leaves	10
1 cup	cocoa or other sorbet	250 mL

1. Peel clementines, separate segments and place in baking dish.

2. In a small saucepan, combine sugar and water and bring to a boil over medium-high heat, stirring to dissolve sugar. Pour over clementines in dish and stir in basil leaves. Cover and refrigerate until chilled, 4 to 6 hours.

3. To serve, spoon clementines with syrup and basil leaves into individual serving dishes. Top with a quenelle or scoop of sorbet.

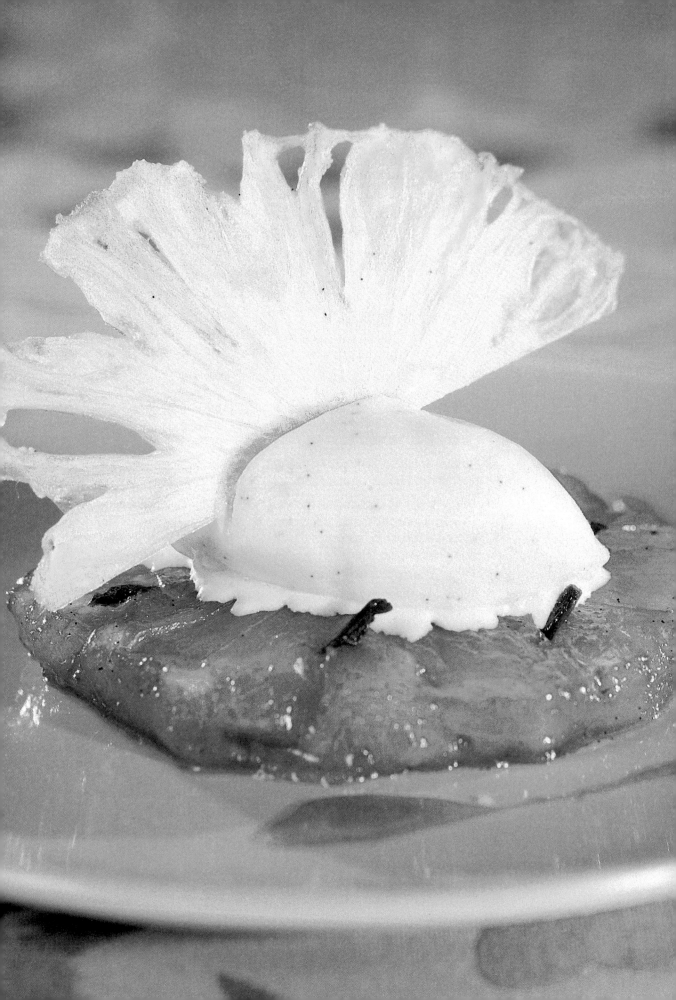

Peppered Strawberry Tulips

Serves 4

Preparation time
45 minutes

Chilling time
30 minutes

Cooking time
20 minutes

- Preheat oven to 400°F (200°C)
- Thin cardboard
- Large baking sheets, lined with silicone liners or parchment paper

2 cups	strawberries, cut into quarters	500 mL
3 tbsp	granulated sugar, divided	45 mL
	Juice of ½ orange	
	Juice of 1 lime	
	Freshly ground black pepper	
½ cup	heavy or whipping (35%) cream	125 mL

Tulips

¼ cup	egg whites	60 mL
¼ cup	granulated sugar	60 mL
⅓ cup	all-purpose flour	75 mL
¼ cup	melted butter	60 mL

1. In a bowl, combine strawberries, 2 tbsp (30 mL) of the sugar, orange juice, lime juice and pepper to taste. Cover and refrigerate for at least 30 minutes or for up to 8 hours.

2. *Tulips:* In a bowl, whisk together egg whites and sugar until frothy. Stir in flour and butter until smooth.

3. Cut a flower shape, about 6 inches (15 cm) in diameter from cardboard to use as a template. Place template on prepared baking sheet and spread a very thin coating of batter inside flower cutout. Carefully lift template. Repeat with remaining batter, leaving at least 2 inches (5 cm) between flowers (only shape flowers on one baking sheet at a time).

4. Bake, one sheet at a time, in preheated oven just until flower starts to brown around the edges and top is set, about 10 minutes. Using a spatula while cookie is hot, lift off baking sheet and place over an inverted bowl or ramekin. Carefully shape around bowl. Let cool completely. Repeat with remaining batter.

5. To serve, in a chilled bowl, whip cream and remaining 1 tbsp (15 mL) of sugar to form soft peaks.

6. Place cooled tulips on serving plates. Spoon strawberries into tulips and top with whipped cream.

Figs with Port

Serves 4

Preparation time
20 minutes

Cooking time
20 minutes

Tip

Serve figs and syrup over frozen yogurt or ice cream. Dulce de leche ice cream is a particularly good match.

½ tsp	oil	2 mL
3	star anise	3
1	whole clove	1
1	piece (2 inches/5 cm) cinnamon stick	1
¾ cup	granulated sugar	175 mL
⅔ cup	port	150 mL
2 tbsp	honey	30 mL
1	vanilla bean	1
1 lb	fresh figs, stems trimmed	500 g

1. In a saucepan, heat oil over medium-low heat. Add star anise, clove and cinnamon stick and heat, stirring, until fragrant, about 2 minutes. Add sugar, port and honey.

2. Cut vanilla bean in half lengthwise and scrape seeds into pan. Add pod to pan. Increase heat to medium and bring to a boil, stirring to dissolve sugar.

3. Add figs. Reduce heat and simmer until figs are translucent, about 20 minutes (do not let boil). Using a slotted spoon, transfer figs to a heatproof bowl.

4. Increase heat to medium-high and boil cooking liquid until reduced and syrupy. Discard vanilla pod. Pour over figs and let cool.

Prickly Pears with Rum

Serves 4

Preparation time
30 minutes

Chilling time
6 hours

Cooking time
5 minutes

• **Shallow baking dish**

6 tbsp	granulated sugar, divided	90 mL
¾ cup	water	175 mL
⅓ cup	rum	75 mL
4	prickly pears	4
¾ cup	heavy or whipping (35%) cream	175 mL

1. In a saucepan, combine ¼ cup (60 mL) of the sugar, water and rum. Bring to a boil over medium-high heat, stirring to dissolve sugar. Transfer to baking dish and let cool.

2. Peel prickly pears and cut into ½-inch (1 cm) thick rounds. Add to dish and spoon syrup over to coat evenly. Cover and refrigerate for 6 hours.

3. Just before serving, in a chilled bowl, whip cream with remaining 2 tbsp (30 mL) of sugar until soft peaks form.

4. Spoon figs and syrup into individual bowls and top with whipped cream.

Dates with Mascarpone

Serves 4			
	4 oz	mascarpone cheese	125 g
	2 tbsp	confectioner's (icing) sugar	30 mL
	½ cup	heavy or whipping (35%) cream	125 mL
	16	Medjool dates	16

Preparation time
20 minutes

Chilling time
30 minutes

See photo, opposite

1. In a bowl, mash together mascarpone and confectioner's sugar.

2. In a chilled bowl, whip cream to form soft peaks. Fold into mascarpone mixture.

3. Slit dates lengthwise without cutting in half. Remove pits. Fill cavity with mascarpone mixture. Cover and refrigerate until chilled, about 30 minutes, or for up to 8 hours before serving.

Date Squares

**Makes
16 squares**

Preparation time
30 minutes

Cooking time
30 minutes

- 8-inch (20 cm) square metal baking pan, greased

Date Filling

1 lb	pitted dates, chopped	500 g
¾ cup	hot water	175 mL
¼ cup	packed brown sugar	60 mL
1 tsp	freshly squeezed lemon juice	5 mL
1 tsp	grated orange zest	5 mL

Base and Topping

1½ cups	all-purpose flour	375 mL
1½ cups	quick-cooking rolled oats	375 mL
1 cup	packed brown sugar	250 mL
Pinch	salt	Pinch
1 cup	unsalted butter, cut into small pieces	250 mL

1. *Date Filling:* In a saucepan, combine dates, hot water and brown sugar. Bring to a boil over medium heat, stirring often. Reduce heat and boil gently, stirring often, until dates are very soft and paste-like, 5 to 10 minutes.

2. Remove from heat and stir in lemon juice and orange zest. Let cool completely.

3. Preheat oven to 350°F (180°C).

4. *Base and Topping:* In a bowl, combine flour, oats, brown sugar and salt. Add butter and work into flour mixture with your hands or a wooden spoon until mixture clumps together.

5. Press half of the crumb mixture into prepared baking pan. Spread filling over base, then cover with remaining crumb mixture, pressing gently.

6. Bake in preheated oven until golden around the edges and topping is firm, about 30 minutes. Let cool slightly in pan on a rack. Cut into squares, then let cool completely.

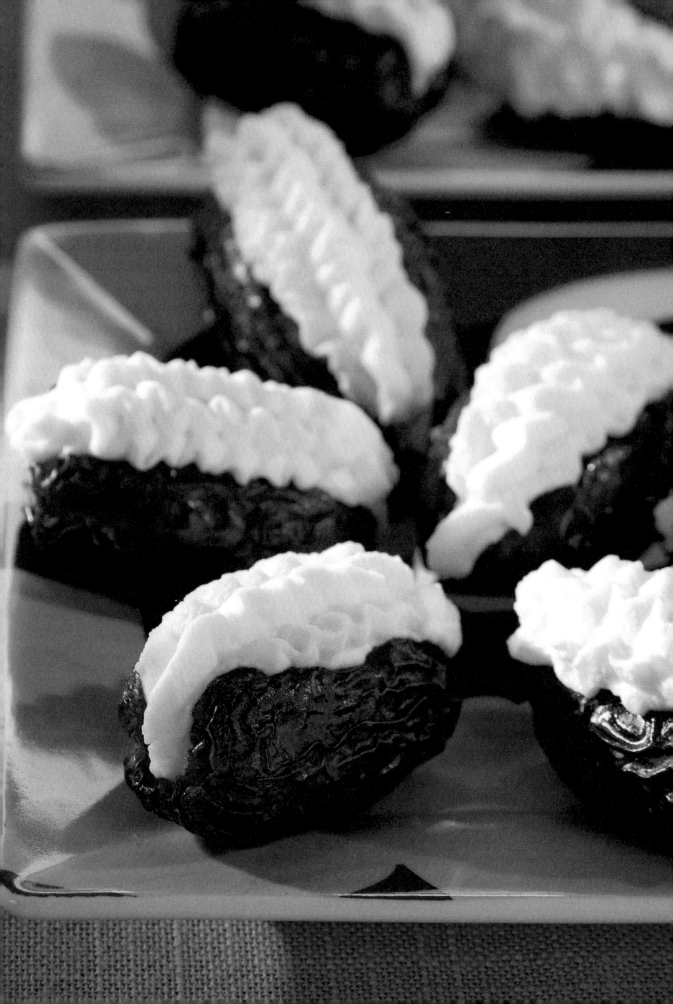

Raspberry Puffs

Serves 4

Preparation time
50 minutes

Cooking time
40 minutes

Chilling time
4 hours

- Preheat oven to 400°F (200°C)
- Pastry bag with plain tip

14 oz	puff pastry	400 g
	All-purpose flour	

Sabayon

3	egg yolks	3
1/4 cup	granulated sugar	60 mL
6 tbsp	dry white wine	90 mL
1/2 cup	heavy or whipping (35%) cream	125 mL
2 cups	raspberries	500 mL
2 tbsp	confectioner's (icing) sugar	30 mL

1. Cut pastry in half (if necessary). On a floured surface, roll out one half of pastry into a large rectangle, 12 by 9 inches (30 by 23 cm). Cut into 6 equal rectangles and place on a baking sheet, at least 1/2 inch (1 cm) apart. Prick all over with a fork.

2. Bake in preheated oven until golden, puffed and crispy, about 20 minutes. Let cool on a wire rack. Repeat with remaining pastry to make 12 rectangles in total.

3. *Sabayon:* In a stainless steel bowl, whisk together egg yolks and sugar until frothy. Set bowl over a saucepan of simmering water and cook, whisking vigorously and constantly, until sugar is dissolved. Gradually whisk in wine. Cook, whisking, until very airy and thick enough to coat the back of a wooden spoon, about 10 minutes. Transfer to a cool bowl, place plastic wrap directly on the surface and refrigerate until chilled, about 4 hours.

4. In a chilled bowl, whip cream until soft peaks form. Fold into chilled sabayon.

5. To assemble, place 4 of the pastry rectangles on individual serving plates. Arrange 2 rows of raspberries on top of each rectangle. Scoop sabayon into pastry bag and pipe between raspberries. Top with another pastry rectangle and repeat with raspberries and sabayon. Top with remaining pastry rectangles. Sprinkle with confectioner's sugar. Serve immediately or refrigerate for up to 1 hour.

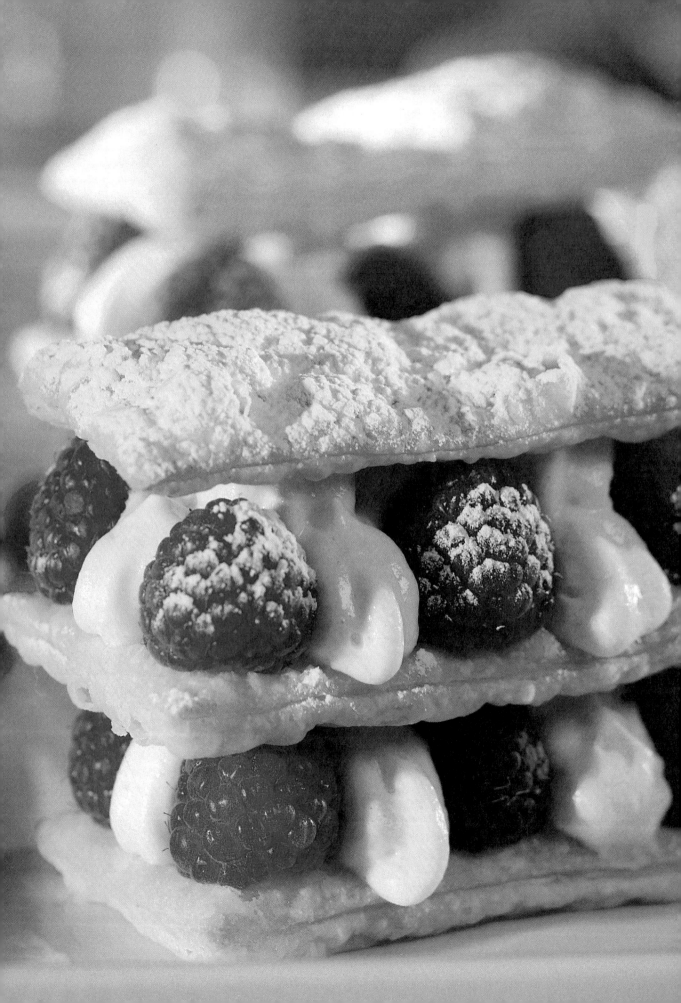

Persimmons Stuffed with Rice Pudding

Serves 4

Preparation time
20 minutes

Cooking time
45 minutes

- Preheat oven to 300°F (150°C)
- Ovenproof saucepan

¼ cup	honey	60 mL
2 tbsp	butter	30 mL
4	firm Fuyu persimmons with stems attached	4

Rice Pudding

½ cup	short-grain rice	125 mL
2 cups	milk	500 mL
½	vanilla bean	½
3 tbsp	granulated sugar	45 mL
¼ cup	currants or raisins	60 mL
1	egg yolk	1
	Butter	

1. In ovenproof saucepan, bring honey and butter to a boil over medium heat. Boil, swirling pan often, until caramelized. Add persimmons.

2. Bake in preheated oven, basting often, until persimmons are slightly softened, about 25 minutes. Let cool.

3. *Rice Pudding:* In a pot of boiling water, boil rice for 2 minutes. Drain and rinse under cold water. Drain well.

4. Place milk in a deep saucepan. Cut vanilla bean in half lengthwise and scrape seeds into milk. Add pod to milk. Bring to a boil over medium-high heat, stirring often. Stir in rice, sugar and currants. Reduce heat to low, cover and simmer, stirring occasionally, until rice is tender, 25 to 30 minutes. Whisk in egg yolk and butter to taste. Let cool slightly. Discard vanilla pod.

5. To serve, trim about ¾ inch (2 cm) off the top of each persimmon. Set aside. Trim bottoms so persimmons sit level, if necessary. Scoop out pulp from top, leaving a ½-inch (1 cm) thick wall. Chop persimmon pulp and stir into rice pudding.

6. Place hollowed persimmons onto individual serving plates. Fill with rice pudding and replace tops of persimmons as lids.

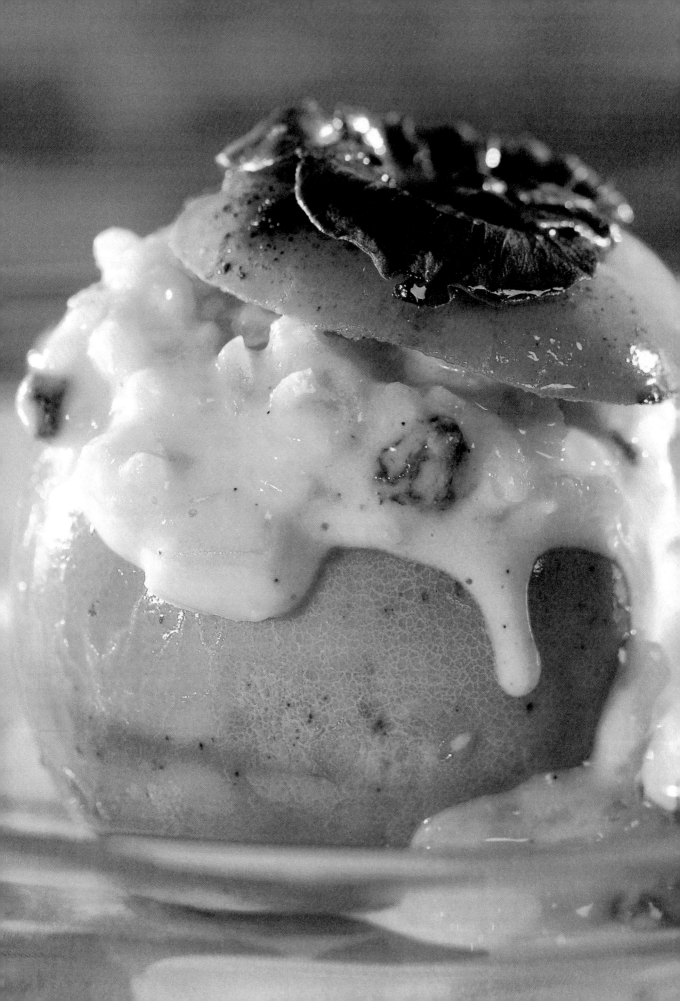

Vanilla Panna Cotta

See photo, opposite

Serves 4

Preparation time
15 minutes

Cooking time
5 minutes

Chilling time
4 hours

Tip

This dessert is delicious with a mixture of plain fresh fruit.

● **Four ½- to ¾-cup (125 to 175 mL) ramekins**

1 tbsp	agar powder	15 mL
2 cups	table (18%) or half-and-half (10%) cream	500 mL
¼ tsp	stevia powder	1 mL
½	vanilla bean, slit lengthwise	½

1. In a saucepan, sprinkle agar powder over cream. Let stand for 5 minutes.

2. Stir in stevia. Scrape vanilla seeds into saucepan and add pod. Bring to a simmer over medium heat, stirring often. Simmer, stirring, until agar is dissolved, about 2 minutes. Discard vanilla pod. Pour into ramekins and let cool. Cover and refrigerate until set, about 4 hours, or for up to 2 days.

Banana Chocolate Cake

Serves 12

Preparation time
30 minutes

Cooking time
50 minutes

● **Preheat oven to 350°F (180°C)**

● **13- by 9-inch (33 by 23 cm) metal cake pan, buttered and floured**

3 cups	all-purpose flour	750 mL
2 tsp	ground cinnamon	10 mL
½ tsp	ground cardamom	2 mL
Pinch	salt	Pinch
¾ cup	granulated sugar	175 mL
¾ cup	packed brown sugar	175 mL
½ cup	butter	125 mL
2	eggs	2
1 tsp	baking soda	5 mL
¼ cup	sour cream	60 mL
2 cups	mashed ripe bananas	500 mL
7 oz	chocolate, coarsely chopped	210 g

1. In a bowl, combine flour, cinnamon, cardamom and salt.

2. In a large bowl, using an electric mixer, beat granulated sugar, brown sugar and butter until light and fluffy. Beat in eggs, one at a time, beating well between each addition.

3. In a small bowl, stir baking soda into sour cream. Beat into sugar mixture. Beat in bananas. Using a spatula or wooden spoon, stir in flour mixture just until blended. Gently stir in chocolate. Spread into prepared pan.

4. Bake in preheated oven until a tester inserted in the center comes out clean, about 50 minutes. Let cool in pan on a wire rack for 10 minutes, then turn out onto rack to cool completely.

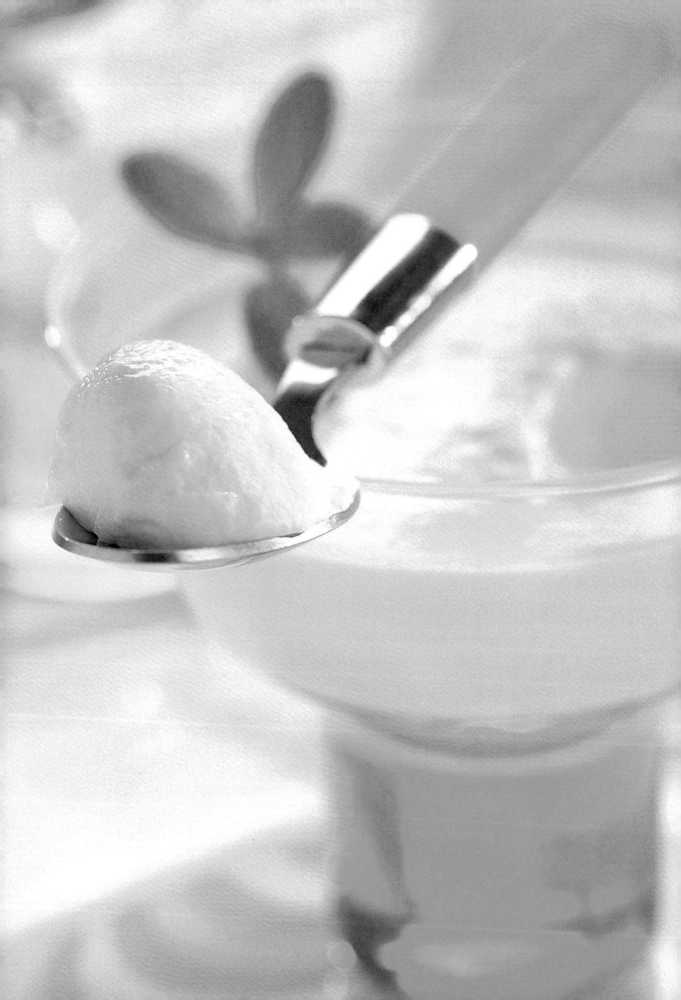

Lemon Pound Cake

Makes 10 to
12 slices

Preparation time
20 minutes

Cooking time
1 hour 10 minutes

● Preheat oven to 350°F (180°C)
● 9- by 5-inch (23 by 12.5 cm) metal loaf pan, buttered and floured

2⅓ cups	all-purpose flour	575 mL
1 tbsp	baking powder	15 mL
4	eggs, separated	4
2 cups	granulated sugar	500 mL
¾ cup + 2 tbsp	butter, softened	205 mL
	Zest of 2 lemons	
½ cup	freshly squeezed lemon juice	125 mL
1 cup	milk	250 mL

1. In a bowl, combine flour and baking powder. Set aside.

2. In a large bowl, using an electric mixer, beat egg yolks, sugar and butter until creamy. Beat in lemon zest and lemon juice.

3. Using a wooden spoon, alternately stir flour mixture into butter mixture alternately with milk, making 3 additions of flour and 2 of milk, until just blended.

4. In another bowl, using an electric mixer with clean beaters or a whisk, beat egg whites to form stiff peaks. Fold into batter just until blended. Spread into prepared loaf pan.

5. Bake in preheated oven for 10 minutes. Reduce temperature to 325°F (160°C) and bake loaf until a tester inserted in the center comes out clean, about 1 hour. Let cool in pan on a wire rack for 20 minutes, then turn out onto rack to cool completely.

Grapefruit Granita

Serves 8 to 10

Preparation time
20 minutes

Cooking time
10 minutes

Freezing time
6 hours

2 cups	granulated sugar	500 mL
2½ cups	water	625 mL
2½ cups	freshly squeezed grapefruit juice	625 mL
1¼ cups	vodka or other 80-proof spirit	300 mL

1. In a saucepan, bring sugar and water to a boil over medium heat, stirring to dissolve sugar. Transfer syrup to a bowl and let cool.

2. Strain grapefruit juice into syrup and stir in vodka. Transfer to a shallow freezer-proof container and freeze until firm, about 6 hours, or for up to 2 days.

3. To serve, using a large spoon, scrape granita into chilled serving dishes.

Cherry Clafoutis

Serves 4

Preparation time
30 minutes

Cooking time
25 minutes

- Preheat oven to 350°F (180°C)
- Four 1-cup (250 mL) ramekins, buttered and dusted with flour

¼ cup	ground almonds (almond flour or meal)	60 mL
1 cup	heavy or whipping (35%) cream	250 mL
1	egg	1
1	egg yolk	1
¼ cup	granulated sugar	60 mL
1 tsp	all-purpose flour	5 mL
2 cups	pitted sweet cherries	500 mL
	Confectioner's (icing) sugar	

1. In a small dry skillet, toast ground almonds over medium heat, stirring constantly, until golden and fragrant, about 3 minutes. Transfer to a bowl and stir in cream.

2. In another bowl, whisk together egg, egg yolk and sugar until frothy. Whisk in flour, then cream mixture, until well blended.

3. Divide cherries evenly among prepared ramekins. Pour cream mixture evenly overtop.

4. Bake in preheated oven until golden around the edges, puffed and just set, about 25 minutes. Serve hot, sprinkled with confectioner's sugar.

Citrus Vanilla Marmalade

Makes about
3½ cups
(875 mL)

Preparation time
45 minutes

Cooking time
1 hour

Chilling time
24 hours

Tip

As the marmalade reduces and thickens in Step 4, you may need to reduce the heat occasionally to keep it at a simmer.

- Two pint (500 mL) canning jars, sterilized (see Tips, page 260)

2 lbs	navel oranges	1 kg
2	lemons	2
1	vanilla bean	1
3 cups	granulated sugar	750 mL

1. Scrub oranges and lemons under running water. Using a vegetable peeler, peel off colored part of zest in strips, being careful to avoid bitter white pith. Cut zest into very thin strips and place in a saucepan.

2. Remove remaining peel and all white pith from oranges and lemons. Cut fruit into segments, discarding membranes and seeds and reserving any juice. Add fruit and juice to saucepan. Cut vanilla bean in half lengthwise and scrape seeds into pan. Add pod to pan and stir in sugar.

3. Place a small plate in freezer to check gel.

4. Bring to a boil over medium heat, stirring to dissolve sugar. Reduce heat and simmer, stirring often, until reaches gel stage, about 1 hour. To test gel, spoon ½ tsp (2 mL) mixture onto chilled plate and freeze for 1 minute. Slowly push drop on plate with fingertip and it should wrinkle. Continue cooking and testing until gel wrinkles. Skim off any foam.

5. Discard vanilla pod. Pour marmalade into hot, sterilized jar. Cover and refrigerate until set, about 1 day. Store for up to 1 month.

Apricot Marmalade

Makes about 4 cups (1 L)

Preparation time
30 minutes

Cooking time
1 hour

Chilling time
24 hours

See photo, opposite

- Two pint (500 mL) or four 8-oz (250 mL) canning jars, sterilized (see Tips, page 260)

2 lbs	fresh apricots, chopped	1 kg
2½ cups	granulated sugar	625 mL
	Juice of 1 lemon	

1. Place a small plate in freezer to check gel.

2. In a large saucepan, combine apricots, sugar and lemon juice. Bring to a boil over medium-high heat, stirring to dissolve sugar.

3. Reduce heat and boil gently, stirring often, until mixture reaches gel stage, about 1 hour. To test gel, spoon ½ tsp (2 mL) mixture onto chilled plate and freeze for 1 minute. Slowly push drop on plate with fingertip and it should wrinkle. Continue cooking and testing until gel wrinkles.

4. Pour marmalade into hot, sterilized jar and let cool. Cover and refrigerate until set, about 1 day. Store for up to 1 month.

Anise-Scented Kumquat Marmalade

Makes about 4 cups (1 L)

Preparation time
30 minutes

Cooking time
1 hour 30 minutes

Chilling time
24 hours

- Candy/deep-fry thermometer
- Two pint (500 mL) or four 8-oz (250 mL) canning jars, sterilized (see Tips, page 260)

2 lbs	kumquats	1 kg
3 cups	granulated sugar	750 mL
1⅓ cups	water	325 mL
2	star anise	2
1 tbsp	freshly squeezed lemon juice	15 mL

1. Trim off blossom end from kumquats. Cut kumquats into quarters and discard seeds.

2. Place kumquats in a saucepan and add cold water to cover. Bring to a boil over high heat. Drain well and return to pot. Add fresh water to cover and repeat three more times (this removes the bitterness). Drain well.

3. In a clean saucepan, combine sugar, water and star anise. Bring to a boil over medium-high heat, stirring to dissolve sugar. Boil until mixture reaches 230°F (110°C).

4. Place a small plate in freezer to check gel.

5. Stir kumquats and lemon juice into sugar mixture. Reduce heat and boil gently, stirring often, until kumquats are translucent and mixture reaches gel stage, 10 to 15 minutes. To test gel, spoon ½ tsp (2 mL) mixture onto chilled plate and freeze for 1 minute. Slowly push drop on plate with fingertip and it should wrinkle. Continue cooking and testing until gel wrinkles.

6. Pour marmalade into hot, sterilized jar and let cool. Cover and refrigerate until set, about 1 day. Store for up to 1 month.

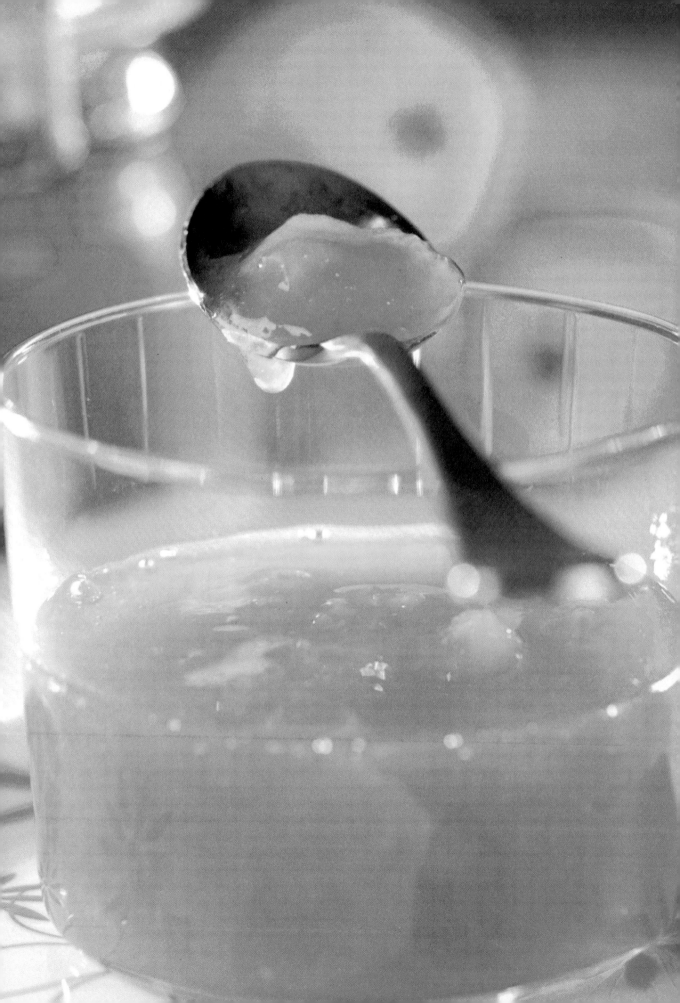

Berry Soup

Serves 4

Preparation time
10 minutes

Chilling time
30 minutes

See photo, opposite

Tip

This soup is
a marvelous
accompaniment to
Blancmange (below).

½ cup	granulated sugar	125 mL
2 cups	water	500 mL
2 tsp	finely chopped fresh mint	10 mL
¾ cup	strawberries	175 mL
½ cup	blueberries	125 mL
½ cup	raspberries	125 mL
½ cup	blackberries	125 mL
	Fresh mint leaves	

1. In a small saucepan, combine sugar and water and bring to a boil over medium-high heat, stirring to dissolve sugar. Remove from heat and stir in finely chopped mint. Let cool completely.

2. In a bowl, combine strawberries, blueberries, raspberries and blackberries. Pour mint syrup over top. Cover and refrigerate for at least 30 minutes or for up to 8 hours.

3. To serve, spoon berries and syrup into individual serving dishes and garnish with mint leaves.

Blancmange

Serves 4

Preparation time
20 minutes

Chilling time
1 hour

See photo, opposite

Variation

This blancmange can
be served with Berry
Soup (above).

2 tsp	agar powder	10 mL
1½ cups	heavy or whipping (35%) cream, divided	375 mL
2	vanilla beans	2
⅓ cup	granulated sugar	75 mL

1. In a bowl, sprinkle agar powder over 2 tbsp (30 mL) of the cream. Let stand for 5 minutes.

2. Place ½ cup (125 mL) of the remaining cream in a bowl and refrigerate.

3. Place remaining cream in a saucepan. Cut vanilla beans in half lengthwise and scrape seeds into cream in saucepan. Add pods to saucepan. Heat over low heat until cream is steaming.

4. Stir sugar into cream. Increase heat to medium and bring to a boil, stirring to dissolve sugar. Stir in soaked agar mixture until dissolved. Transfer to a bowl and let cool completely.

5. Remove vanilla pods from cream mixture. Whip reserved chilled cream to firm peaks and fold into cooled cream mixture. Spoon into individual serving dishes. Cover and refrigerate until set, about 1 hour, or for up to 1 day.

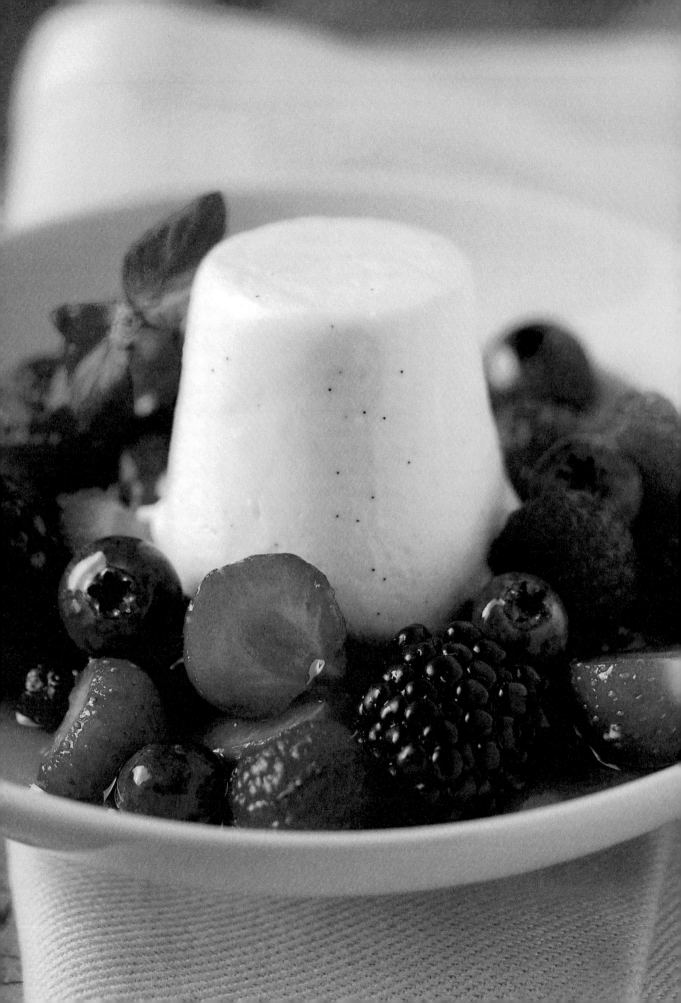

Apple Strudel

Serves 4

Preparation time
1 hour 10 minutes

Chilling time
30 minutes

Cooking time
45 minutes

● Baking sheet, buttered or lined with parchment paper

Dough

1½ cups	all-purpose flour	375 mL
Pinch	salt	Pinch
1	egg	1
⅓ cup	butter, softened	75 mL
⅓ cup	water	75 mL
¼ cup	bread crumbs	60 mL

Filling

⅔ cup	raisins	150 mL
	Boiling water	
5	apples, peeled and diced	5
½ cup	granulated sugar	125 mL
¼ cup	pine nuts	60 mL
1 tsp	ground cinnamon	5 mL
¼ cup	rum	60 mL

Topping

1	egg, beaten	1
2 tsp	melted butter	10 mL
2 tbsp	granulated sugar	30 mL

1. *Dough:* In a bowl, combine flour and salt and make a well in the center. Add egg, butter and water to well and stir until dough gathers. On a floured surface, knead lightly until smooth. Press into a disk, wrap and refrigerate for 30 minutes.

2. Preheat oven to 350°F (180°C).

3. *Filling:* In a bowl, cover raisins with boiling water and let soak until plump, about 10 minutes. Drain well and pat dry.

4. In a bowl, combine raisins, apples, sugar, pine nuts, cinnamon and rum.

5. To assemble, knead bread crumbs into dough if dough feels too moist. On a floured surface, roll out dough into a 16- by 10-inch (40 by 25 cm) rectangle.

6. Spoon filling in center of the dough in a rectangle, leaving about a 2½-inch (6 cm) border along each long side and a 1½-inch (4 cm) border at each narrow end. Fold one long edge toward center over filling. Brush edge with beaten egg. Fold remaining long edge toward the center, overlapping opposite edge slightly and enclosing filling. Pinch edge to seal and brush with egg. Fold up both ends, pinch edges to seal and brush with egg.

7. Carefully transfer to baking sheet, seam side down. Brush all over with melted butter, then remaining egg. Sprinkle with sugar.

8. Bake in preheated oven until pastry is golden and crisp and apples are tender, about 45 minutes. Serve warm or let cool completely.

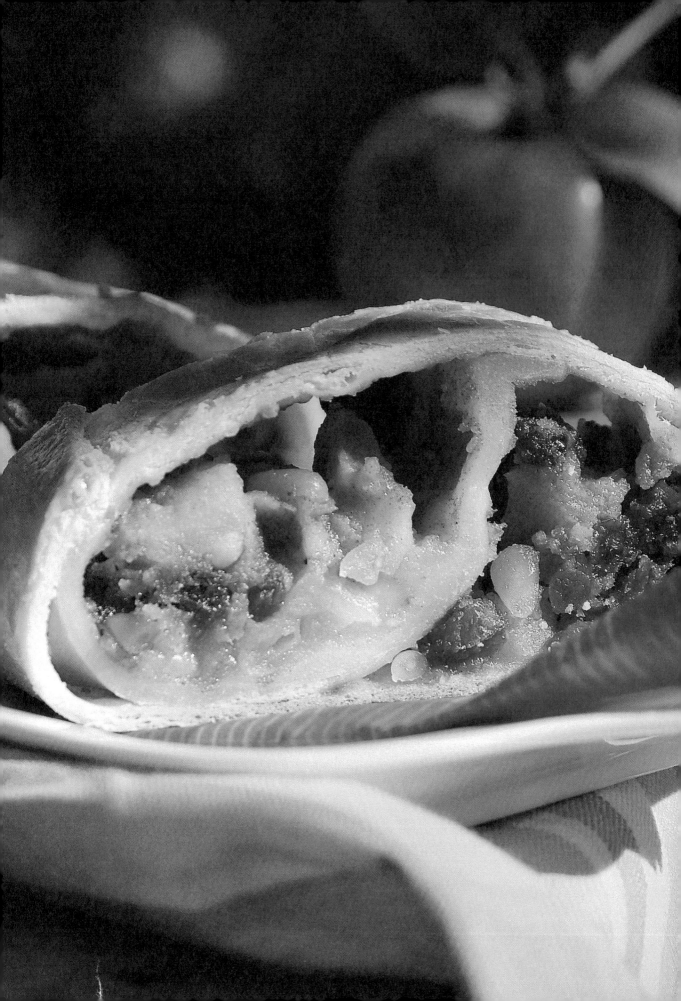

Fig and Almond Tart

Serves 4

Preparation time
40 minutes

Cooking time
20 minutes

See photo, opposite

• **Preheat oven to 400°F (200°C)**

¼ cup	butter, softened	60 mL
3½ tbsp	granulated sugar	52 mL
1	egg	1
½ cup	finely chopped almonds	125 mL
2 tbsp	all-purpose flour, sifted	30 mL
8 oz	puff pastry dough	250 g
12	fresh figs, thinly sliced	12
2 tbsp	pine nuts	30 mL
2 tbsp	granulated sugar	30 mL

1. In a bowl, using an electric mixer, beat butter and sugar until fluffy. Beat in egg until blended. Stir in almonds and flour.

2. On a floured surface, roll out puff pastry into a very thin rectangle. Place on a baking sheet.

3. Spread almond mixture over rectangle, leaving a ½-inch (1 cm) border along all the edges. Arrange fig slices on top of almond mixture, overlapping as necessary.

4. Bake in preheated oven for 9 minutes. Sprinkle with pine nuts and granulated sugar. Bake until pastry is crisp and golden, about 9 minutes longer. Let cool slightly and serve warm or let cool completely.

Egg Custard

Serves 4

Preparation time
30 minutes

Cooking time
35 minutes

• **6- to 8-cup (1.5 to 2 L) glass baking dish**
• **Roasting pan**

4 cups	milk	1 L
1 cup	granulated sugar, divided	250 mL
1	vanilla bean, slit lengthwise	1
8	eggs	8
	Boiling water	

1. In a saucepan, combine milk and ¾ cup (175 mL) of the sugar. Scrape seeds from vanilla bean into milk and add pod. Bring to a boil over medium heat, stirring often. Remove from heat and let cool for 30 minutes. Discard vanilla pod.

2. Preheat oven to 300°F (150°C).

3. In a bowl, beat eggs with remaining sugar until pale and thick. Gradually whisk in milk mixture. Pour into baking dish.

4. Place dish in roasting pan and place in preheated oven. Pour in boiling water to come halfway up sides of dish for a bain-marie. Bake until custard is just set, about 35 minutes. Remove baking dish from bain-marie and let cool slightly on a rack. Serve warm or refrigerate until chilled.

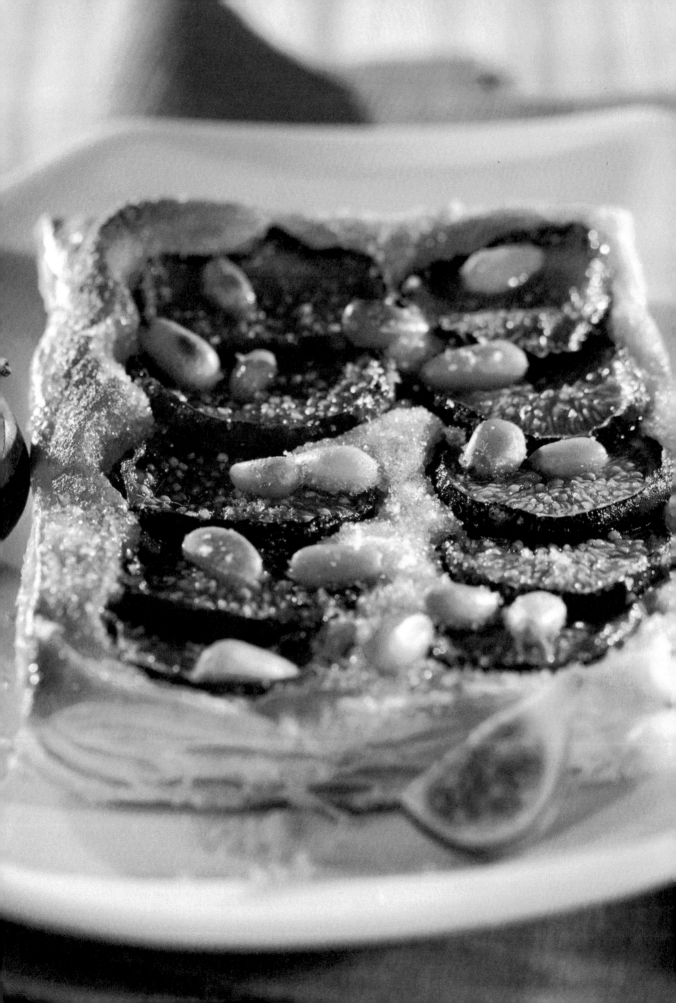

Apricot and Lavender Tart

• Preheat oven to 400°F (200°C)
• Large baking sheet, lined with parchment paper

Frangipane

2 tbsp	butter, softened	30 mL
1/4 cup	confectioner's (icing) sugar	60 mL
1	egg	1
1/2 cup	ground almonds (almond flour or meal)	125 mL
10 oz	puff pastry dough	300 g
12	apricots, cut in half	12
	Fresh lavender (see Tips, page 54)	

1. *Frangipane:* In a bowl, using an electric mixer, beat butter and confectioner's sugar until creamy. Beat in eggs, one at a time, beating well between each addition. Beat in ground almonds. Cover and refrigerate.

2. On a floured surface, roll out puff pastry dough in a square or a circle about 11 inches (28 cm) in diameter and about 1/8-inch (3 mm) thick. Cut four 5-inch (12.5 cm) circles from dough. Discard scraps. Lightly prick pastry circles with a fork and place on prepared baking sheet.

3. Divide frangipane among pastry circles and spread to evenly coat. Place 6 apricot halves, cut side down, on each. Sprinkle with lavender flowers.

4. Bake in preheated oven until pastry is golden and crisp and apricots are tender, 20 to 25 minutes.

Prunes Poached in Spiced Wine

10 oz	prunes	300 g
1 1/2 cups	red wine	375 mL
2	whole cloves	2
1	piece (4 inches/10 cm) cinnamon stick	1
1	star anise	1
	Finely grated zest of 1 lemon	
	Finely grated zest of 1 orange	
	Granulated sugar	

1. In a saucepan, combine prunes and wine. Pour in enough water to almost cover prunes. Add cloves, cinnamon stick, star anise, lemon zest and orange zest. Stir in sugar to taste (do not add too much, as it will become concentrated and prunes are sweet).

2. Bring to a simmer over medium heat, stirring occasionally. Reduce heat and simmer, stirring occasionally, until prunes are plump and tender, about 15 minutes. Let cool to room temperature.

Index

(v) = variation

Library and Archives Canada Cataloguing in Publication

Brotto, Igor
 The vegetarian kitchen table cookbook : 275 delicious recipes / Igor Brotto and Olivier Guiriec.

Includes index.
Translation of: Le grand livre de la cuisine végétarienne.
ISBN 978-0-7788-0293-8

 1. Vegetarian cooking. 2. Cookbooks. I. Guiriec, Olivier II. Title.

TX837.B7613 2012   641.5'636   C2011-907459-1